Contagious Diseases

SOURCEBOOK

Third Edition

Health Reference Series

Third Edition

Contagious Diseases
SOURCEBOOK

Basic Consumer Health Information about Diseases Spread from Person to Person through Direct Physical Contact, Airborne Transmissions, Sexual Contact, or Contact with Blood or Other Body Fluids, including Pneumococcal, Staphylococcal, and Streptococcal Diseases, Colds, Ebola, HIV, Influenza, Tuberculosis, Zika Virus, and Others

Along with Facts about Self-Care and Over-The-Counter Medications, Antibiotics and Drug Resistance, Disease Prevention, Vaccines, and Bioterrorism, a Glossary, and a Directory of Resources for More Information

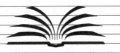

OMNIGRAPHICS

615 Griswold, Ste. 901, Detroit, MI 48226

Bibliographic Note

Because this page cannot legibly accommodate all the copyright notices, the Bibliographic Note portion of the Preface constitutes an extension of the copyright notice.

* * *

Health Reference Series
Keith Jones, *Managing Editor*

***

OMNIGRAPHICS

A PART OF RELEVANT INFORMATION

***

Copyright © 2016 Omnigraphics
ISBN 978-0-7808-1488-2
E-ISBN 978-0-7808-1487-5

Library of Congress Cataloging-in-Publication Data

Names: Omnigraphics, Inc.

Title: Contagious diseases sourcebook: basic consumer health information about diseases spread from person to person through direct physical contact, airborne transmissions, sexual contact, or contact with blood or other body fluids, including pneumococcal, staphylococcal, and streptococcal diseases, colds, influenza, lice, measles, mumps, tuberculosis, and others; along with facts about self-care and over-the-counter medications, antibiotics and drug resistance, disease prevention, vaccines, and bioterrorism, a glossary, and a directory of resources for more information.

Description: Third edition. | Detroit, MI: Omnigraphics, [2016] | Series: Health reference series | Includes bibliographical references and index.

Identifiers: LCCN 2016034737 (print) | LCCN 2016035672 (ebook) | ISBN 9780780814882 (hardcover: alk. paper) | ISBN 9780780814875 (ebook) | ISBN 9780780814875 (eBook)

Subjects: LCSH: Communicable diseases--Popular works.

Classification: LCC RC113 .C664 2016 (print) | LCC RC113 (ebook) | DDC 616.9--dc23

LC record available at https://lccn.loc.gov/2016034737

Table of Contents

Part I: What You Need to Know about Germs

Part II: Types of Contagious Diseases

Part III: Self-Treatment for Contagious Diseases

Part IV: Medical Diagnosis and Treatment of Contagious Diseases

Part V: Preventing Contagious Diseases

Part VI: Additional Help and Information

Preface

About This Book

Contagious diseases occur when microbes—bacteria, viruses, and fungi—are passed from person to person. Vaccination programs and other prevention measures have successfully reduced the number of new cases of many contagious diseases. However, in many industrialized countries where communicable disease mortality has greatly decreased over the past century, the return of old communicable diseases, the emergence of new ones, and the evolution of antimicrobial resistance that have made treatments less effective continues to present a challenge, and infectious disease remains a major public health concern in the United States and around the world.

Contagious Diseases Sourcebook, Third Edition, provides updated information about microbes that are spread from person to person and the diseases they cause, including influenza, lice infestation, smallpox, measles, staphylococcal and streptococcal infections, tuberculosis, and others. The types of diagnostic tests and treatments available from medical professionals are explained, and self-care practices for familiar symptoms, such as common cold and sore throat are described. Antibiotic resistance, the role of handwashing in preventing the spread of disease, and recommendations and controversies surrounding vaccination programs are also described. The book concludes with a glossary of related terms and a directory of additional resources.

How to Use This Book

This book is divided into parts and chapters. Parts focus on broad areas of interest. Chapters are devoted to single topics within a part.

Part I: What You Need to Know about Germs describes various types of microbes and different kinds of infections. It also explains how the immune system responds to germs and how diseases can be transmitted from person to person. Public health issues are also discussed, including the practice of screening internationally adopted children for contagious diseases and the threat of bioterrorism.

Part II: Types of Contagious Diseases provides facts about specific diseases of concern—from adenovirus to Zika virus—in individual, alphabetically arranged chapters.

Part III: Self-Treatment for Contagious Diseases discusses frequently used remedies for common illnesses and disease symptoms. Facts about the proper use of over-the-counter (OTC) medications are also explained, along with a chapter focusing on the dangers associated with drug interactions. The part concludes with information about the use of probiotics, herbal and dietary supplements, and other forms of complementary and alternative medicines for contagious diseases.

Part IV: Medical Diagnosis and Treatment of Contagious Diseases explains the tests and procedures used to identify the presence of microbial infection and viruses associated with colds, influenza, and other diseases. Antibiotics, antivirals, and other prescription medications are also discussed. The growing problem of antimicrobial resistance—the way microbes change to counteract the effectiveness of drug treatments—is explained, along with directions for combating the resistance.

Part V: Preventing Contagious Diseases offers information about a simple practice that is a key element in the fight against the spread of germs—handwashing. It provides information on vaccines, another effective tool for halting the spread of disease. It provides vaccine recommendations for children, adolescents, and adults and also addresses problems associated with vaccines, the vaccine adverse event reporting system, and the difficulties that can arise as a result of vaccine misinformation. It concludes by discussing quarantine and isolation for controlling contagious diseases.

Part VI: Additional Help and Information provides a glossary of terms related to contagious diseases and a directory of resources for additional information.

Bibliographic Note

This volume contains documents and excerpts from publications issued by the following U.S. government agencies: Centers for Disease Control and Prevention (CDC); Federal Bureau of Prisons (BOP); FLU. gov; Genetics Home Reference (GHR); National Center for Complementary and Integrative Health (NCCIH); National Heart, Lung, and Blood Institute (NHLBI); National Institute of Allergy and Infectious Diseases (NIAID); National Institute of Diabetes and Digestive and Kidney Diseases (NIDDK); National Institutes of Health (NIA); *NIH News in Health*; Office on Women's Health (OWH); U.S. Department of Health and Human Services (HHS); U.S. Department of Veterans Affairs (VA); and U.S. Food and Drug Administration (FDA).

In addition, this volume contains copyrighted documents from the following organization: The Nemours Foundation

It may also contain original material produced by Omnigraphics and reviewed by medical consultants.

About the Health Reference Series

The *Health Reference Series* is designed to provide basic medical information for patients, families, caregivers, and the general public. Each volume takes a particular topic and provides comprehensive coverage. This is especially important for people who may be dealing with a newly diagnosed disease or a chronic disorder in themselves or in a family member. People looking for preventive guidance, information about disease warning signs, medical statistics, and risk factors for health problems will also find answers to their questions in the *Health Reference Series*. The *Series*, however, is not intended to serve as a tool for diagnosing illness, in prescribing treatments, or as a substitute for the physician/patient relationship. All people concerned about medical symptoms or the possibility of disease are encouraged to seek professional care from an appropriate health care provider.

A Note about Spelling and Style

Health Reference Series editors use *Stedman's Medical Dictionary* as an authority for questions related to the spelling of medical terms and the *Chicago Manual of Style* for questions related to grammatical structures, punctuation, and other editorial concerns. Consistent adherence is not always possible, however, because the individual volumes within the *Series* include many documents from a wide variety of different producers, and the editor's primary goal is to present material from each source as accurately as is possible. This sometimes means that information in different chapters or sections may follow other guidelines and alternate spelling authorities.

Medical Review

Omnigraphics contracts with a team of qualified, senior medical professionals who serve as medical consultants for the *Health Reference Series*. As necessary, medical consultants review reprinted and originally written material for currency and accuracy. Citations including the phrase, "Reviewed (month, year)" indicate material reviewed by this team. Medical consultation services are provided to the *Health Reference Series* editors by:

Dr. Vijayalakshmi, MBBS, DGO, MD
Dr. K. Sivanandham, MBBS, DCH, MS (Research), PhD

Our Advisory Board

We would like to thank the following board members for providing initial guidance on the development of this series:

- Dr. Lynda Baker, Associate Professor of Library and Information Science, Wayne State University, Detroit, MI

- Nancy Bulgarelli, William Beaumont Hospital Library, Royal Oak, MI

- Karen Imarisio, Bloomfield Township Public Library, Bloomfield Township, MI

- Karen Morgan, Mardigian Library, University of Michigan-Dearborn, Dearborn, MI

- Rosemary Orlando, St. Clair Shores Public Library, St. Clair Shores, MI

Health Reference Series *Update Policy*

The inaugural book in the *Health Reference Series* was the first edition of *Cancer Sourcebook* published in 1989. Since then, the *Series* has been enthusiastically received by librarians and in the medical community. In order to maintain the standard of providing high-quality health information for the layperson the editorial staff at Omnigraphics felt it was necessary to implement a policy of updating volumes when warranted.

Medical researchers have been making tremendous strides, and it is the purpose of the *Health Reference Series* to stay current with the most recent advances. Each decision to update a volume is made on an individual basis. Some of the considerations include how much new information is available and the feedback we receive from people who use the books. If there is a topic you would like to see added to the update list, or an area of medical concern you feel has not been adequately addressed, please write to:

Managing Editor
Health Reference Series
Omnigraphics
615 Griswold, Ste. 901
Detroit, MI 48226

Part One

What You Need to Know about Germs

Chapter 1

Understanding Microbes (Germs)

Chapter Contents

Section 1.1

What Are Microbes?

This section contains text excerpted from the following sources:
Text in this section begins with excerpts from "Microbes," National
Institute of Allergy and Infectious Diseases (NIAID), July 9, 2015;
Text under the heading "Bacteria" is excerpted from "Understanding
Microbes in Sickness and in Health," National Institute of
Allergy and Infectious Diseases (NIAID), September 1, 2009.
Reviewed August 2016.

Microbes are tiny **organisms**—too tiny to see without a microscope,
yet they are abundant on Earth. They live everywhere—in air, soil,
rock, and water. Some live happily in searing heat, while others thrive
in freezing cold. Some microbes need oxygen to live, but others do not.
These microscopic organisms are found in plants and animals as well
as in the human body.

Some microbes cause **disease** in humans, plants, and animals.
Others are essential for a healthy life, and we could not exist without
them. Indeed, the relationship between microbes and humans is del-
icate and complex. In this section, we will learn that some microbes
keep us healthy while others can make us sick.

Most microbes belong to one of four major groups: bacteria, viruses,
fungi, or protozoa. A common word for microbes that cause disease
is "germs." Some people refer to disease-causing microbes as "bugs."
"I've got the flu bug," for example, is a phrase you may hear during
the wintertime to describe an influenza virus **infection**.

Since the 19th century, we have known that microbes cause **infectious diseases.** Near the end of the 20th century, researchers began
to learn that microbes also contribute to many chronic diseases and
illnesses. Mounting scientific evidence strongly links microbes to some
forms of cancer, coronary artery disease, diabetes, multiple sclerosis,
and chronic lung diseases.

Bacteria

Microbes belonging to the bacteria group are made up of only one
cell. Under a microscope, bacteria look like balls, rods, or spirals.

4

Bacteria are so small that a line of 1,000 could fit across the eraser of a pencil. Life in any form on Earth could not exist without these tiny cells.

Scientists have discovered fossilized remains of bacteria that date back more than 3.5 billion years, placing them among the oldest living things on Earth. Bacteria can inhabit a variety of environments, including extremely cold and hot areas.

- Psychrophiles, or cold-loving bacteria, can live in temperatures as cold as those found in the Arctic and Antarctic.

- Thermophiles are heat-loving bacteria that can live in high temperatures, such as in the hot springs of Yellowstone National Park in Wyoming.

- Extreme thermophiles, or hyperthermophiles, can thrive at 235°F near volcanic vents on the ocean floor.

Many bacteria, however, prefer the milder temperature of the healthy human body.

Like humans, some bacteria (aerobic bacteria) need oxygen to survive. Others (anaerobic bacteria) do not. Amazingly, some can adapt to new environments by learning to survive with or without oxygen.

Like all living cells, each bacterium requires food for energy and building materials. There are countless numbers of bacteria on Earth—most are harmless, and many are even beneficial to humans. In fact, less than 1 percent of bacteria cause diseases in humans. For example, harmless anaerobic bacteria, such as *Lactobacilli acidophilus*, live in our intestines, where they help digest food, destroy disease-causing microbes, fight cancer cells, and give the body needed vitamins.

Healthy food products, such as yogurt, sauerkraut, and cheese, are made using bacteria.

Some bacteria, however, produce poisons called toxins, which can make us sick. For example, botulism, a severe form of food poisoning, affects the nerves and is caused by toxins from *Clostridium botulinum* bacteria.

Are Toxins Always Harmful?

Under certain circumstances, bacterial toxins can be helpful. Several vaccines that keep us from getting sick are made from bacterial toxins. For example, one type of pertussis vaccine, which protects infants and children from pertussis (whooping cough), contains toxins from *Bordetella pertussis* bacteria. This vaccine is safe and effective and causes fewer reactions than other types of pertussis vaccines.

Viruses

Viruses are among the smallest microbes, much smaller even than bacteria. Viruses, however, are not cells. They consist of one or more **molecules** of **DNA** or **RNA**, which contain the virus' **genes** surrounded by a **protein** coat. Viruses can be rod-shaped, sphere-shaped, or multisided. Some viruses look like tadpoles.

Unlike most bacteria, most viruses do cause disease because they invade living, normal cells, such as those in your body. Once inside the cells, they multiply and produce other viruses like themselves. Each virus is very particular about which cell it attacks. Various human viruses specifically attack particular cells in your body's organs, systems, or **tissues**, such as the liver, respiratory system, or blood.

Although types of viruses behave differently, most survive by taking over the machinery that makes a cell work. Briefly, when a piece of a virus, called a virion, comes in contact with a cell it likes, it may attach to special landing sites on the surface of that cell. From there, the virus may inject molecules into the cell, or the cell may swallow the virion. Once inside the cell, viral molecules such as DNA or RNA direct the cell to make new virus offspring. That's how a virus infects a cell.

Viruses can even "infect" bacteria. These viruses, called bacteriophages, may help researchers develop alternatives to **antibiotic** medicines for preventing and treating bacterial infections.

Many viral infections do not result in disease. For example, by the time most people in the United States become adults, they have been infected by cytomegalovirus (CMV). Most people infected with CMV, however, do not develop CMV-disease symptoms. Other viral infections can result in deadly diseases such as acquired immune deficiency syndrome (AIDS) or Ebola hemorrhagic fever.

Fungi

A fungus is actually a primitive plant. Fungi can be found in air, in soil, on plants, and in water. Thousands, perhaps millions, of different types of fungi exist on Earth. The most familiar ones to us are mushrooms, yeast, mold, and mildew. Some live in the human body, usually without causing illness.

Fungal diseases are called mycoses. Mycoses can affect your skin, nails, body hair, internal organs such as your lungs, and body systems such as your nervous system. *Aspergillus fumigatus* fungi, for example, can cause aspergillosis, a lung disease.

Some fungi have made our lives easier. Penicillin and other antibiotics, which can kill harmful bacteria in our bodies, are made from fungi. Other fungi, such as certain yeasts, also can be helpful. For example, when a warm liquid, such as water, and a food source, such as sugar, are added to certain yeasts, the fungus ferments. The process of fermentation is essential for making healthy foods like some breads and cheeses.

Protozoa

Protozoa are a group of microscopic one-celled animals. Protozoa can be **parasites** or predators. In humans, protozoa usually cause disease.

Some protozoa, like plankton, live in water environments and serve as food for marine animals, such as some kinds of whales. Protozoa also can be found on land in decaying matter and in soil, but they must have a moist environment to survive. Termites wouldn't be able to do such a good job of digesting wood without these **microorganisms** in their guts.

Malaria is caused by a protozoan parasite. Another protozoan parasite, *Toxoplasma gondii*, causes toxoplasmosis, or toxo, in humans. This is an especially troublesome infection in pregnant women because of its effects on the fetus, and in people with **HIV**/AIDS or other disorders of the immune system.

Table 1.1. Microbes in the Healthy Human Body

Microbes in the Healthy Human Body*	
Ear (outer)	Aspergillus (fungus)
Skin	Candida (fungus)
Small intestine	Clostridium
Intestines	*E. coli*
Vagina	*Gardnerella vaginalis*
Stomach	*Lactobacillus*
Urethra	Mycobacterium
Nose	*Staphylococcus aureus*
Mouth	*Streptococcus salivarius*
Large intestine	*Trichomonas hominis* (protozoa)

*A selection of usually harmless microbes, some of which help keep our bodies functioning normally. If their numbers become unbalanced, however, these microbes may make us sick. All are bacteria, unless otherwise noted.

Section 1.2

Microbes Can Cause Different Kinds of Infections

This section includes text excerpted from "Microbes,"
National Institute of Allergy and Infectious Diseases (NIAID),
November 3, 2010. Reviewed August 2016.

Microbes Infections

Microbes can cause different kinds of infections. Some disease-causing microbes can make you very sick quickly and then not bother you again. Some can last for a long time and continue to damage tissues. Others can last forever, but you won't feel sick anymore, or you will feel sick only once in a while. Most infections caused by microbes fall into three major groups:

- Acute infections
- Chronic infections
- Latent infections

Acute Infections

Acute infections are usually severe and last a short time. They can make you feel very uncomfortable, with signs and symptoms such as tiredness, achiness, coughing, and sneezing. The common cold is such an infection. The signs and symptoms of a cold can last for 2 to 24 days (but usually a week), though it may seem like a lot longer. Once your body's immune system has successfully fought off one of the many different types of rhinoviruses or other viruses that may have caused your cold, the cold doesn't come back. If you get another cold, it's probably because you have been infected with other cold-causing viruses.

Chronic Infections

Chronic infections usually develop from acute infections and can last for days to months to a lifetime. Sometimes people are unaware they are infected but still may be able to transmit the germ to others. For example, hepatitis C, which affects the liver, is a chronic viral infection. In fact, most people who have been infected with the hepatitis C virus don't know it until they have a blood test that shows antibodies to the virus. Recovery from this infection is rare—about 85 percent of infected people become chronic carriers of the virus. In addition, serious signs of liver damage, like cirrhosis or cancer, may not appear until as long as 20 years after the infection began.

Latent Infections

Latent infections are "hidden" or "silent" and may or may not cause symptoms again after the first acute episode. Some infectious microbes, usually viruses, can "wake up"—become active again but not always causing symptoms—off and on for months or years. When these microbes are active in your body, you can transmit them to other people. Herpes simplex viruses, which cause genital herpes and cold sores, can remain latent in nerve cells for short or long periods of time, or forever.

Chickenpox is another example of a latent infection. Before the chickenpox vaccine became available in the 1990s, most children in the United States got chickenpox. After the first acute episode, usually when children are very young, the *Varicella zoster* virus goes into hiding in the body. In many people, it emerges many years later when they are older adults and causes a painful disease of the nerves called herpes zoster, or shingles.

Researchers are studying what turns these microbial antics off and on and are looking for ways to finally stop the process.

Diseases and Infections Caused by Microbes

The table below shows some common diseases and infections and their microbial causes.

Table 1.2. Diseases and Infections Caused by Microbes

	Bacteria	Fungus	Protozoa	Virus
Athlete's foot		♦		
Chickenpox				♦
Common cold				♦
Diarrheal diseases	♦		♦	♦

Table 1.2. Continued

	Bacteria	Fungus	Protozoa	Virus
Flu (Influenza)				◆
Genital herpes				◆
Malaria			◆	
Meningitis	◆			◆
Pneumonia	◆	◆		◆
Sinusitis	◆	◆		
Skin diseases	◆	◆	◆	◆
Tuberculosis	◆			
Urinary tract infection	◆			
Vaginal infections	◆	◆	◆	
Viral hepatitis				◆

Emerging and Re-Emerging Microbes

With the arrival of antibiotics and modern vaccines, as well as improved sanitation and hygiene, many diseases that formerly posed an urgent threat to public health were brought under control or largely eliminated. As a result, by the mid-20th century some scientists thought that medical science had conquered infectious diseases.

Despite these public health advances, new microbes emerge and old microbes re-emerge just as they have throughout history. Several pressures contribute to the emergence of diseases, such as

- Redistribution of human populations

- Rapid global travel

- Changes in the way we use land

- Ecological, environmental, and technological changes

Practices such as the misuse of antibiotic medicines also contribute to disease emergence.

In addition, unsanitary conditions in animal agriculture and increasing commerce in exotic animals (for food and as pets) have contributed to the rise in opportunity for animal microbes to jump from animals to humans. From time to time, with the right combination of selective pressures, a formerly harmless microbe found in humans or animals can evolve into a pathogen that can cause a major outbreak of human disease. These pressures are shaping the evolution of microbes and bringing people into closer and more frequent contact with pathogens.

Emerging Microbes

Scientists usually define emerging microbes as those that have appeared only recently in a population or have existed but are rapidly increasing in incidence or geographic range. Recent examples of such disease-causing microbes are methicillin-resistant *Staphylococcus aureus* (MRSA) bacteria, West Nile virus, and 2009 H1N1 influenza virus.

Some newly emerging/emerged microbes

- 2009 H1N1 influenza virus

- Ebola virus

- H5N1 avian influenza virus

- Marburg virus

- MRSA bacteria

- Multidrug-resistant and extensively drug-resistant tuberculosis bacteria

- Nipah virus

- SARS virus

- West Nile virus

- Zika virus

Re-Emerging Microbes

The reappearance of microbes that had been conquered successfully or controlled by medicines and vaccines is distressing to the scientific and medical communities, as well as to the public. One major cause of disease re-emergence is that many microbes responsible for causing these diseases are becoming resistant to the drugs used to treat them. Some examples of re-emerging infectious diseases that are of significant public health concern are dengue, malaria, tuberculosis (TB), and polio.

Section 1.3

Preventing Microbial Diseases

This section contains text excerpted from the following sources: Text under the heading "You Can Prevent Catching or Passing on Germs" is excerpted from "Microbes Prevention," National Institute of Allergy and Infectious Diseases (NIAID), November 3, 2010. Reviewed August 2016; Text under the heading "Some Vaccine-Preventable Infectious Diseases" is excerpted from "Understanding Microbes," National Institute of Allergy and Infectious Diseases (NIAID), September 1, 2009. Reviewed August 2016.

You Can Prevent Catching or Passing on Germs

Handwashing

Handwashing is one of the simplest, easiest, and most effective ways to prevent getting or passing on many germs. Amazingly, it is also one of the most overlooked. Healthcare experts recommend scrubbing your hands vigorously for at least 15 seconds with soap and water, about as long as it takes to recite the English alphabet. This will wash away cold and flu viruses and staph and strep bacteria as well as many other disease causing microbes.

It is especially important to wash your hands

- Before preparing or eating food
- After coughing or sneezing
- After using the bathroom
- After changing a diaper

Healthcare providers should be especially conscientious about washing their hands before and after examining any patient. Workers in childcare and eldercare settings, too, should be vigilant about hand washing around those in their care.

Medicines

There are medicines on the market that help prevent you from getting infected by germs. For example, you can prevent getting the flu by taking an antiviral medicine. Vaccines, however, are the best defense against influenza viruses.

Under specific circumstances, your healthcare provider may prescribe antibiotics to protect you from getting certain bacteria such as *Mycobacterium tuberculosis*, which causes tuberculosis (TB). Healthcare experts usually advise people traveling to areas where malaria is present to take antiparasitic medicines to prevent possible infection.

Vaccines

In 1796, Edward Jenner laid the foundation for modern vaccines by discovering one of the basic principles of immunization. He had used a relatively harmless microbe, cowpox virus, to bring about an immune response that would help protect people from getting infected by the related but deadly smallpox virus.

Dr. Jenner's discovery helped researchers find ways to ease human disease suffering worldwide. By the beginning of the 20th century, doctors were immunizing patients with vaccines for diphtheria, typhoid fever, and smallpox.

Today, safe and effective vaccines prevent childhood diseases, including measles, whooping cough, chickenpox, and the form of meningitis caused by *Haemophilus influenzae* type B (Hib) virus.

Vaccines, however, are not only useful for young children. Adolescents and adults should get vaccinated regularly for tetanus and diphtheria. A vaccine to prevent meningococcal meningitis is recommended for all adolescents. In addition, adults who never had diseases such as measles or chickenpox during childhood or who never received vaccines to prevent them should consider being immunized. Childhood diseases can be far more serious in adults.

If you travel or plan to travel outside the United States, getting the immunizations that are recommended for your destination(s) is very important. Vaccines can prevent yellow fever, polio, typhoid fever, hepatitis A, cholera, rabies, and other diseases that are more prevalent abroad than in this country.

Some Vaccine-Preventable Infectious Diseases

- Bacterial meningitis
- Chickenpox
- Cholera
- Diphtheria
- *Haemophilus influenzae* type B (Hib)
- Hepatitis A
- Hepatitis B

- Influenza (flu)
- Measles
- Mumps
- Pertussis (whooping cough)
- Pneumococcal pneumonia
- Polio
- Rabies
- Shingles
- Tetanus (lockjaw)
- Yellow fever

Some People Are Immune to Certain Diseases

We become immune to germs through natural and artificial means. As long ago as the 5th century B.C., Greek doctors noticed that people who had recovered from the plague would never get it again—they seemed to have become immune or resistant to the germ. You can become immune, or develop **immunity**, to a microbe in several ways.

The first time **T cells** and **B cells** in your **immune system** meet up with an **antigen**, such as a virus or bacterium, they prepare the immune system to destroy the antigen. Because the immune system often can remember its enemies, those cells become active if they meet that particular antigen again. This is called naturally acquired immunity.

Another example of naturally acquired immunity occurs when a pregnant woman passes **antibodies** to her unborn baby. Babies are born with weak **immune responses**, but they are protected from some diseases for their first few months of life by antibodies received from their mothers before birth. Babies who are nursed also receive antibodies from breast milk that help protect their digestive tracts.

Artificial immunity can come from vaccines. **Immunization** with vaccines is a safe way to get protection from germs. Some vaccines contain microorganisms or parts of microorganisms that have been weakened or killed. If you get this type of vaccine, those microorganisms (or their parts) will start your body's immune response, which will demolish the foreign invader but not make you sick. This is a type of artificially acquired immunity.

Immunity can be strong or weak and short-or long-lived, depending on the type of antigen, the amount of antigen, and the route by which it enters your body. When faced with the same antigen, some people's immune system will respond forcefully, others feebly, and some not at all.

The genes you inherit also can influence your likelihood of getting a disease. In simple terms, the genes you get from your parents can influence how your body reacts to certain microbes.

Section 1.4

General Symptoms, Diagnosis, and Treatment of Microbial Diseases

This section contains text excerpted from the following sources: Text under the heading "When You Should Go to the Doctor" is excerpted from "Symptoms of Microbes," National Institute of Allergy and Infectious Diseases (NIAID), November 3, 2010. Reviewed August 2016; Text under the heading "Infectious Diseases Are Treated in Many Ways" is excerpted from "Understanding Microbes," National Institute of Allergy and Infectious Diseases (NIAID), September 1, 2009. Reviewed August 2016.

When You Should Go to the Doctor

Generally, you should consult your healthcare provider if you have or think you may have an infectious disease. These trained professionals can determine whether you have been infected, determine the seriousness of your infection, and give you the best advice for treating or preventing disease.

Some infectious diseases, such as the common cold, usually do not require a visit to your doctor. They often last a short time and are not life-threatening, or there is no specific treatment. We've all heard the advice to rest and drink plenty of liquids to treat colds. Unless there are complications, most victims of colds find that their immune systems successfully fight off the viral culprits. In fact, the coughing and sneezing that make you feel miserable are part of your immune system's way of fighting off the culprits.

If, however, you have other conditions in which your immune system doesn't function properly, you should be in contact with your healthcare provider whenever you suspect you have any infectious disease, even the common cold. Such conditions can include asthma and immune deficiency diseases like acquired immune deficiency syndrome (AIDS).

In addition, some common, usually mild infectious diseases, such as chickenpox or seasonal flu, can cause serious harm in very young children and the elderly.

You Should Call a Healthcare Provider Immediately If...

- You have been bitten by an animal
- You are having difficulty breathing
- You have a cough that has lasted for more than a week
- You have a fever higher than 100°F
- You have episodes of rapid heartbeat
- You have a rash (especially if you have a fever at the same time)
- You have swelling
- You suddenly start having difficulty with seeing (blurry vision, for example)
- You have been vomiting

Infectious Diseases Are Diagnosed in Many Ways

Sometimes your healthcare provider can diagnose an infectious disease by listening to your medical history and doing a physical exam. For example, listening to you describe what happened and any symptoms you have noticed plays an important part in helping your doctor find out what's wrong.

Blood and urine tests are other ways to diagnose an infection. A laboratory expert can sometimes see the offending microbe in a sample of blood or urine viewed under a microscope. One or both of these tests may be the only way to determine what caused the infection, or they may be used to confirm a diagnosis.

In another type of test, your healthcare provider will take a sample of blood or other body fluid, such as vaginal secretion, and then put it into a special container called a Petri dish to see whether any microbe "grows." This test is called a culture. Lab workers usually can identify certain bacteria, such as chlamydia, and viruses, such as herpes simplex, using this method.

X-rays, scans, and biopsies (taking a tiny sample of tissue from the infected area and inspecting it under a microscope) are among other tools your healthcare provider can use to make an accurate diagnosis.

All of the above procedures are relatively safe, and some can be done in your healthcare provider's office or a clinic. Others pose a higher risk to you because they involve procedures that go inside your body. One such invasive procedure is taking a biopsy from an internal organ. For example, one way a doctor can diagnose *Pneumocystis carinii* pneumonia, a lung disease caused by a fungus, is by doing a biopsy on lung tissue and then examining the sample under a microscope.

Infectious Diseases Are Treated in Many Ways

How an infectious disease is treated depends on the microbe that caused it and sometimes on the age and medical condition of the person who is sick. Certain diseases are not treated at all, but are allowed to run their course, with the immune system doing its job alone. Some diseases, such as the common cold, are treated only to relieve the symptoms. Others, such as strep throat, are treated to destroy the offending microbe as well as to relieve symptoms.

By Your Immune System

Your immune system has an arsenal of ways to fight off invading microbes. Most begin with B and T cells and antibodies whose sole purpose is to keep your body healthy. Some of these cells sacrifice their lives to rid you of disease and restore your body to a healthy state. Some microbes normally present in your body also help destroy microbial invaders. For example, normal, good bacteria, such as *lactobacillus* in your digestive system, help destroy germs that find their way there.

Other important ways your body reacts to an infection include fever and coughing and sneezing.

Fever

Fever is one of your body's special ways of fighting an infectious disease. Many microbes are very sensitive to temperature changes and cannot survive in temperatures higher than normal body heat, which is usually around 98.6°F. Your body uses fever to destroy influenza viruses, for example.

Coughing and Sneezing

Another tool in your immune system's reaction to invading disease-causing microbes is mucus production. Coughing and sneezing help mucus move those germs out of your body efficiently and quickly.

Other methods your body may use to fight off an infectious disease include

- Inflammation
- Vomiting

- Diarrhea
- Fatigue
- Cramping

By Your Healthcare Provider

For Bacteria

The last century saw an explosion in our knowledge about how microbes work and in our methods of treating infectious diseases. For example, the discovery of antibiotics to treat and cure many bacterial diseases was a major breakthrough in medical history. Healthcare providers, however, sometimes prescribe antibiotics unnecessarily for a variety of reasons, including pressure from patients with viral diseases such as the flu.

Because antibiotics have been prescribed too often or prescribed for the wrong diseases for many years, some bacteria have become resistant to the killing effects of these drugs. This resistance, commonly called antibiotic or drug resistance, has become a very serious problem, especially in hospital settings.

Bacteria that are not killed by the antibiotic become strong enough to resist the same medicine the next time it is given. Because bacteria multiply so rapidly, changed or mutated bacteria that resist antibiotics will quickly outnumber those that can be destroyed by those same drugs.

For Viruses

Viral diseases can be very difficult to treat because viruses live inside your body's cells, where they are protected from medicines in the bloodstream. Researchers developed the first antiviral drug in the late 20th century. The drug, acyclovir, was first approved by the Food and Drug Administration to treat herpes simplex virus infections. Only a few other antiviral medicines are available to prevent and treat viral infections and diseases.

Healthcare providers treat HIV infection with a group of powerful medicines that can keep the virus in check. Known as highly active antiretroviral therapy, or HAART, this treatment has improved and lengthened the lives of many suffering from this deadly infection.

Viral diseases should never be treated with antibiotics. Sometimes a person with a viral disease will develop a bacterial disease as a complication of the initial viral disease. For example, children with chickenpox often scratch the itchy skin lesions (sores) caused by the virus. Bacteria such as *Staphylococcus* can enter those lesions and cause a bacterial infection. The healthcare provider may then prescribe an antibiotic to destroy the bacteria. The antibiotic, however, will not destroy the chickenpox virus, only the staph bacteria.

Although safe and effective treatments and cures for most viral diseases have eluded researchers, there are safe vaccines to protect us from viral infections and diseases.

For Fungi

Medicines applied directly to the infected area are available by prescription and over the counter to treat skin and nail fungal infections. Unfortunately, many people have had limited success with them. Very powerful oral antifungal medicines are available only to treat systemic (within the body) fungal infections, such as histoplasmosis. Healthcare providers usually prescribe oral antifungal medicines with caution because all of them, even the milder ones for skin and nail fungi, can have very serious side effects.

For Protozoa

Diseases caused by protozoan parasites are among the leading causes of death and disease in tropical and subtropical regions of the world. Developing countries within these areas contain three-quarters of the world's population, and their people suffer the most from these diseases. Currently, there are no vaccines that can control parasitic diseases.

In many cases, controlling the insects that transmit these diseases is difficult because of pesticide resistance, concerns regarding environmental damage, and lack of adequate public health systems to apply existing insect-control methods. Thus, disease control relies heavily on the availability of medicines. Healthcare providers usually use antiparasitic medicines to treat protozoal infections. Unfortunately, there are very few medicines that fight protozoa, and some of those are either harmful to humans or are becoming ineffective.

The fight against the protozoan *Plasmodium falciparum*, the cause of the most deadly form of malaria, is a good example. This protozoan has become resistant to most of the medicines currently available to destroy it. A major focus of malaria research is on developing a vaccine to prevent people from getting the disease in the first place. In the meantime, many worldwide programs hope to eventually control malaria by keeping people from contact with infected mosquitoes or preventing infection if contact can't be avoided.

19

Chapter 2

The Immune System and Its Functions

Overview of the Immune System

Function

The overall function of the immune system is to prevent or limit infection. An example of this principle is found in immunocompromised people, including those with genetic immune disorders, immune-debilitating infections like acquired immune deficiency syndrome (AIDS), and even pregnant women, who are susceptible to a range of microbes that typically do not cause infection in healthy individuals.

The immune system can distinguish between normal, healthy cells and unhealthy cells by recognizing a variety of "danger" cues called danger-associated molecular patterns (DAMPs). Cells may be unhealthy because of infection or because of cellular damage caused by non-infectious agents like sunburn or cancer. Infectious microbes such as viruses and bacteria release another set of signals recognized by the immune system called pathogen-associated molecular patterns (PAMPs).

When the immune system first recognizes these signals, it responds to address the problem. If an immune response cannot be activated when there is sufficient need, problems arise, like infection. On the

This chapter includes text excerpted from "Immune System," National Institute of Allergy and Infectious Diseases (NIAID), December 30, 2013.

other hand, when an immune response is activated without a real threat or is not turned off once the danger passes, different problems arise, such as allergic reactions and autoimmune disease.

The immune system is complex and pervasive. There are numerous cell types that either circulate throughout the body or reside in a particular tissue. Each cell type plays a unique role, with different ways of recognizing problems, communicating with other cells, and performing their functions. By understanding all the details behind this network, researchers may optimize immune responses to confront specific issues, ranging from infections to cancer.

Location

All immune cells come from precursors in the bone marrow and develop into mature cells through a series of changes that can occur in different parts of the body.

Skin: The skin is usually the first line of defense against microbes. Skin cells produce and secrete important antimicrobial proteins, and immune cells can be found in specific layers of skin.

Bone marrow: The bone marrow contains stems cells that can develop into a variety of cell types. The common myeloid progenitor stem cell in the bone marrow is the precursor to innate immune cells—neutrophils, eosinophils, basophils, mast cells, monocytes, dendritic cells, and macrophages—that are important first-line responders to infection.

The common lymphoid progenitor stem cell leads to adaptive immune cells—B cells and T cells—that are responsible for mounting responses to specific microbes based on previous encounters (immunological memory). Natural killer (NK) cells also are derived from the common lymphoid progenitor and share features of both innate and adaptive immune cells, as they provide immediate defenses like innate cells but also may be retained as memory cells like adaptive cells. B, T, and NK cells also are called lymphocytes.

Bloodstream: Immune cells constantly circulate throughout the bloodstream, patrolling for problems. When blood tests are used to monitor white blood cells, another term for immune cells, a snapshot of the immune system is taken. If a cell type is either scarce or overabundant in the bloodstream, this may reflect a problem.

Thymus: T cells mature in the thymus, a small organ located in the upper chest.

Lymphatic system: The lymphatic system is a network of vessels and tissues composed of lymph, an extracellular fluid, and lymphoid organs, such as lymph nodes. The lymphatic system is a conduit for travel and communication between tissues and the bloodstream. Immune cells are carried through the lymphatic system and converge in lymph nodes, which are found throughout the body.

Lymph nodes are a communication hub where immune cells sample information brought in from the body. For instance, if adaptive immune cells in the lymph node recognize pieces of a microbe brought in from a distant area, they will activate, replicate, and leave the lymph node to circulate and address the pathogen. Thus, doctors may check patients for swollen lymph nodes, which may indicate an active immune response.

Spleen: The spleen is an organ located behind the stomach. While it is not directly connected to the lymphatic system, it is important for processing information from the bloodstream. Immune cells are enriched in specific areas of the spleen, and upon recognizing blood-borne pathogens, they will activate and respond accordingly.

Mucosal tissue: Mucosal surfaces are prime entry points for pathogens, and specialized immune hubs are strategically located in mucosal tissues like the respiratory tract and gut. For instance, Peyer's patches are important areas in the small intestine where immune cells can access samples from the gastrointestinal tract.

Features of an Immune Response

An immune response is generally divided into innate and adaptive immunity. Innate immunity occurs immediately, when circulating innate cells recognize a problem. Adaptive immunity occurs later, as it relies on the coordination and expansion of specific adaptive immune cells. Immune memory follows the adaptive response, when mature adaptive cells, highly specific to the original pathogen, are retained for later use.

Innate Immunity

Innate immune cells express genetically encoded receptors, called Toll-like receptors (TLRs), which recognize general danger-or pathogen-associated patterns. Collectively, these receptors can broadly recognize viruses, bacteria, fungi, and even non-infectious problems. However, they cannot distinguish between specific strains of bacteria or viruses.

There are numerous types of innate immune cells with specialized functions. They include neutrophils, eosinophils, basophils, mast cells, monocytes, dendritic cells, and macrophages. Their main feature is the ability to respond quickly and broadly when a problem arises, typically leading to inflammation. Innate immune cells also are important for activating adaptive immunity. Innate cells are critical for host defense, and disorders in innate cell function may cause chronic susceptibility to infection.

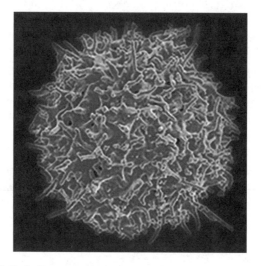

Figure 2.1. *A T Cell, Part of Adaptive Immunity That Provides Immune Memory*

Adaptive Immunity

Adaptive immune cells are more specialized, with each adaptive B or T cell bearing unique receptors, B-cell receptors (BCRs) and T-cell receptors (TCRs), that recognize specific signals rather than general patterns. Each receptor recognizes an antigen, which is simply any molecule that may bind to a BCR or TCR. Antigens are derived from a variety of sources including pathogens, host cells, and allergens. Antigens are typically processed by innate immune cells and presented to adaptive cells in the lymph nodes.

The genes for BCRs and TCRs are randomly rearranged at specific cell maturation stages, resulting in unique receptors that may potentially recognize anything. Random generation of receptors allows the immune system to respond to new or unforeseen problems. This concept is especially important because environments may frequently change, for instance when seasons change or a person relocates, and pathogens are constantly evolving to survive. Because BCRs and TCRs are so specific, adaptive cells may only recognize one strain of a particular pathogen, unlike innate cells, which recognize broad classes of pathogens. In fact, a group of adaptive cells that recognize the same strain will likely recognize different areas of that pathogen.

If a B or T cell has a receptor that recognizes an antigen from a pathogen and also receives cues from innate cells that something is wrong, the B or T cell will activate, divide, and disperse to address the problem. B cells make antibodies, which neutralize pathogens, rendering them harmless. T cells carry out multiple functions, including killing infected cells and activating or recruiting other immune cells. The adaptive response has a system of checks and balances to prevent unnecessary activation that could cause damage to the host. If a B or T cell is auto-reactive, meaning its receptor recognizes antigens from the body's own cells, the cell will be deleted. Also, if a B or T cell does not receive signals from innate cells, it will not be optimally activated.

Immune memory is a feature of the adaptive immune response. After B or T cells are activated, they expand rapidly. As the problem resolves, cells stop dividing and are retained in the body as memory cells. The next time this same pathogen enters the body, a memory cell is already poised to react and can clear away the pathogen before it establishes itself.

Vaccination

Vaccination, or immunization, is a way to train your immune system against a specific pathogen. Vaccination achieves immune memory without an actual infection, so the body is prepared when the virus or bacterium enters. Saving time is important to prevent a pathogen from establishing itself and infecting more cells in the body.

An effective vaccine will optimally activate both the innate and adaptive response. An immunogen is used to activate the adaptive immune response so that specific memory cells are generated. Because BCRs and TCRs are unique, some memory cells are simply better at eliminating the pathogen. The goal of vaccine design is to select immunogens that will generate the most effective and efficient memory response against a particular pathogen. Adjuvants, which are important for activating innate immunity, can be added to vaccines to optimize the immune response. Innate immunity recognizes broad patterns, and without innate responses, adaptive immunity cannot be optimally achieved.

Chapter 3

Immunodeficiency and Contagious Diseases

Primary Immune Deficiency Diseases (PIDDs)

There are more than 200 different forms of primary immune deficiency diseases (PIDDs) affecting only about 500,000 people in the United States. These rare genetic diseases may be chronic, debilitating, and costly. Since the 1970s, National Institute of Allergy and Infectious Diseases (NIAID)-supported investigators have been examining the causes and complications of PIDDs to improve the lives of patients and families. NIAID aims to improve diagnosis, explore new treatments and preventions for PIDDs, and facilitate genetic counseling. It is home to the Primary Immune Deficiency Clinic, which provides diagnoses and disease management recommendations to patients and families whose lives are touched by PIDDs.

Types of Primary Immune Deficiency Diseases

Autoimmune Lymphoproliferative Syndrome (ALPS)

In ALPS, unusually high numbers of white blood cells called lymphocytes accumulate in the lymph nodes, liver, and spleen, which can

---

This chapter includes text excerpted from "Primary Immune Deficiency Diseases (PIDDs)," National Institute of Allergy and Infectious Diseases (NIAID), December 5, 2015.

27

lead to enlargement of these organs. ALPS can cause numerous auto-immune problems, including low levels of red blood cells, clot-forming platelets, and infection-fighting white blood cells called neutrophils.

Autoimmune Polyglandular Syndrome Type 1 (APS-1)

APS-1 causes a diverse range of symptoms, including autoimmunity against different types of organs and candidiasis, a fungal infection caused by Candida yeast. The disease also is called autoimmune poly-endocrinopathy-candidiasis-ectodermal dystrophy (APECED).

CARD9 Deficiency and Other Syndromes of Susceptibility to Candidiasis

CARD9 deficiency results in susceptibility to fungal infections like candidiasis, which is caused by the yeast fungus Candida. Typically, Candida and other fungi are present on the skin and do not cause severe problems in healthy people.

Chronic Granulomatous Disease (CGD)

CGD occurs when white blood cells called phagocytes are unable to kill certain bacteria and fungi, and mutations in one of five different genes may cause this disease. People with CGD have increased sus-ceptibility to infections.

Common Variable Immunodeficiency (CVID)

CVID is caused by a variety of different genetic abnormalities that result in a defect in the capability of immune cells to produce normal amounts of antibodies. People with CVID experience frequent bacterial or viral infections of the upper airway, sinuses, and lungs.

Congenital Neutropenia Syndromes

Congenital neutropenia syndromes are a group of disorders char-acterized by low levels of neutrophils—white blood cells necessary for combating infections—from birth.

CTLA4 Deficiency

CTLA4 deficiency impairs normal regulation of the immune system, resulting in excessive numbers of immune cells called lymphocytes, autoimmunity, low levels of antibodies, and recurrent infections. The disease is characterized by infiltration of immune cells into the gut, lungs, bone marrow, central nervous system, kidneys, and possibly other organs.

DOCK8 Deficiency

DOCK8 deficiency is named after the mutated gene responsible for the disease. The genetic defect causes decreased numbers and defective function of immune cells, which lead to recurrent infections.

GATA2 Deficiency

GATA2 deficiency can manifest as five distinct syndromes. There is a wide variety of symptoms, including severe infections, respiratory problems, hearing loss, leg swelling, and cancer. Symptoms can appear early in childhood but also later on in life.

Glycosylation Disorders with Immunodeficiency

Glycosylation refers to the attachment of sugars to proteins, a normal process required for the healthy function of cells. Defects in glycosylation can disrupt the immune system, resulting in immunodeficiency.

Hyper-Immunoglobulin E Syndrome (Job's Syndrome)

Hyper-IgE syndrome (HIES), also called Job's Syndrome, results from mutations in a gene that encodes a signaling molecule called STAT3. People with HIES experience recurrent infections of the skin and lungs caused by bacteria.

Hyper-Immunoglobulin M (Hyper-IgM) Syndromes

Hyper-IgM syndromes are conditions in which the immune system fails to produce normal immunoglobulin A (IgA), IgG, and IgE antibodies but can produce normal or elevated IgM. Infants with a hyper-IgM syndrome usually develop severe respiratory infections within the first year of life.

Interferon Gamma, Interleukin 12, Interleukin 23 Deficiencies

Interferon gamma, interleukin 12, and interleukin 23 are key signals that raise an alert against bacteria and other infectious microbes.

People with deficiencies in one or more of these pathways are susceptible to infections caused by bacteria and viruses.

Leukocyte Adhesion Deficiency (LAD)

LAD occurs when immune cells called phagocytes are unable to move to the site of an infection. This inability to fight germs results in recurrent, life-threatening infections, and poor wound healing.

NF-κB Essential Modifier (NEMO) Mutations

People with mutations in the NEMO gene cannot "turn on" certain genes, especially those involved in inflammation and the immune response. People with NEMO mutations are highly susceptible to infections with mycobacteria.

PI3 Kinase Disease

PI3 Kinase disease is caused by genetic mutations that overactivate an important immune system signaling pathway. This causes a chain reaction of problems, disrupting the normal development of infection-fighting B and T cells. People with the disease have a weakened immune system and experience frequent bacterial and viral infections.

PLCG2-Associated Antibody Deficiency and Immune Dysregulation (PLAID)

PLAID and PLAID-like diseases are rare immune disorders with overlapping features, and an allergic response to cold, called cold urticaria, is the most distinct symptom.

Severe Combined Immunodeficiency (SCID)

Severe Combined Immunodeficiency (SCID) is a group of rare, life-threatening disorders caused by mutations in different genes involved in the development and function of infection-fighting T and B cells. Infants with SCID appear healthy at birth but are highly susceptible to severe infections.

Warts, Hypogammaglobulinemia, Infections, and Myelokathexis Syndrome (WHIMS)

People with WHIM syndrome have low levels of infection-fighting white blood cells, especially neutrophils, in their bloodstreams.

This deficiency predisposes them to frequent infections and persistent warts.

Wiskott-Aldrich Syndrome (WAS)

People with WAS have problems with their infection-fighting B and T cells and clot-forming platelets. This can result in prolonged episodes of bleeding, recurrent bacterial and fungal infections, and an increased risk of cancers and autoimmune diseases.

X-Linked Agammaglobulinemia (XLA)

XLA is caused by an inability to produce B cells or immunoglobulins (antibodies), which are made by B cells. People with XLA develop frequent infections of the ears, throat, lungs, and sinuses.

X-Linked Lymphoproliferative Disease (XLP)

XLP primarily affects boys and is characterized by a life-long vulnerability to Epstein-Barr virus (EBV), a common type of herpesvirus. Boys with XLP are healthy until they are exposed to EBV. Then, they can become seriously ill and experience swollen lymph nodes, an enlarged liver and spleen, hepatitis, and lymphoma, a type of cancer.

Genetics and Inheritance

PIDDs are caused by genetic abnormalities that prevent the body from developing normal immune responses.

All of the body's cells contain instructions on how to do their jobs. These instructions are packaged into 23 pairs of chromosomes—22 pairs of numbered chromosomes, called autosomes, and one pair of sex chromosomes (XX for girls and XY for boys). One chromosome in each pair is inherited from the person's mother and the other from the father. Each chromosome contains many genes, which are made up of DNA, the carrier of genetic information. Errors, or mutations, in genes can cause diseases such as PIDDs.

Genetic mutations sometimes appear randomly. For example, de novo, or "new," mutations occur as a result of a mutation in the egg or sperm of one of the parents or in the fertilized egg itself. In these cases, the affected person does not have a family history of disease.

Most often, genetic mutations run in families. Several types of inherited mutations can cause PIDDs.

Autosomal Dominant

To develop an autosomal dominant disease, a person needs an abnormal gene from only one parent, even if the matching gene from the other parent is normal. A parent with an autosomal dominant disease has a 50 percent chance of having a child with the condition. The chance of one child inheriting the mutation is independent of whether his or her siblings have the mutation. In other words, if the first two children in a family have the mutation, the third child still has a 50 percent chance of inheriting it.

Autosomal Recessive

Two copies of an abnormal gene—one from each parent—must be present for an autosomal recessive disease to develop. Typically, both parents of an affected child carry one abnormal gene and are unaffected by the disease because the normal gene on the other chromosome continues to function. In this case, each child has a 25 percent, or one in four, chance of being affected by the disease. Each child also has a 50 percent chance of inheriting one copy of the mutated gene. People who inherit one abnormal gene copy will not develop the disease, but they can pass the mutation on to their children.

X-Linked Recessive

X-linked recessive diseases are caused by genes located on the X chromosome. Boys have only one copy of X-linked genes because they have one X chromosome. If a boy inherits a disease-causing mutation in a gene located on the X chromosome, he will develop the disease.

Girls usually do not develop X-linked recessive diseases because they have two X chromosomes and would need to inherit two abnormal copies of the gene—one from each parent—to be affected by the disease. Even if a girl carries the mutated gene on one X chromosome, the normal gene on the other X chromosome continues to function and she remains unaffected by the disease. Women who inherit one abnormal gene copy can pass the mutated gene on to their children.

Talking to Your Doctor

We rely on our immune system to fight harmful bacteria or viruses—either on its own or with the help of antibiotics or antivirals—every day. Most of us recover quickly from infectious illnesses, and our immune system helps protect us from repeat infections in the future.

People with primary immune deficiency diseases (PIDDs), however, have defects in one or more parts of their immune system. They often cannot overcome infections, even with the aid of medicine.

Are You or Your Child at Risk for a PIDD?

- Do you get multiple, serious infections that are difficult to treat within a year?

- Have you had bacterial infections that don't get better, even after you've taken antibiotics?

- When you are sick, do you need to go to the hospital and/or receive intravenous antibiotics to get well?

- Do you have a family history of primary immune deficiency?

If you answered "yes" to any of these questions, you may be at risk for a PIDD. Consult with your doctor to get tested for an immune deficiency.

What to Ask Your Doctor

- Based on my medical and family history, am I at risk for an immune deficiency?

- What tests will be performed to determine my diagnosis, and how long will it take to get the results back?

- What precautions should I take to reduce my risk of infection?

- Should I see a specialist?

To diagnose a potential immune deficiency, your doctor will need to take a blood sample and send it to a lab for an initial screening test. If that test shows that you may be at risk for a PIDD, you'll need additional testing.

What to Bring to Your Doctor's Appointment

- A current list of medicines you have taken in the past and their effects.

- Specific questions you want to have answered.

- A journal to write down answers to your questions or to take notes.

Chapter 4

Common Variable Immune Deficiency

Common variable immunodeficiency (CVID) is a disorder that impairs the immune system. People with CVID are highly susceptible to infection from foreign invaders such as bacteria, or more rarely, viruses and often develop recurrent infections, particularly in the lungs, sinuses, and ears. Pneumonia is common in people with CVID. Over time, recurrent infections can lead to chronic lung disease. Affected individuals may also experience infection or inflammation of the gastrointestinal tract, which can cause diarrhea and weight loss. Abnormal accumulation of immune cells causes enlarged lymph nodes (lymphadenopathy) or an enlarged spleen (splenomegaly) in some people with CVID. Immune cells can accumulate in other organs, forming small lumps called granulomas.

Approximately 25 percent of people with CVID have an autoimmune disorder, which occurs when the immune system malfunctions and attacks the body's tissues and organs. The blood cells are most frequently affected by autoimmune attacks in CVID; the most commonly occurring autoimmune disorders are immune thrombocytopenia purpura, which is an abnormal bleeding disorder caused by a decrease in platelets, and autoimmune hemolytic anemia, which results in premature destruction of red blood cells. Other autoimmune disorders

This chapter includes text excerpted from "Common Variable Immune Deficiency," Genetics Home Reference (GHR), National Institutes of Health (NIH), June 28, 2016.

such as rheumatoid arthritis can occur. Individuals with CVID also have a greater than normal risk of developing certain types of cancer, including a cancer of immune system cells called non-Hodgkin lymphoma and less frequently, stomach (gastric) cancer.

People with CVID may start experiencing signs and symptoms of the disorder anytime between childhood and adulthood; most people with CVID are diagnosed in their twenties or thirties. The life expectancy of individuals with CVID varies depending on the severity and frequency of illnesses they experience. Most people with CVID live into adulthood.

There are many different types of CVID that are distinguished by genetic cause. People with the same type of CVID may have varying signs and symptoms.

Frequency

CVID is estimated to affect 1 in 25,000 to 1 in 50,000 people worldwide, although the prevalence can vary across different populations.

Genetic Changes

The cause in CVID is unknown in approximately 90 percent of cases. It is likely that this condition is caused by both environmental and genetic factors. While the specific environmental factors are unclear, the genetic influences in CVID are believed to be mutations in genes that are involved in the development and function of immune system cells called B cells. B cells are specialized white blood cells that help protect the body against infection. When B cells mature, they produce special proteins called antibodies (also known as immunoglobulins). These proteins attach to foreign particles, marking them for destruction. Mutations in the genes associated with CVID result in dysfunctional B cells that cannot make sufficient amounts of antibodies.

In about 10 percent of cases, a genetic cause for CVID is known. Mutations in at least 13 genes have been associated with CVID. The most frequent mutations occur in the *TNFRSF13B* gene. The protein produced from this gene plays a role in the survival and maturation of B cells and in the production of antibodies. *TNFRSF13B* gene mutations disrupt B cell function and antibody production, leading to immune dysfunction. Other genes associated with CVID are also involved in the function and maturation of immune system cells, particularly of B cells; mutations in these genes account for only a small percentage of cases.

All individuals with CVID have a shortage (deficiency) of two or three specific antibodies. Some have a deficiency of the antibodies called immunoglobulin G (IgG) and immunoglobulin A (IgA), while others, in addition to lacking IgG and IgA, are also deficient in immunoglobulin M (IgM). A shortage of these antibodies makes it difficult for people with this disorder to fight off infections. Abnormal and deficient immune responses over time likely contribute to the increased cancer risk. In addition, vaccines for diseases such as measles and influenza do not provide protection for people with CVID because they cannot produce an antibody response.

Inheritance Pattern

Most cases of CVID are sporadic and occur in people with no apparent history of the disorder in their family. These cases probably result from a complex interaction of environmental and genetic factors.

In rare cases, CVID is inherited in an autosomal recessive pattern, which means both copies of a gene in each cell have mutations. The parents of an individual with an autosomal recessive condition each carry one copy of the mutated gene, but they typically do not show signs and symptoms of the condition.

In a few cases, this condition is inherited in an autosomal dominant pattern, which means one copy of an altered gene in each cell is sufficient to cause the disorder.

When CVID is caused by mutations in the *TNFRSF13B* gene, it is often sporadic and the result of a new mutation in the gene that occurs during the formation of reproductive cells (eggs or sperm) or in early embryonic development. When *TNFRSF13B* gene mutations are inherited, they can cause either autosomal dominant CVID or autosomal recessive CVID.

Not all individuals who inherit a gene mutation associated with CVID will develop the disease. In many cases, affected children have an unaffected parent who has the same mutation. Additional genetic or environmental factors are likely needed for the disorder to occur.

Other Names for This Condition

- common variable hypogammaglobulinemia
- common variable immunodeficiency
- immunodeficiency, common variable

37

Chapter 5

Transmission of Contagious Diseases

Chapter Contents

Section 5.1

Transmission of Microbes That Cause Contagious Diseases

This section includes text excerpted from "Microbes," National Institute of Allergy and Infectious Diseases (NIAID), July 25, 2014.

According to healthcare experts, infectious diseases caused by microbes are responsible for more deaths worldwide than any other single cause. They estimate the annual cost of medical care for treating infectious diseases in the United States alone is about $120 billion.

The science of microbiology explores how microbes work and how to control them. It seeks ways to use that knowledge to prevent and treat the diseases microbes cause. The 20th century saw an extraordinary increase in our knowledge about microbes. Microbiologists and other researchers had many successes in learning how microbes cause certain infectious diseases and how to combat those microbes.

Unfortunately, microbes are much better at adapting to new environments than are people. Having existed on Earth for billions of years, microbes are constantly challenging human newcomers with ingenious new survival tactics.

- Many microbes are developing new properties to resist drug treatments that once effectively destroyed them. Drug resistance has become a serious problem worldwide.

- Changes in the environment have put certain human populations in contact with newly identified microbes that cause diseases we have never seen before, or that previously occurred only in isolated populations.

- Newly emerging diseases are a growing global health concern. Since 1976, scientists have identified approximately 30 new pathogens, such as HIV.

Some Ways Microbes Are Transmitted

Some Microbes Can Travel through the Air

You can transmit microbes to another person through the air by coughing or sneezing. These are common ways to get viruses that cause colds or flu, or the bacteria that cause tuberculosis. Interestingly, international airplane travel can expose you to germs not common in your own country.

Close Contact Can Pass Germs to Another Person

Scientists have identified more than 500 types of bacteria that live in our mouths. Some keep the oral environment healthy, while others cause problems like gum disease. One way you can transmit oral bacteria is by kissing.

Microbes such as HIV, herpes simplex virus type 2, which causes genital herpes, and *Neisseria gonorrhoeae* bacteria, which causes gonorrhea, are examples of germs that you can pass to another during sexual intercourse.

You Can Pick up and Spread Germs by Touching Infectious Material

A common way for some microbes to enter the body, especially when caring for young children, is through unintentionally passing feces from hand to mouth or the mouths of young children. Infant diarrhea is often spread in this way. Daycare workers, for example, can pass diarrhea-causing rotavirus or *Giardia lamblia* (protozoa) from one baby to the next between diaper changes and other childcare practices.

It also is possible to pick up cold viruses from shaking someone's hand or from touching contaminated surfaces, such as a doorknob or computer keyboard.

A Healthy Person Can Carry Germs and Pass Them onto Others

The story of "Typhoid Mary" is a famous example from medical history about how a person can pass germs on to others, yet not be affected by those germs. The germs in this case were *Salmonella typhi* bacteria, which cause typhoid fever and are usually spread through food or water.

41

In the early 20th century, Mary Mallon, an Irish immigrant, worked as a cook for several New York City families. More than half of the first family she worked for came down with typhoid fever. Through a clever deduction, a researcher determined that the disease was caused by the family cook. He concluded that although Mary had no symptoms of the disease, she probably had had a mild typhoid infection sometime in the past. Though not sick, she still carried the *Salmonella* bacteria and was able to spread them to others through the food she prepared.

Germs from Your Household Pet Can Make You Sick

You can catch a variety of germs from animals, especially household pets. The rabies virus, which can infect cats and dogs, is one of the most serious and deadly of these microbes. Fortunately, rabies vaccine prevents animals from getting rabies. Vaccines also protect people from accidentally getting the virus from an animal. In addition, vaccines prevent people who already have been exposed to the virus, such as through an animal bite, from getting sick.

Dog and cat saliva can contain any of more than 100 different germs that can make you sick. *Pasteurella* bacteria, the most common, can be transmitted through bites that break the skin causing serious, and sometimes fatal, diseases such as meningitis. Meningitis is inflammation of the lining of the brain and spinal cord.

Warm-blooded animals are not the only ones that can cause you harm. Pet reptiles such as turtles, snakes, and iguanas can give *Salmonella* bacteria to their unsuspecting owners.

You Can Get Microbes from Tiny Critters

Mosquitoes may be the most common carriers, also called vectors, of pathogens. The female anopheles mosquito, which causes malaria, picks up the malarial parasite from an infected person during a blood meal. When the mosquito takes a blood meal on an uninfected person, the parasites are transmitted to the new host, starting another human infection.

Fleas that pick up *Yersinia pestis* bacteria from rodents can then transmit plague to humans.

Ticks, which are more closely related to crabs than to insects, are another common vector. The tiny deer tick can infect humans with *Borrelia burgdorferi*, the bacterium that causes Lyme disease, which the tick picks up from mice.

Some Microbes in Food or Water Could Make You Sick

Every year, millions of people worldwide become ill from eating contaminated foods. Although many cases of foodborne illness or "food poisoning" are not reported, the Centers for Disease Control and Prevention (CDC) estimates there are 76 million cases of such illnesses in the United States each year. In addition, CDC estimates 325,000 hospitalizations and 5,000 deaths are related to foodborne diseases each year. Microbes can cause these illnesses, some of which can be fatal if not treated properly.

Poor manufacturing processes or poor food preparation can allow microbes to grow in food and subsequently infect you. *Escherichia coli* (E. coli) bacteria sometimes persist in food products such as undercooked hamburger meat and unpasteurized fruit juice. These bacteria can have deadly consequences in vulnerable people, especially children and the elderly.

Cryptosporidia are bacteria found in human and animal feces. These bacteria can get into lake, river, and ocean water from sewage spills, animal waste, and water runoff. Millions can be released from infectious fecal matter. People who drink, swim in, or play in infected water can get sick.

People, including babies, with diarrhea caused by *Cryptosporidia* or other diarrhea-causing microbes such as *Giardia* and *Salmonella*, can infect others while using swimming pools, water parks, hot tubs, and spas.

Transplanted Animal Organs May Harbor Germs

Researchers are investigating the possibility of transplanting animal organs, such as pig hearts, into people. They, however, must guard against the risk that those organs also may transmit microbes that were harmless to the animal into humans, where they may cause disease.

How You Can Protect Yourself from Microbes

We become immune to germs through natural and artificial means. As long ago as the 5th century B.C., Greek doctors noticed that people who had recovered from the plague would never get it again—they seemed to have become immune or resistant to the germ. You can become immune, or develop immunity, to a microbe in several ways. The first time T cells and B cells in your immune system meet up with an antigen, such as a virus or bacterium, they prepare the immune system to destroy the antigen.

Naturally Acquired Immunity

Because the immune system often can remember its enemies, those cells become active if they meet that particular antigen again. This is called naturally acquired immunity.

Another example of naturally acquired immunity occurs when a pregnant woman passes antibodies to her unborn baby. Babies are born with weak immune responses, but they are protected from some diseases for their first few months of life by antibodies received from their mothers before birth. Babies who are nursed also receive antibodies from breast milk that help protect their digestive tracts.

Artificial Immunity

Artificial immunity can come from vaccines. Immunization with vaccines is a safe way to get protection from germs. Some vaccines contain microorganisms or parts of microorganisms that have been weakened or killed. If you get this type of vaccine, those microorganisms (or their parts) will start your body's immune response, which will demolish the foreign invader but not make you sick. This is a type of artificially acquired immunity.

Immunity can be strong or weak and short-or long-lived, depending on the type of antigen, the amount of antigen, and the route by which it enters your body. When faced with the same antigen, some people's immune system will respond forcefully, others feebly, and some not at all.

The genes you inherit also can influence your likelihood of getting a disease. In simple terms, the genes you get from your parents can influence how your body reacts to certain microbes.

Section 5.2

Preventing the Transmission of Sexually Transmitted Disease

This section includes text excerpted from "How You Can Prevent
Sexually Transmitted Diseases," Centers for Disease Control
and Prevention (CDC), March 31, 2016.

Abstinence

The most reliable way to avoid infection is to not have sex (i.e.,
anal, vaginal or oral).

Vaccination

Vaccines are safe, effective, and recommended ways to prevent
hepatitis B and human papillomavirus (HPV). HPV vaccines for males
and females can protect against some of the most common types of
HPV. It is best to get all three doses (shots) before becoming sexually
active. However, HPV vaccines are recommended for all teen girls and
women through age 26 and all teen boys and men through age 21, who
did not get all three doses of the vaccine when they were younger. You
should also get vaccinated for hepatitis B if you were not vaccinated
when you were younger.

Reduce Number of Sex Partners

Reducing your number of sex partners can decrease your risk for
STDs. It is still important that you and your partner get tested, and
that you share your test results with one another.

Mutual Monogamy

Mutual monogamy means that you agree to be sexually active with
only one person, who has agreed to be sexually active only with you.
Being in a long-term mutually monogamous relationship with an uninfected partner is one of the most reliable ways to avoid STDs. But you

must both be certain you are not infected with STDs. It is important to have an open and honest conversation with your partner.

Use Condoms

Correct and consistent use of the male latex condom is highly effective in reducing STD transmission. Use a condom every time you have anal, vaginal or oral sex.

If you have latex allergies, synthetic non-latex condoms can be used. But it is important to note that these condoms have higher breakage rates than latex condoms. Natural membrane condoms are not recommended for STD prevention.

Section 5.3

Risk of Infectious Disease from Blood Transfusion

This section contains text excerpted from the following sources: Text beginning with the heading "What Is a Blood Transfusion?" is excerpted from "What Is a Blood Transfusion?" National Heart, Lung, and Blood Institute (NHLBI), January 30, 2012. Reviewed August 2016; Text beginning with the heading "What Are the Risks of a Blood Transfusion?" is excerpted from "What Are the Risks of a Blood Transfusion?" National Heart, Lung, and Blood Institute (NHLBI), January 30, 2012. Reviewed August 2016.

What Is a Blood Transfusion?

A blood transfusion is a safe, common procedure in which blood is given to you through an intravenous (IV) line in one of your blood vessels.

Blood transfusions are done to replace blood lost during surgery or due to a serious injury. A transfusion also may be done if your body can't make blood properly because of an illness.

During a blood transfusion, a small needle is used to insert an IV line into one of your blood vessels. Through this line, you receive healthy blood. The procedure usually takes 1 to 4 hours, depending on how much blood you need.

Blood transfusions are very common. Each year, almost 5 million Americans need a blood transfusion. Most blood transfusions go well. Mild complications can occur. Very rarely, serious problems develop.

Important Information about Blood

The heart pumps blood through a network of arteries and veins throughout the body. Blood has many vital jobs. It carries oxygen and other nutrients to your body's organs and tissues. Having a healthy supply of blood is important to your overall health.

Blood is made up of various parts, including red blood cells, white blood cells, platelets, and plasma. Blood is transfused either as whole blood (with all its parts) or, more often, as individual parts.

Blood Types

Every person has one of the following blood types: A, B, AB or O. Also, every person's blood is either Rh-positive or Rh-negative. So, if you have type A blood, it's either A positive or A negative.

The blood used in a transfusion must work with your blood type. If it doesn't, antibodies (proteins) in your blood attack the new blood and make you sick.

Type O blood is safe for almost everyone. About 40 percent of the population has type O blood. People who have this blood type are called universal donors. Type O blood is used for emergencies when there's no time to test a person's blood type.

People who have type AB blood are called universal recipients. This means they can get any type of blood.

If you have Rh-positive blood, you can get Rh-positive or Rh-negative blood. But if you have Rh-negative blood, you should only get Rh-negative blood. Rh-negative blood is used for emergencies when there's no time to test a person's Rh type.

Blood Banks

Blood banks collect, test, and store blood. They carefully screen all donated blood for possible infectious agents, such as viruses, that could make you sick.

Blood bank staff also screen each blood donation to find out whether it's type A, B, AB, or O and whether it's Rh-positive or Rh-negative.

Getting a blood type that doesn't work with your own blood type will make you very sick. That's why blood banks are very careful when they test the blood.

To prepare blood for a transfusion, some blood banks remove white blood cells. This process is called white cell or leukocyte reduction. Although rare, some people are allergic to white blood cells in donated blood. Removing these cells makes allergic reactions less likely.

Not all transfusions use blood donated from a stranger. If you're going to have surgery, you may need a blood transfusion because of blood loss during the operation. If it's surgery that you're able to schedule months in advance, your doctor may ask whether you would like to use your own blood, rather than donated blood.

If you choose to use your own blood, you will need to have blood drawn one or more times prior to the surgery. A blood bank will store your blood for your use.

Alternatives to Blood Transfusions

Researchers are trying to find ways to make blood. There's currently no man-made alternative to human blood. However, researchers have developed medicines that may help do the job of some blood parts.

For example, some people who have kidney problems can now take a medicine called erythropoietin that helps their bodies make more red blood cells. This means they may need fewer blood transfusions.

Surgeons try to reduce the amount of blood lost during surgery so that fewer patients need blood transfusions. Sometimes they can collect and reuse the blood for the patient.

What Are the Risks of a Blood Transfusion?

Most blood transfusions go very smoothly. However, mild problems and, very rarely, serious problems can occur.

Allergic Reactions

Some people have allergic reactions to the blood given during transfusions. This can happen even when the blood given is the right blood type.

Allergic reactions can be mild or severe. Symptoms can include:

- Anxiety
- Chest and/or back pain

- Trouble breathing

- Fever, chills, flushing, and clammy skin

- A quick pulse or low blood pressure

- Nausea (feeling sick to the stomach)

A nurse or doctor will stop the transfusion at the first signs of an allergic reaction. The healthcare team determines how mild or severe the reaction is, what treatments are needed, and whether the transfusion can safely be restarted.

Viruses and Infectious Diseases

Some infectious agents, such as HIV, can survive in blood and infect the person receiving the blood transfusion. To keep blood safe, blood banks carefully screen donated blood.

The risk of catching a virus from a blood transfusion is very low.

- HIV. Your risk of getting HIV from a blood transfusion is lower than your risk of getting killed by lightning. Only about 1 in 2 million donations might carry HIV and transmit HIV if given to a patient.

- Hepatitis B and C. The risk of having a donation that carries hepatitis B is about 1 in 205,000. The risk for hepatitis C is 1 in 2 million. If you receive blood during a transfusion that contains hepatitis, you'll likely develop the virus.

- Variant Creutzfeldt-Jakob disease (vCJD). This disease is the human version of Mad Cow Disease. It's a very rare, yet fatal brain disorder. There is a possible risk of getting vCJD from a blood transfusion, although the risk is very low. Because of this, people who may have been exposed to vCJD aren't eligible blood donors.

Fever

You may get a sudden fever during or within a day of your blood transfusion. This is usually your body's normal response to white blood cells in the donated blood. Over-the-counter fever medicine usually will treat the fever.

Some blood banks remove white blood cells from whole blood or different parts of the blood. This makes it less likely that you will have a reaction after the transfusion.

Iron Overload

Getting many blood transfusions can cause too much iron to build up in your blood (iron overload). People who have a blood disorder like thalassemia, which requires multiple transfusions, are at risk for iron overload. Iron overload can damage your liver, heart, and other parts of your body.

If you have iron overload, you may need iron chelation therapy. For this therapy, medicine is given through an injection or as a pill to remove the extra iron from your body.

Lung Injury

Although it's unlikely, blood transfusions can damage your lungs, making it hard to breathe. This usually occurs within about 6 hours of the procedure.

Most patients recover. However, 5 to 25 percent of patients who develop lung injuries die from the injuries. These people usually were very ill before the transfusion.

Doctors aren't completely sure why blood transfusions damage the lungs. Antibodies (proteins) that are more likely to be found in the plasma of women who have been pregnant may disrupt the normal way that lung cells work. Because of this risk, hospitals are starting to use men's and women's plasma differently.

Acute Immune Hemolytic Reaction

Acute immune hemolytic reaction is very serious, but also very rare. It occurs if the blood type you get during a transfusion doesn't match or work with your blood type. Your body attacks the new red blood cells, which then produce substances that harm your kidneys.

The symptoms include chills, fever, nausea, pain in the chest or back, and dark urine. The doctor will stop the transfusion at the first sign of this reaction.

Delayed Hemolytic Reaction

This is a much slower version of acute immune hemolytic reaction. Your body destroys red blood cells so slowly that the problem can go unnoticed until your red blood cell level is very low.

Both acute and delayed hemolytic reactions are most common in patients who have had a previous transfusion.

Graft-Versus-Host Disease

Graft-versus-host disease (GVHD) is a condition in which white blood cells in the new blood attack your tissues. GVHD usually is fatal. People who have weakened immune systems are the most likely to get GVHD.

Symptoms start within a month of the blood transfusion. They include fever, rash, and diarrhea. To protect against GVHD, people who have weakened immune systems should receive blood that has been treated so the white blood cells can't cause GVHD.

Section 5.4

Contagious Diseases Transmission on Airplanes and Cruise Ships

This section contains text excerpted from the following sources: Text beginning with the heading "In-Flight Transmission of Communicable Diseases" is excerpted from "Air Travel," Centers for Disease Control and Prevention (CDC), July 10, 2015; Text beginning with the heading "Illnesses and Injury aboard Cruise Ships" is excerpted from "Cruise Ship Travel," Centers for Disease Control and Prevention (CDC), July 10, 2015.

In-Flight Transmission of Communicable Diseases

Communicable diseases may be transmitted to other travelers during air travel; therefore, people who are acutely ill, or still within the infectious period for a specific disease, should delay their travel until they are no longer contagious. Travelers should be up-to-date on routine vaccinations and receive destination-specific vaccinations before travel. Travelers should be reminded to wash their hands frequently and thoroughly (or use an alcohol-based hand sanitizer containing ≥60% alcohol), especially after using the toilet and before preparing or eating food, and to cover their noses and mouths when coughing or sneezing.

If a passenger with a communicable disease is identified as having flown on a particular flight (or flights), passengers who may have been exposed may be contacted by public health authorities for possible screening or prophylaxis. When necessary, public health authorities will obtain contact information from the airline for potentially exposed travelers so they may be contacted and offered intervention. Notifying a passenger of potential exposure to a communicable disease during a flight is facilitated if he or she has provided the airline with accurate and up-to-date contact information.

Centers for Disease Control and Prevention (CDC) has the authority to restrict travel for people who are contagious with a communicable disease that poses a public health threat during travel if 1) they plan to travel by commercial air (domestically or internationally) or travel internationally by other means and 2) are not adhering to or are unaware of public health recommendations.

Tuberculosis

Mycobacterium tuberculosis is transmitted from person to person via airborne respiratory droplet nuclei. Although the risk of transmission onboard aircraft is low, CDC recommends conducting passenger contact investigations for flights ≥8 hours if the person with tuberculosis (TB) is sputum smear positive for acid-fast bacilli and has cavitation on chest radiograph or has multidrug-resistant TB. People known to have active TB disease should not travel by commercial air (or any other commercial means) until they are determined to be noninfectious. State health department TB controllers are valuable resources for advice.

Neisseria Meningitidis

Meningococcal disease (caused by *Neisseria meningitidis*) is transmitted by direct contact with respiratory droplets and secretions and can be rapidly fatal. Therefore, close contacts need to be quickly identified and provided with prophylactic antimicrobial agents. Antimicrobial prophylaxis should be considered for any of the following:

- Household member traveling with the ill traveler

- Travel companion with very close contact

- Passenger seated directly next to the ill traveler on flights ≥8 hours

Measles

Measles (rubeola) is a viral illness transmitted by respiratory droplets or direct contact, but it can also be spread via airborne routes. Most measles cases diagnosed in the United States are imported from countries where measles is endemic. Travelers should ensure they are immune to measles before travel. Infants aged 6–11 months who will be traveling overseas should receive 1 dose of measles-mumps-rubella (MMR) vaccine before travel. However, this dose will not count as part of the recommended immunization schedule of 2 doses, which begins at age 12–15 months. An ill traveler is considered infectious during a flight of any duration if he or she traveled during the 4 days before rash onset through 4 days after rash onset. Flight-related contact investigations are initiated as quickly as possible so post-exposure prophylaxis may be provided to susceptible travelers. MMR vaccine given within 72 hours of exposure or immune globulin given within 6 days of exposure may prevent measles or decrease its severity.

Influenza

Transmission of the influenza virus aboard aircraft has been documented, but data are limited. Transmission is thought to be primarily due to large droplets; therefore, passengers seated closest to the source patient are believed to be most at risk for exposure. Influenza vaccine is routinely recommended each year for all people aged ≥6 months who do not have contraindications.

Disinsection

To reduce the accidental spread of mosquitoes and other vectors via airline cabins and luggage compartments, a number of countries require disinsection of all inbound flights. The World Health Organization (WHO) and the International Civil Aviation Organization specify 2 approaches for aircraft disinsection:

- Spraying the aircraft cabin with an aerosolized insecticide (usually 2% phenothrin) while passengers are on board.

- Treating the aircraft's interior surfaces with a residual insecticide while the aircraft is empty.

Some countries use a third method, in which aircraft are sprayed with an aerosolized insecticide while passengers are not on board.

Disinsection is not routinely done on incoming flights to the United States. Although disinsection, when done appropriately, was declared safe by WHO in 1995, there is still much debate about the safety of the agents and methods used. Guidelines for disinsection have been updated for the revised International Health Regulations. Many countries, including the United States, reserve the right to increase the use of disinsection in case of increased threat of vector or disease spread.

Illnesses and Injury Aboard Cruise Ships

Cruise ship medical clinics deal with a wide variety of illnesses and injuries. Approximately 3%–11% of conditions reported to cruise ship infirmaries are urgent or an emergency. Approximately 95% of illnesses are treated or managed onboard, and 5% require evacuation and shoreside consultation for medical, surgical, and dental problems. Approximately half of passengers who seek medical care are older than 65 years. Most (69%–88%) passenger dispensary visits are due to medical conditions, of which respiratory (19%–29%) and gastrointestinal (GI) (9%–10%) illnesses are the most frequently reported diagnoses. Approximately 10%–25% of passengers report sea sickness, and injuries (typically from slips, trips, or falls) account for 12%–18% of medical visits. Death rates for cruise ship passengers, most often from cardiovascular events, range from 0.6 to 9.8 deaths per million passenger-nights.

The most frequently documented cruise ship outbreaks involve respiratory infections (influenza and Legionnaires' disease), GI infections (norovirus), and vaccine-preventable diseases other than influenza, such as rubella and varicella (chickenpox). To reduce the risk of onboard introduction of communicable diseases by embarking passengers, ships may conduct pre embarkation medical screening to identify ill passengers before boarding.

The following measures should be encouraged to limit the introduction and spread of communicable diseases on cruise ships:

- Passengers and their clinicians should consult CDC's Travelers' Health website before travel for updates on outbreaks and travel health notices.

- Passengers ill with communicable diseases before a voyage should delay travel until they are no longer contagious.

- Passengers who become ill during the voyage should seek care in the ship's infirmary to receive clinical management, facilitate infection control measures, and maximize reporting of potential public health events.

Specific Health Risks

Gastrointestinal Illness

CDC's Vessel Sanitation Program (VSP) conducts twice-yearly, unannounced inspections of ships carrying ≥13 passengers with international itineraries that call on U.S. seaports. In spite of good cruise ship environmental health standards and high VSP inspection scores, outbreaks of gastroenteritis on cruise ships continue to occur. More than 90% of GI outbreaks investigated by VSP with a confirmed cause are due to norovirus. Characteristics of norovirus that facilitate outbreaks are a low infective dose, easy person-to-person transmissibility, prolonged viral shedding, no long-term immunity, and the organism's ability to survive routine cleaning procedures. From 2005 through 2009, approximately 27 outbreaks of norovirus infections occurred on cruise ships each year. To reduce the spread of norovirus on cruise ships, passengers should be counseled on the following:

- Information on cruise ship norovirus outbreaks is available at www.cdc.gov/nceh/vsp.

- Passengers should wash their hands with soap and water often, especially before eating and after using the restroom.

- Passengers who develop a GI illness, even if symptoms are mild, should promptly call the ship's medical center and follow cruise ship guidance regarding isolation and other infection control measures. If no medical center exists, contact the ship's master to report GI illness.

Gastrointestinal (GI) outbreaks on cruise ships from food and water sources have also been associated with *Salmonella* spp., *enterotoxigenic Escherichia coli, Shigella spp., Vibrio* spp.*, Staphylococcus aureus, Clostridium perfringens, Cyclospora cayetanensis,* and *hepatitis* A and E viruses.

Respiratory Illness

Influenza

Influenza seasons in the Northern and Southern Hemispheres typically occur at opposite times of the year. Since passengers and crew originate from all regions of the world, shipboard outbreaks of influenza A and B can occur year-round, and travelers on cruise ships can be exposed to strains circulating in different parts of the world. Using

2008–2011 surveillance data, CDC found a mean rate of influenza like illness (defined as temperature ≥100°F plus cough or sore throat) of 0.065 cases per 1,000 person-nights, without a detectable seasonal pattern.

During outbreaks, travelers can expect onboard control measures such as isolation of ill people, antiviral treatment of ill people, surveillance for new cases, and prophylaxis of contacts who are at high risk for complications. The following measures are recommended to reduce the spread of influenza aboard cruise ships:

- Clinicians should provide cruise travelers, particularly those at high risk for influenza complications, with the current seasonal influenza vaccine (if available) ≥2 weeks before travel.

- Passengers at high risk for influenza complications should discuss antiviral treatment and chemoprophylaxis with their healthcare provider before travel.

- Passengers should practice good respiratory hygiene and cough etiquette.

- Passengers should report their respiratory illness to the infirmary promptly and follow isolation recommendations, if indicated.

Legionnaires' Disease

Legionnaires' disease is a severe pneumonia caused by inhalation or possibly aspiration of warm, aerosolized water containing *Legionella* organisms. The organism is not transmitted from person to person. Contaminated ships' whirlpool spas and potable water supply systems are the most commonly implicated sources of shipboard *Legionella* outbreaks. Improvements in ship design and standardization of water disinfection have reduced the risk of *Legionella* growth and colonization.

Symptom onset is typically 2–10 days after exposure, and older travelers (≥65 years) and those with underlying medical conditions are at increased risk for infection. Most cruise ships can perform *Legionella* urine antigen testing. People with suspected Legionnaires' disease require prompt antibiotic treatment.

More than 20%–25% of all Legionnaires' disease reported to CDC is travel-associated. Clusters of Legionnaires' disease associated with hotel or cruise ship travel are difficult to identify, because travelers often disperse from the source of infection before symptoms begin.

In evaluating cruise travelers for Legionnaires' disease, clinicians should do the following:

- Obtain a thorough travel history of all destinations from 10 days before symptom onset (to assist in the identification of potential source of exposure).

- Collect urine for antigen testing.

- Collect respiratory secretions for culture, which is essential for identifying the pathogen.

- Inform CDC of any travel-associated Legionnaires' disease cases by sending an email to travellegionella@cdc.gov.

Vaccine-Preventable Diseases (VPDs)

Although most cruise ship passengers are from countries with routine vaccination programs (such as the United States and Canada), many crew members originate from developing countries with low immunization rates. Outbreaks of measles, rubella, and, most commonly, varicella have been reported on cruise ships. Preventive measures to reduce the spread of VPDs aboard cruise ships should be followed:

- Crew members should have documented proof of immunity to VPDs.

- Passengers, especially older passengers (>65 years) and immuno-compromised people, should be up-to-date with routine vaccinations before travel, as well as any required or recommended vaccinations specific for their destinations.

- Women of childbearing age should be immune to rubella before cruise ship travel.

Vectorborne Diseases

Cruise ship port visits may include countries where vector borne diseases, such as malaria, dengue, yellow fever, and Japanese encephalitis are endemic. New diseases might surface in unexpected locations. For example, chikungunya was reported in late 2013 for the first time in the Caribbean (with subsequent spread throughout the Caribbean and in several North, Central, and South American countries), and outbreaks of Zika were reported in the Western Pacific in the first half of 2014. Yellow fever vaccination certificates may be required by some countries for entry.

Passengers should follow recommendations for avoiding mosquito bites and vector borne infections:

- Use an effective insect repellent

- While indoors, remain in well-screened or air-conditioned areas

- When outdoors, wear long-sleeved shirts, long pants, boots, and hats

- Take antimalarial chemoprophylaxis if needed

Other Health Concerns

Stresses of cruise ship travel include varying weather and environmental conditions, as well as unaccustomed changes in diet and physical activity. Foreign travel may increase the likelihood of risk-taking behaviors such as alcohol misuse, drug use, and unsafe sex. In spite of modern stabilizer systems, seasickness is a common complaint (affecting up to one-fourth of travelers)

Chapter 6

Screening Internationally Adopted Children for Contagious Diseases

Travel Preparation for Adoptive Parents and Their Families

A pre-travel visit is strongly recommended for prospective adoptive parents. In preparation, the travel health provider must know the disease risks in the adopted child's country of origin and the medical and social histories of the adoptee (if available), as well as which family members will be traveling, their immunization and medical histories, the season of travel, the length of stay in the country, and the itinerary while in country.

Family members who remain at home, including extended family, should be current on their routine immunizations. Protection against measles, varicella, tetanus, diphtheria, pertussis, hepatitis A, hepatitis B, and polio must be ensured for everyone who will be in the house-hold or in close contact by providing care for the adopted child. Measles immunity or 2 doses of measles-mumps-rubella (MMR) vaccine separated by ≥28 days should be documented for all people born in or after 1957. Varicella vaccine should be given to those without a history

This chapter includes text excerpted from "International Adoption," Centers for Disease Control and Prevention (CDC), July 10, 2015.

of varicella disease or documentation of 2 doses of varicella vaccine ≥3 months apart. Adults who have not received the tetanus-diphtheria-acellular pertussis (Tdap) vaccine, including adults >65 years old, should receive a single dose of Tdap to protect against *Bordetella pertussis* in addition to tetanus and diphtheria. Unprotected family members and close contacts of the adopted child should be immunized against hepatitis A virus (HAV) before the child's arrival. Most adult family members and caretakers will need to be immunized with hepatitis B vaccine, since it has only been routinely given since 1990. If the adopted child is from a polio-endemic area, family members and caretakers should ensure they have completed the recommended age-appropriate polio vaccine series. A one-time inactivated polio booster for adults who have completed the primary series in the past is recommended if they are traveling to these areas and can be considered for adults who remain at home but who will be in close contact caring for the child.

Prospective adoptive parents and any children traveling with them should receive advice on travel safety, food safety, immunization, malaria chemoprophylaxis, diarrhea prevention and treatment, and other travel-related health issues, as outlined elsewhere in this book. Instructions on car seats, injury prevention, food safety, and air travel apply equally to the adoptive child, so the travel health provider should also be familiar with and provide information on these child-specific issues.

Overseas Medical Examination of the Adopted Child

All immigrants, including children adopted internationally by US citizens, must undergo a medical examination in their country of origin, performed by a physician designated by the Department of State. The medical examination is used primarily to detect diseases or risk behaviors that may make the immigrant ineligible for a visa. Prospective adoptive parents should not rely on this medical examination to detect all possible disabilities and illnesses. Laboratory results from the country of origin may be unreliable. This examination should not replace the evaluation that is recommended once the child comes to the United States.

Follow-Up Medical Examination after Arrival in the United States

The adopted child should have a medical examination within two weeks of arrival in the United States or earlier if the child has fever, anorexia, diarrhea, vomiting, or other medical concerns. Items to consider during medical examination of an adopted child include the following:

- Temperature (fever requires further investigation)
- General appearance: alert, interactive
- Anthropometric measurements: weight/age, height/age, weight/height, head circumference/age, body mass index
- Facial features: length of palpebral fissures, philtrum, upper lip (fetal alcohol syndrome: short palpebral fissures, thin upper lip, indistinct philtrum)
- Hair: texture, color
- Eyes: jaundice, pallor, strabismus, visual acuity screen
- Ears: hearing screen, otitis media
- Mouth: palate, teeth
- Neck: thyroid (enlargement secondary to hypothyroidism, iodine deficiency)
- Heart: murmurs
- Chest: symmetry, Tanner stage breasts
- Abdomen: liver or spleen enlargement
- Skin: Mongolian spots, scars, bacillus Calmette-Guérin (BCG) scar, birthmarks, molluscum contagiosum, tinea capitis, tinea corporis
- Lymph nodes: enlargement suggestive of TB or other infections
- Back: scoliosis
- Genitalia: Tanner stage, presence of both testicles, findings of sexual abuse

In addition, all children should receive a developmental screening by a clinician with experience in child development to determine if immediate referrals should be made for a more detailed neuro-developmental examination and therapies. Further evaluation will depend on the country of origin, the age of the child, previous living conditions, nutritional status, developmental status, and the adoptive family's specific questions. Concerns raised during the pre adoption medical review may dictate further investigation.

Screening for Infectious Diseases

The current panel of tests for infectious diseases recommended by the American Academy of Pediatrics (AAP) for screening internationally adopted children is as follows:

- HAV serologic testing (IgG and IgM)

- Hepatitis B virus (HBV) serologic testing (repeat at 6 months if negative)

- Hepatitis C antibody

- Syphilis serologic testing (treponemal and non-treponemal testing)

- HIV 1 and 2 serologic testing

- Complete blood cell count with differential and red blood cell indices

- Stool examination for ova and parasites (3 specimens)

- Stool examination for *Giardia intestinalis and Cryptosporidium antigen* (1 specimen)

- Tuberculin skin test (TST) (all ages) or interferon-γ release assay (IGRA) (for children >5 years of age) (repeat at 6 months if negative)

Additional screening tests may be useful, depending on the child's country of origin or specific risk factors. These screens may include Chagas disease serologic tests, malaria smears, or serologic testing for schistosomiasis, strongyloidiasis, and filariasis.

Gastrointestinal Parasites

Gastrointestinal parasites are commonly seen in international adoptees, but the prevalence varies by birth country and age. The highest rates of infection have been reported from Ukraine and Ethiopia and increase with older age. G. *intestinalis* is the most common parasite identified. Three stool samples collected in the early morning, 2–3 days apart and placed in a container with preservative are recommended for ova and parasite analysis. Only one of these samples needs to be analyzed for *Giardia* antigen and *Cryptosporidium* antigen. Although theoretically possible, transmission of intestinal parasites from internationally adopted children to family and school contacts has not been reported; however, good hand hygiene is recommended to prevent infection. Stool samples should be cultured for enteric bacterial pathogens for any child with fever and bloody diarrhea. Unlike refugees, internationally adopted children are not treated for parasites before departure.

Hepatitis A

HAV serology (IgG and IgM) should be considered for all internationally adopted children to identify children who may be acutely infected and shedding virus and to make decisions regarding HAV immunization. In 2007 and early 2008, multiple cases of hepatitis A secondary to exposure to newly arrived internationally adopted children were reported in the United States. Some of these cases involved extended family members who were not living in the household. Identification of acutely infected toddlers new to the United States is necessary to prevent further transmission. If a child is found to have acute infection, HAV vaccine or immunoglobulin can be given to close contacts to prevent infection. In addition, it is cost effective to identify children with past infection with serologic testing since they would not need to receive the HAV vaccine.

Hepatitis B

All internationally adopted children should be screened for HBV infection with serology for hepatitis B surface antigen (HBsAg) and hepatitis B surface antibody to determine past or current infection and protection from vaccination. HBV infection has been reported in 1%–5% of newly arrived adoptees. Because of widespread use of the HBV vaccine, the prevalence of HBV infection has decreased over the years. Children found to be positive for HBsAg should be retested 6 months later to determine if the child has a chronic infection. Results of a positive HBsAg test should be reported to the state health department. HBV is highly transmissible within the household. All members of households adopting children with chronic HBV infection must be immunized and should have follow-up antibody titers to determine whether levels consistent with immunity have been achieved. Children with chronic HBV infection should receive additional tests for HBV e antigen, HBV e antibody, hepatitis D virus antibody, viral load, and liver function. They should be vaccinated for hepatitis A if they are not immune. They should also have a consultation with a pediatric gastroenterologist. Repeat screening at 6 months after arrival should be done on all children who initially test negative for HBV surface antibody.

Hepatitis C

Routine screening for hepatitis C virus (HCV) should be considered, since most children with HCV infection are asymptomatic, screening for risk factors is not possible, effective treatments are available, and close follow-up of infected patients is needed to identify long-term complications. Antibody testing with an EIA should be done for screening. Since maternal antibody may be present in children <18 months of age, PCR testing should be done if the EIA is positive. Children with HCV infection should be referred to a gastroenterologist for further evaluation, management, and treatment.

Syphilis

Screening for *Treponema pallidum* is recommended for all internationally adopted children. Initial screening is done with both non-treponemal and treponemal tests. Treponemal tests remain positive for life in most cases even after successful treatment and are specific for treponemal diseases, which include syphilis and other diseases (such as yaws, pinta, and bejel) that can be seen in some countries. In children with a history of syphilis, the child's initial evaluation, treatment (antibiotic type and treatment duration), and follow-up testing are rarely available; therefore, a full evaluation for disease must be undertaken and anti treponemal treatment given dependent upon the results.

Chagas Disease

Screening for Chagas disease should be considered for children arriving from a country cndcmic for Chagas disease. Chagas disease is endemic throughout much of Mexico, Central America, and South America. The risk of Chagas disease varies by region within endemic countries. Although the risk of Chagas disease is likely low in adopted children from endemic countries, treatment of infected children is effective. Serologic testing when the child is aged 9–12 months will avoid possible false-positive results from maternal antibody. Testing by PCR can be done in children <9 months of age. If a child tests positive for Chagas disease, the child should be referred to a specialist for further evaluation and management.

Malaria

Routine screening for malaria is not recommended for internationally adopted children. However, thick and thin malaria smears should be obtained immediately for any febrile child newly arrived from a malaria-endemic area.

Tuberculosis

All internationally adopted children should be screened for tuberculosis (TB) after arriving in the United States. Internationally adopted children are at 4–6 times the risk for TB than their U.S.-born peers. The TST is indicated for all children, regardless of their BCG status. TST results must be interpreted carefully for internationally adopted children; guidelines may be found in the bibliography. For children aged ≥5 years, IGRA (such as QuantiFERON-TB Gold) is an acceptable screening alternative to the TST. IGRA has the advantage of not requiring a follow-up visit for testing or requiring individual interpretation of results (although results may be termed "indeterminate" by the laboratory). In addition, they appear to be more specific than the TST for *Mycobacterium tuberculosis* infection in children who have had BCG vaccination. The TST remains the most widely used screening test for TB in children. A chest radiograph and complete physical examination to assess for pulmonary and extrapulmonary TB are indicated for all children with positive TB screening results. Hilar lymphadenopathy is a more sensitive finding for TB in young children than are pulmonary infiltrates or cavitation. A repeat TST 3–6 months after arrival is recommended for children who initially test negative. Children who have a positive TST or IGRA result but have no evidence of active disease have latent tuberculosis infection (LTBI) and should generally be treated with isoniazid for 9 months. In consultation with TB experts, a shorter-course LTBI treatment regimen may be considered if active disease is found, every effort should be made to isolate the organism and determine sensitivities, particularly if the child is from a region of the world with a high rate of multidrug-resistant TB.

Eosinophilia

A complete blood count with a differential should be done on all internationally adopted children. An eosinophil count >450 cells/mm3 in an internationally adopted child may warrant further evaluation. Intestinal parasite screening will identify some helminths that may cause eosinophilia. Further investigation of the eosinophilia might include serologic evaluation for *Strongyloides stercoralis, Toxocara canis, Ancylostoma spp.,* and *Trichinella spiralis*. For children arriving from countries endemic for Schistosoma spp. and filariasis, serologic testing should be done for these diseases as well.

Screening for Noninfectious Diseases

Several screening tests for noninfectious diseases should be performed in all or in select internationally adopted children. All children should have a complete blood count with a differential, hemoglobin electrophoresis, and G6PD deficiency screening. Serum levels of thyroid-stimulating hormone and lead should be measured in all internationally adopted children. Testing for serum levels of iron, iron-binding capacity, transferrin, ferritin, and total vitamin D 25 hydroxy should be considered. In certain circumstances, neurologic and psychological testing may also be considered.

Chapter 7

Bioterrorism: Disease Used as a Weapon

Chapter Contents

Section 7.1

Bioterrorism Overview

This section includes text excerpted from "Bioterrorism," Centers for Disease Control and Prevention (CDC), January 14, 2016.

A biological attack, or bioterrorism, is the intentional release of viruses, bacteria, or other germs that can sicken or kill people, livestock, or crops. *Bacillus anthracis*, the bacteria that causes anthrax, is one of the most likely agents to be used in a biological attack.

The Threat

We do not know if or when another anthrax attack might occur. However, federal agencies have worked for years with health departments across the country to plan and prepare for an anthrax attack. If such an emergency were to occur in the United States, Centers for Disease Control and Prevention (CDC) and other federal agencies would work closely with local and state partners to coordinate a response.

Why Would Anthrax Be Used as a Weapon?

If a bioterrorist attack were to happen, *Bacillus anthracis*, the bacteria that causes anthrax, would be one of the biological agents most likely to be used. Biological agents are germs that can sicken or kill people, livestock, or crops. Anthrax is one of the most likely agents to be used because:

- Anthrax spores are easily found in nature, can be produced in a lab, and can last for a long time in the environment.

- Anthrax makes a good weapon because it can be released quietly and without anyone knowing. The microscopic spores could be put into powders, sprays, food, and water. Because they are so small, you may not be able to see, smell, or taste them.

- Anthrax has been used as a weapon before.

Anthrax has been used as a weapon around the world for nearly a century. In 2001, powdered anthrax spores were deliberately put into letters that were mailed through the U.S. postal system. Twenty-two people, including 12 mail handlers, got anthrax, and five of these 22 people died.

How Dangerous Is Anthrax?

A subset of select agents and toxins have been designated as Tier 1 because these biological agents and toxins present the greatest risk of deliberate misuse with significant potential for mass casualties or devastating effect to the economy, critical infrastructure, or public confidence, and pose a severe threat to public health and safety. *Bacillus anthracis* is a Tier 1 agent.

B. anthracis is a select agent. The possession, use, or transfer of *B. anthracis* is regulated by the Division of Select Agents and Toxins (DSAT), located in CDC's Office of Public Health Preparedness and Response.

What Might an Anthrax Attack Look Like?

An anthrax attack could take many forms. For example, it could be placed in letters and mailed, as was done in 2001, or it could be put into food or water. Anthrax also could be released into the air from a truck, building, or plane. This type of attack would mean the anthrax spores could easily be blown around by the wind or carried on people's clothes, shoes, and other objects. It only takes a small amount of anthrax to infect a large number of people.

If anthrax spores were released into the air, people could breathe them in and get sick with anthrax. Inhalation anthrax is the most serious form and can kill quickly if not treated immediately. If the attack were not detected by one of the monitoring systems in place in the United States, it might go unnoticed until doctors begin to see unusual patterns of illness among sick.

Section 7.2

Strategic National Stockpile of Medicine

This section includes text excerpted from "Office of Public Health Preparedness and Response," Centers for Disease Control and Prevention (CDC), June 17, 2016.

What Is Strategic National Stockpile (SNS)

Centers for Disease Control and Prevention's (CDC) Strategic National Stockpile (SNS) has large quantities of medicine and medical supplies to protect the American public if there is a public health emergency (terrorist attack, flu outbreak, earthquake) severe enough to cause local supplies to run out. Once Federal and local authorities agree that the SNS is needed, medicines will be delivered to any state in the United States in time for them to be effective. Each state has plans to receive and distribute SNS medicine and medical supplies to local communities as quickly as possible.

What Should You Know about the Medicines in the SNS?

- The medicine in the SNS is FREE for everyone.

- The SNS has stockpiled enough medicine to protect people in several large cities at the same time.

- Federal, state, and local community planners are working together to ensure that the SNS medicines will be delivered to the affected area to protect you and your family if there is a terrorist attack.

How Will You Get Your Medicine If the SNS Is Delivered to Your Area?

- Local communities are prepared to receive SNS medicine and medical supplies from the state to provide to everyone in the community who needs them.

- Find out about how to get medicine to protect you and your family by watching TV, listening to the radio, reading the newspaper, checking the community Website on the Internet or learning from trusted community leaders.

Helping State and Local Jurisdictions Prepare for a National Emergency

An act of terrorism (or a large scale natural disaster) targeting the U.S. civilian population will require rapid access to large quantities of pharmaceuticals and medical supplies. Such quantities may not be readily available unless special stockpiles are created. No one can anticipate exactly where a terrorist will strike and few state or local governments have the resources to create sufficient stockpiles on their own. Therefore, a national stockpile has been created as a resource for all.

In 1999 Congress charged the U.S. Department of Health and Human Services (HHS) and the Centers for Disease Control and Prevention (CDC) with the establishment of the National Pharmaceutical Stockpile (NPS). The mission was to provide a re-supply of large quantities of essential medical materiel to states and communities during an emergency within twelve hours of the federal decision to deploy.

The Homeland Security Act of 2002 tasked the Department of Homeland Security (DHS) with defining the goals and performance requirements of the Strategic National Stockpile (SNS) Program, as well as managing the actual deployment of assets. Effective on 1 March 2003, the NPS became the SNS Program managed jointly by DHS and HHS. With the signing of the BioShield legislation, the SNS Program was returned to HHS for oversight and guidance. The SNS Program works with governmental and non-governmental partners to upgrade the nation's public health capacity to respond to a national emergency. Critical to the success of this initiative is ensuring capacity is developed at federal, state, and local levels to receive, stage, and dispense SNS assets.

The Cities Readiness Initiative (CRI) of CDC's SNS was established in 2004 and focuses on enhancing preparedness in the nation's largest cities and metropolitan statistical areas, where more than 50% of the U.S. population resides. Through CRI, state and large metropolitan public health departments have developed plans to respond to a large-scale bioterrorist event by dispensing antibiotics to the entire population of an identified MSA within 48 hours.

A National Repository of Life-Saving Pharmaceuticals and Medical Supplies

The SNS is a national repository of antibiotics, chemical antidotes, antitoxins, life-support medications, IV administration, airway maintenance supplies, and medical/surgical items. The SNS is designed to supplement and re-supply state and local public health agencies in the event of a national emergency anywhere and at anytime within the United States or its territories.

The SNS is organized for flexible response. The first line of support lies within the immediate response 12-hour Push Packages. These are caches of pharmaceuticals, antidotes, and medical supplies designed to provide rapid delivery of a broad spectrum of assets for an ill defined threat in the early hours of an event. These Push Packages are positioned in strategically located, secure warehouses ready for immediate deployment to a designated site within 12 hours of the federal decision to deploy SNS assets.

If the incident requires additional pharmaceuticals and/or medical supplies, follow-on vendor managed inventory (VMI) supplies will be shipped to arrive within 24 to 36 hours. If the agent is well defined, VMI can be tailored to provide pharmaceuticals, supplies and/or products specific to the suspected or confirmed agent(s). In this case, the VMI could act as the first option for immediate response from the SNS Program.

Determining and Maintaining SNS Assets

To determine and review the composition of the SNS Program assets, HHS and CDC consider many factors, such as current biological and/or chemical threats, the availability of medical materiel, and the ease of dissemination of pharmaceuticals. One of the most significant factors in determining SNS composition, however, is the medical vulnerability of the U.S. civilian population.

The SNS Program ensures that the medical materiel stock is rotated and kept within potency shelf-life limits. This involves quarterly quality assurance/quality control checks (QA/QC's) on all 12-hour Push Packages, annual 100% inventory of all 12-hour Push Package items, and inspections of environmental conditions, security, and overall package maintenance.

Supplementing State and Local Resources

During a national emergency, state, local, and private stocks of medical materiel will be depleted quickly. State and local first responders and health officials can use the SNS to bolster their response to a national emergency, with a 12-hour Push Package, VMI, or a combination of both, depending on the situation. The SNS is not a first response tool.

Rapid Coordination and Transport

- The SNS Program is committed to have 12-hour Push Packages delivered anywhere in the United States or its territories within 12 hours of a federal decision to deploy. The 12-hour Push Packages have been configured to be immediately loaded onto either trucks or commercial cargo aircraft for the most rapid transportation. Concurrent to SNS transport, the SNS Program will deploy its Stockpile Service Advance Group (SSAG). The SSAG staff will coordinate with state and local officials so that the SNS assets can be efficiently received and distributed upon arrival at the site.

Section 7.3

U.S. Preparedness for Health Emergencies from Bioterrorism (Anthrax)

This section includes text excerpted from "Anthrax," Centers for Disease Control and Prevention (CDC), September 1, 2015.

Hopefully, an attack involving anthrax will never happen in the United States. However, there are steps that you and your family can take to help prepare if an anthrax emergency ever did happen. If such an emergency were to occur in the United States, Centers for Disease Control and Prevention (CDC) and other federal agencies would be ready to respond.

What CDC Is Doing to Prepare

CDC is working with other federal agencies and health departments across the country to prepare for an anthrax attack. Activities include:

73

- Providing funds and guidance to help health departments strengthen their abilities to respond to all types of public health incidents and build more resilient communities.

- Providing training in emergency response for the public health workforce and healthcare providers, as well as leaders in the public and private sector.

- Coordinating response activities and providing resources to health departments through the CDC Emergency Operations Center.

- Regulating the possession, use, and transfer of biological agents and toxins that could pose a severe threat to public health and safety through the CDC Select Agent Program.

- Promoting science and practices to strengthen preparedness and response activities.

- Ensuring that the United States has enough laboratories that can quickly conduct tests when anthrax is suspected.

- Working with hospitals, laboratories, emergency response teams, and healthcare providers to make sure they have the medicine and supplies they would need if an anthrax attack occurred.

- Developing guidance to protect the health and safety of workers who would be responding during an anthrax emergency.

Worker Safety

During an anthrax event, certain workers could be exposed to *B. anthracis* either during the initial attack or when responding to the emergency. The workers that could be at risk include mail handlers (if spores are sent through the mail), law enforcement personnel, healthcare workers, decontamination workers, and critical infrastructure workers who could be exposed to airborne (aerosolized) spores, depending on how the spores were disseminated.

Chapter 8

Nationally Notifiable Infectious Diseases: Protecting the Public Health

National Notifiable Diseases Surveillance System

The National Notifiable Diseases Surveillance System (NNDSS) is a nationwide collaboration that enables all levels of public health—local, state, territorial, federal, and international—to share notifiable disease-related health information. Public health uses this information to monitor, control, and prevent the occurrence and spread of state-reportable and nationally notifiable infectious and noninfectious diseases and conditions.

NNDSS is a multifaceted program that includes the surveillance system for collection, analysis, and sharing of health data. It also includes policies, laws, electronic messaging standards, people, partners, information systems, processes, and resources at the local, state, territorial, and national levels.

This chapter includes text excerpted from "National Notifiable Diseases Surveillance System," Centers for Disease Control and Prevention (CDC), December 27, 2015.

Supporting Public Health Surveillance in Jurisdictions and at CDC

Notifiable disease surveillance begins at the level of local, state, and territorial public health departments (also known as jurisdictions). Jurisdictional laws and regulations mandate reporting of cases of specified infectious and noninfectious conditions to health departments. The health departments work with healthcare providers, laboratories, hospitals, and other partners to obtain the information needed to monitor, control, and prevent the occurrence and spread of these health conditions. In addition, health departments notify about the occurrence of certain conditions.

The CDC Division of Health Informatics and Surveillance (DHIS) supports NNDSS by receiving, securing, processing, and providing nationally notifiable infectious diseases data to disease-specific CDC programs. DHIS also supports local, state, and territorial public health departments in helping them collect, manage, and submit case notification data to CDC for NNDSS. DHIS provides this support through funding, health information exchange standards and frameworks, electronic health information systems, and technical support through the NNDSS web site, tools, and training. Together, DHIS and the CDC programs prepare annual summaries of infectious and noninfectious diseases and conditions, which are published in the CDC *Morbidity and Mortality Weekly Report*.

These programs collaborate with the Council of State and Territorial Epidemiologists (CSTE) to determine which conditions reported to local, state, and territorial public health departments are nationally notifiable. The CDC programs, in collaboration with subject matter experts in CSTE and in health departments, determine what data elements are included in national notifications. Health departments participating in NNDSS voluntarily submit infectious disease data to DHIS and also submit some data directly to CDC programs.

CDC Programs Responsible for National Surveillance, Prevention, and Control of Infectious and Noninfectious Conditions

- Center for Global Health (CGH)

- National Center for Chronic Disease Prevention and Health Promotion (NCCDPHP)

- National Center for Emerging and Zoonotic Infectious Diseases (NCEZID)

- National Center for Environmental Health (NCEH)

- National Center for HIV/AIDS, Viral Hepatitis, STD, and TB Prevention (NCHHSTP)

- National Center for Immunization and Respiratory Diseases (NCIRD)

- National Institute for Occupational Safety and Health (NIOSH)

NNDSS Modernization Initiative

With the evolution of technology and data and exchange standards, CDC now has the opportunity to strengthen and modernize the infrastructure supporting NNDSS. As part of the CDC Surveillance Strategy the NNDSS Modernization Initiative (NMI) is underway to enhance the system's ability to provide more comprehensive, timely, and higher quality data than ever before for public health decision making.

Through this multi-year initiative, CDC seeks to increase the robustness of the NNDSS technological infrastructure so that it is based on interoperable, standardized data and exchange mechanisms.

NNDSS Data Sources and Reporting

Integrated surveillance information systems in reporting jurisdictions that are based on the National Electronic Disease Surveillance System (NEDSS) architectural standards are primary data sources for NNDSS. Jurisdictions use these information systems to create and send standards-based case notifications to CDC for NNDSS. Currently, case notifications can be sent using three different standards; CDC's NNDSS Modernization Initiative will provide a single, new standard to transmit data to CDC.

Connecting the Healthcare System to Public Health

By encouraging the use of standards-based public health surveillance systems and helping to support these systems, NEDSS helps public health agencies accept the electronic data exchanges from the healthcare system to public health departments.

NEDSS standards help connect the healthcare system to public health departments and those health departments to CDC by

- providing leadership and resources to local, state, and territorial public health departments to adopt standards-based systems needed to support national disease surveillance strategy;

- defining the content—such as clinical disease information, risk factor information, lab confirmation results, and patient demographics—of data messages sent by using the Health Level Seven (HL7) messaging standard;

- implementing content standards that the healthcare industry currently uses (for example, LOINC as the standard for transmitting laboratory test names and SNOMED as the standard for transmitting test results) for increased interoperability between public health departments and the healthcare industry; and

- providing the NEDSS Base System (NBS), a CDC-developed information system, to help reporting jurisdictions manage reportable disease data and send notifiable diseases data to CDC.

NEDSS Base System

NBS is a CDC-developed integrated information system that helps local, state, and territorial public health departments manage reportable disease data and send notifiable disease data to CDC.

NBS provides a tool to support the public health investigation workflow and to process, analyze, and share disease-related health information. NBS also provides reporting jurisdictions with a NEDSS-compatible information system to transfer epidemiologic, laboratory, and clinical data efficiently and securely over the Internet.

Built and maintained by CDC, NBS integrates data from many sources on multiple public health conditions to help local, state, and territorial public health officials identify and track cases of disease over time. This capability allows public health to provide appropriate interventions to help limit the severity and spread of disease.

NBS facilitates the adoption of national consensus standards used across public health and healthcare—including vocabulary standards such as LOINC, SNOMED, and RXNORM and messaging standards such as HL7—and helps local, state, and territorial public health departments use standards when sending information to CDC about notifiable diseases and conditions.

To date, 22 health departments (19 states; Washington, DC; Guam; and U.S. Virgin Islands) use NBS to manage public health investigations and transfer general communicable disease surveillance data to CDC.

Part Two

Types of Contagious Diseases

Chapter 9

Adenovirus

What Is Adenovirus?[1]

Adenoviruses are very common and come in many types. Depending on the virus type, adenoviruses can cause:

- respiratory (breathing) problems that can include cough, fever, and runny nose
- headache
- sore throat
- eye infections

These symptoms can last up to ten days. Infection with adenovirus can also rarely lead to more serious problems, such as **pneumonia**, **stomach and bowel problems**, and even **death**. Some people who are infected may have to be hospitalized.

Adenovirus infection can be spread from person to person through the air (for example, by sneezing or coughing). It can also be spread by personal contact, such as touching an infected person or handling objects that an infected person has touched.

This chapter contains text excerpted from documents published by two public domain sources. Text under headings marked 1 are excerpted from "Adenovirus VIS," Centers for Disease Control and Prevention (CDC), June 18, 2014; text under headings marked 2 are excerpted from "Adenoviruses," Centers for Disease Control and Prevention (CDC), April 20, 2015.

Two types of adenovirus (Type 4 and Type 7) have caused severe outbreaks of respiratory illness among military recruits.

Symptoms[2]

Adenoviruses can cause a wide range of illnesses such as:

- Common cold
- Sore throat (pharyngitis)
- Bronchitis
- Pneumonia
- Diarrhea
- Pinkeye (conjunctivitis)
- Fever
- Bladder inflammation or infection (cystitis)
- Inflammation of stomach and intestines (gastroenteritis)
- Neurologic disease

Adenoviruses rarely cause serious illness or death. However, infants and people with weakened immune systems, or existing respiratory or cardiac disease, are at higher risk of developing severe illness from an adenovirus infection.

Transmission[2]

Adenoviruses are usually spread from an infected person to others through:

- close personal contact, such as touching or shaking hands
- the air by coughing and sneezing
- touching an object or surface with adenoviruses on it, then touching your mouth, nose, or eyes before washing your hands

Some adenoviruses can spread through an infected person's stool, for example, during diaper changing. Adenovirus can also spread through the water, such as swimming pools, but this is less common.

Sometimes the virus can be shed for months after a person recovers from an adenovirus infection. This "virus shedding" usually occurs without any symptoms, even though the person can still spread adenovirus to other people.

Prevention[2]

There is currently no adenovirus vaccine available to the general public. A vaccine against adenovirus types 4 and 7 was approved by the U.S. Food and Drug Administration (FDA) in March 2011, for U.S. military personnel only.

You can protect yourself and others from adenoviruses and other respiratory illnesses by following a few simple steps:

- Wash your hands often with soap and water.
- Cover your mouth and nose when coughing or sneezing.
- Avoid touching your eyes, nose or mouth with unwashed hands.
- Avoid close contact with people who are sick.
- Stay home when you are sick.

Frequent hand washing is especially important in childcare settings and healthcare facilities. Adenoviruses are resistant to many common disinfectant products and can remain infections for long periods on surfaces, objects, and in water of swimming pools and small lakes. It is important to keep adequate levels of chlorine in swimming pools to prevent outbreaks of conjunctivitis caused by adenoviruses.

Treatment[2]

There is no specific treatment for people with adenovirus infection. Most adenovirus infections are mild and may require only care to help relieve symptoms.

Adenovirus Vaccine[1]

Adenovirus vaccine contains live adenovirus Type 4 and Type 7. It will prevent most illness caused by these two virus types. Adenovirus vaccine comes as **two tablets**, taken orally (by mouth) at the same time. The tablets should be swallowed whole, not chewed or crushed. Adenovirus vaccine may be given at the same time as other vaccines.

Who Should Get Adenovirus Vaccine?

The vaccine is approved for military personnel 17 through 50 years of age. It is recommended by the Department of Defense for **military recruits entering basic training**. It may also be recommended for other military personnel at high risk for adenovirus infection.

Precautions[1]

Some People Should Not Get Adenovirus Vaccine

- Anyone with a severe (life-threatening) allergy to any component of the vaccine. Tell the doctor if you have any severe allergies.

- Pregnant women or nursing mothers.

- Anyone who is unable to swallow the vaccine tablets whole without chewing them.

- Anyone younger than 17 or older than 50 years of age.

Other Precautions

- Talk with a doctor if:

  - you have HIV/AIDS or another disease that affects the immune system, or

  - your immune system is weakened because of cancer or other medical conditions, a transplant, or radiation or drug treatment (such as steroids or cancer chemotherapy).

- Women should not become pregnant for 6 weeks following vaccination.

- Vaccination should be postponed for anyone with vomiting or diarrhea.

- Virus from the vaccine can be shed in the stool for up to 28 days after vaccination. To minimize the risk of spreading vaccine virus to other people during this period, observe proper **personal hygiene**, such as frequent hand washing, especially following bowel movements. This is especially important if you have close contact with children 7 years of age and younger, with anyone having a weakened immune system, or with pregnant women.

What Are the Risks from Adenovirus Vaccine?[1]

A vaccine, like any medicine, could cause a serious reaction. But the risk of a vaccine causing serious harm, or death, is extremely small.

Mild Problems

Several mild problems have been reported within 2 weeks of getting the vaccine:

- headaches, upper respiratory tract infection (about 1 person in 3)
- stuffy nose, sore throat, joint pain (about 1 person in 6)
- abdominal pain, cough, nausea (about 1 person in 7)
- diarrhea (about 1 person in 10)
- fever (about 1 person in 100)

Serious Problems

More serious problems have been reported by about 1 person in 100, within 6 months of vaccination. These problems included:

- blood in the urine or stool
- pneumonia
- inflammation of the stomach or intestines

It is not clear whether these mild or serious problems were caused by the vaccine or occurred after vaccination by chance. As with all vaccines, adenovirus vaccine will continue to be monitored for unexpected or severe problems.

What If There Is a Serious Reaction?[1]

What Should I Look For?

Look for any unusual condition, such as a high fever, severe stomach pain or diarrhea. Signs of an allergic reaction can include difficulty breathing, hoarseness or wheezing, hives, paleness, weakness, a fast heartbeat or dizziness within a few minutes to a few hours after swallowing the tablets.

What Should I Do?

- If you think it is a severe allergic reaction or other emergency that can't wait, call 9-1-1 or get the person to the nearest hospital. Otherwise, call your doctor.
- Afterward, the reaction should be reported to the Vaccine Adverse Event Reporting System (VAERS). Your doctor might file this report, or you can do it yourself through the VAERS website, or by calling **1-800-822-7967.**

VAERS is only for reporting reactions. They do not give medical advice.

Chapter 10

Amebiasis

What Is Amebiasis?

Amebiasis is a disease caused by a one-celled parasite called *Entamoeba histolytica*.

Who Is at Risk for Amebiasis?

Although anyone can have this disease, it is more common in people who live in tropical areas with poor sanitary conditions. In the United States, amebiasis is most common in:

- People who have traveled to tropical places that have poor sanitary conditions.
- Immigrants from tropical countries that have poor sanitary conditions.
- People who live in institutions that have poor sanitary conditions.
- Men who have sex with men.

How Can I Become Infected with E. histolytica?

E. histolytica infection can occur when a person:

- Puts anything into their mouth that has touched the feces (poop) of a person who is infected with *E. histolytica*.

This chapter includes text excerpted from "Parasites-Amebiasis-*Entamoeba histolytica* Infection," Centers for Disease Control and Prevention (CDC), July 20, 2015.

- Swallows something, such as water or food, that is contaminated with *E. histolytica.*

- Swallows *E. histolytica* cysts (eggs) picked up from contaminated surfaces or fingers.

What Are the Symptoms of Amebiasis?

Only about 10% to 20% of people who are infected with *E. histolytica* become sick from the infection. The symptoms are often quite mild and can include loose feces (poop), stomach pain, and stomach cramping. Amebic dysentery is a severe form of amebiasis associated with stomach pain, bloody stools (poop), and fever. Rarely, *E. histolytica* invades the liver and forms an abscess (a collection of pus). In a small number of instances, it has been shown to spread to other parts of the body, such as the lungs or brain, but this is very uncommon.

If I Swallowed E. histolytica, How Quickly Would I Become Sick?

Only about 10% to 20% of people who are infected with *E. histolytica* become sick from the infection. Those people who do become sick usually develop symptoms within 2 to 4 weeks, though it can sometimes take longer.

What Should I Do If I Think I Have Amebiasis?

See your healthcare provider.

How Is Amebiasis Diagnosed?

Your healthcare provider will ask you to submit fecal (poop) samples. Because *E. histolytica* is not always found in every stool sample, you may be asked to submit several stool samples from several different days.

Diagnosis of amebiasis can be very difficult. One problem is that other parasites and cells can look very similar to *E. histolytica* when seen under a microscope. Therefore, sometimes people are told that they are infected with *E. histolytica* even though they are not. *Entamoeba histolytica* and another ameba, *Entamoeba dispar*, which is about 10 times more common, look the same when seen under a microscope. Unlike infection with *E. histolytica*, which sometimes makes people sick, infection with *E. dispar* does not make people sick and therefore does not need to be treated.

If you have been told that you are infected with *E. histolytica* but you are feeling fine, you might be infected with *E. dispar* instead. Unfortunately, most laboratories do not yet have the tests that can tell whether a person is infected with *E. histolytica* or with *E. dispar*. Until these tests become more widely available, it usually is best to assume that the parasite is *E. histolytica*.

A blood test is also available but is only recommended when your healthcare provider thinks that your infection may have spread beyond the intestine (gut) to some other organ of your body, such as the liver. However, this blood test may not be helpful in diagnosing your current illness because the test can be positive if you had amebiasis in the past, even if you are not infected now.

How Is Amebiasis Treated?

Several antibiotics are available to treat amebiasis. Treatment must be prescribed by a physician. You will be treated with only one antibiotic if your *E. histolytica* infection has not made you sick. You probably will be treated with two antibiotics (first one and then the other) if your infection has made you sick.

I Am Going to Travel to a Country That Has Poor Sanitary Conditions. What Should I Eat and Drink There So I Will NOT Become Infected with E. histolytica or Other Such Germs?

The following items are safe to drink:

- Bottled water with an unbroken seal

- Tap water that has been boiled for at least 1 minute

- Carbonated (bubbly) water from sealed cans or bottles

- Carbonated (bubbly) drinks (like soda) from sealed cans or bottles

You can also make tap water safe for drinking by filtering it through an "absolute 1 micron or less" filter and dissolving chlorine, chlorine dioxide, or iodine tablets in the filtered water. "Absolute 1 micron" filters can be found in camping/outdoor supply stores.

The following items may NOT be safe to drink or eat:

• Fountain drinks or any drinks with ice cubes

• Fresh fruit or vegetables that you did not peel yourself

• Milk, cheese, or dairy products that may not have been pasteurized.

• Food or drinks sold by street vendors

Should I Be Concerned about Spreading the Infection to Others?

Yes, but the risk of spreading infection is low if the infected person is treated with antibiotics and practices good personal hygiene. This includes thorough handwashing with soap and water after using the toilet, after changing diapers, and before handling or preparing food.

Chapter 11

Chancroid

The prevalence of chancroid has declined in the United States. When infection does occur, it is usually associated with sporadic outbreaks. Worldwide, chancroid appears to have declined as well, although infection might still occur in some regions of Africa and the Caribbean. Like genital herpes and syphilis, chancroid is a risk factor in the transmission and acquisition of human immunodeficiency virus (HIV) infection.

Diagnostic Considerations

A definitive diagnosis of chancroid requires the identification of *Haemophilus ducrey* on special culture media that is not widely available from commercial sources; even when these media are used, sensitivity is <80%. No U.S. Food and Drug Administration (FDA)-cleared polymerase chain reaction (PCR) test for *H. ducreyi* is available in the United States, but such testing can be performed by clinical laboratories that have developed their own PCR test and have conducted Clinical Laboratory Improvement Amendments (CLIA) verification studies in genital specimens.

The combination of a painful genital ulcer and tender suppurative inguinal adenopathy suggests the diagnosis of chancroid. For both

This chapter includes text excerpted from "Chancroid," Centers for Disease Control and Prevention (CDC), June 4, 2015.

clinical and surveillance purposes, a probable diagnosis of chancroid can be made if all of the following criteria are met:

- the patient has one or more painful genital ulcers

- the clinical presentation, appearance of genital ulcers and, if present, regional lymphadenopathy are typical for chancroid

- the patient has no evidence of *T. pallidum* infection by darkfield examination of ulcer exudate or by a serologic test for syphilis performed at least 7 days after onset of ulcers

- an herpes simplex virus (HSV) PCR test or HSV culture performed on the ulcer exudate is negative

Treatment

Successful treatment for chancroid cures the infection, resolves the clinical symptoms, and prevents transmission to others. In advanced cases, scarring can result despite successful therapy.

Azithromycin and ceftriaxone offer the advantage of single-dose therapy. Worldwide, several isolates with intermediate resistance to either ciprofloxacin or erythromycin have been reported. However, because cultures are not routinely performed, data are limited regarding the current prevalence of antimicrobial resistance.

Other Management Considerations

Men who are uncircumcised and patients with human immunodeficiency virus (HIV) infection do not respond as well to treatment as persons who are circumcised or HIV-negative. Patients should be tested for HIV infection at the time chancroid is diagnosed. If the initial test results were negative, a serologic test for syphilis and HIV infection should be performed three months after the diagnosis of chancroid.

Follow-Up

Patients should be re-examined 3–7 days after initiation of therapy. If treatment is successful, ulcers usually improve symptomatically within 3 days and objectively within 7 days after therapy. If no clinical improvement is evident, the clinician must consider whether:

- the diagnosis is correct

- the patient is coinfected with another sexually transmitted disease (STD)

- the patient is infected with HIV

- the treatment was not used as instructed

- the *H. ducreyi* strain causing the infection is resistant to the prescribed antimicrobial

The time required for complete healing depends on the size of the ulcer; large ulcers might require >2 weeks.

In addition, healing is slower for some uncircumcised men who have ulcers under the foreskin. Clinical resolution of fluctuant lymphadenopathy is slower than that of ulcers and might require needle aspiration or incision and drainage, despite otherwise successful therapy. Although needle aspiration of buboes is a simpler procedure, incision and drainage might be preferred because of reduced need for subsequent drainage procedures.

Management of Sex Partners

Regardless of whether symptoms of the disease are present, sex partners of patients who have chancroid should be examined and treated if they had sexual contact with the patient during the ten days preceding the patient's onset of symptoms.

Special Considerations

Pregnancy

Data suggest ciprofloxacin presents a low risk to the fetus during pregnancy, with a potential for toxicity during breastfeeding. Alternate drugs should be used during pregnancy and lactation. No adverse effects of chancroid on pregnancy outcome have been reported.

HIV Infection

Persons with HIV infection who have chancroid should be monitored closely because they are more likely to experience treatment failure and to have ulcers that heal slowly. Persons with HIV infection might require repeated or longer courses of therapy, and treatment failures can occur with any regimen. Data are limited concerning the therapeutic efficacy of the recommended single-dose azithromycin and ceftriaxone regimens in persons with HIV infection.

Chapter 12

Chickenpox (Varicella)

Chickenpox is a very contagious disease caused by the *Varicella zoster* virus (VZV). It causes a blister-like rash, itching, tiredness, and fever. The rash appears first on the stomach, back and face and can spread over the entire body causing between 250 and 500 itchy blisters. Chickenpox can be serious, especially in babies, adults, and people with weakened immune systems. The best way to prevent chickenpox is to get the chickenpox vaccine.

Signs and Symptoms

Anyone who hasn't had chickenpox or gotten the chickenpox vaccine can get the disease. Chickenpox illness usually lasts about 5–7 days. The classic symptom of chickenpox is a rash that turns into itchy, fluid-filled blisters that eventually turn into scabs. The rash may first show up on the face, chest, and back then spread to the rest of the body, including inside the mouth, eyelids or genital area. It usually takes about one week for all the blisters to become scabs.

Other typical symptoms that may begin to appear 1–2 days before rash include:

- fever

- tiredness

This chapter includes text excerpted from "Chickenpox (Varicella)," Centers for Disease Control and Prevention (CDC), April 11, 2016.

- loss of appetite

- headache

Children usually miss 5–6 days of school or childcare due to chickenpox.

Vaccinated Persons

Some people who have been vaccinated against chickenpox can still get the disease. However, the symptoms are usually milder with fewer red spots or blisters and mild or no fever. Though uncommon, some vaccinated people who get chickenpox will develop illness as serious as chickenpox in unvaccinated persons.

People at Risk for Severe Chickenpox

Some people who get chickenpox may have more severe symptoms and may be at higher risk for complications.

Complications

Complications from chickenpox can occur, but they are not common in healthy people who get the disease. People who may get a serious case of chickenpox and may be at high risk for complications include:

- Infants

- Adolescents

- Adults

- Pregnant women

- People with weakened immune systems because of illness or medications. For example:

  - People with HIV/AIDS or cancer

  - Patients who have had transplants

  - People on chemotherapy, immunosuppressive medications or long-term use of steroids

Serious complications from chickenpox include:

- bacterial infections of the skin and soft tissues in children including Group A streptococcal infections

- pneumonia

- infection or inflammation of the brain (encephalitis, cerebellar ataxia)

- bleeding problems

- bloodstream infections (sepsis)

- dehydration

Some people with serious complications from chickenpox can become so sick that they need to be hospitalized. Chickenpox can also cause death. Some deaths from chickenpox continue to occur in healthy, unvaccinated children and adults. Many of the healthy adults who died from chickenpox contracted the disease from their unvaccinated children.

Transmission

Chickenpox is a very contagious disease caused by the *Varicella zoster* virus. The virus spreads easily from people with chickenpox to others who have never had the disease or been vaccinated. The virus spreads mainly by touching or breathing in the virus particles that come from chickenpox blisters, and possibly through tiny droplets from infected people that get into the air after they breathe or talk, for example.

The *Varicella zoster* virus also causes shingles. Chickenpox can be spread from people with shingles to others who have never had chickenpox or received the chickenpox vaccine. This can happen if a person touches or breathes in virus from shingles blisters. In these cases, a person might develop chickenpox, not shingles.

When Is a Person Contagious?

- A person with chickenpox can spread the disease from 1 to 2 days before they get the rash until all their chickenpox blisters have formed scabs (usually 5–7 days).

- It takes about 2 weeks (from 10 to 21 days) after exposure to a person with chickenpox or shingles for someone to develop chickenpox.

- If a person vaccinated for chickenpox gets the disease, they can still spread it to others.

For most people, getting chickenpox once provides immunity for life. However, for a few people, they can get chickenpox more than once, although this is not common.

Prevention

The best way to prevent chickenpox is to get the chickenpox vaccine. Children, adolescents, and adults should get two doses of chickenpox vaccine. Chickenpox vaccine is very safe and effective at preventing the disease. Most people who get the vaccine will not get chickenpox. If a vaccinated person does get chickenpox, it is usually mild—with fewer red spots or blisters and mild or no fever. The chickenpox vaccine prevents almost all cases of severe disease. For people exposed to chickenpox, call a healthcare provider if the person:

- has never had chickenpox disease and is not vaccinated with the chickenpox vaccine

- is pregnant

- has a weakened immune system caused by disease or medication. For example:

  - People with HIV/AIDS or cancer

  - Patients who have had transplants

  - People on chemotherapy, immunosuppressive medications or long-term use of steroids

Treatment

Treatments at Home for People with Chickenpox

There are several things that can be done at home to help relieve the symptoms and prevent skin infections. Calamine lotion and colloidal oatmeal baths may help relieve some of the itching. Keeping fingernails trimmed short may help prevent skin infections caused by scratching blisters.

Over-the-Counter Medications

Use non-aspirin medications, such as acetaminophen, to relieve fever from chickenpox. Do not use aspirin or aspirin-containing products to relieve fever from chickenpox. The use of aspirin in children with chickenpox has been associated with Reye's syndrome, a severe disease that affects the liver and brain and can cause death.

When to Call the Healthcare Provider

Some people are more likely to have a serious case of chickenpox. Call a healthcare provider if:

1. the person at risk of serious complications:
   - is less than 1 year-old
   - is older than 12 years of age
   - has a weakened immune system
   - is pregnant, or
2. develops any of the following symptoms:
   - fever that lasts longer than 4 days
   - fever that rises above 102°F (38.9°C)
   - any areas of the rash or any part of the body becomes very red, warm, or tender, or begins leaking pus (thick, discolored fluid), since these symptoms may indicate a bacterial infection
   - extreme illness
   - difficult waking up or confused demeanor
   - difficulty walking
   - stiff neck
   - frequent vomiting
   - difficulty breathing
   - severe cough
   - severe abdominal pain
   - rash with bleeding or bruising (hemorrhagic rash)

Treatments Prescribed by Your Doctor for People with Chickenpox

Your healthcare provider can advise you on treatment options. Antiviral medications are recommended for people with chickenpox who are more likely to develop serious disease including:

- otherwise healthy people older than 12 years of age

- people with chronic skin or lung disease
- people receiving steroid therapy
- pregnant women

Acyclovir, an antiviral medication, is licensed for treatment of chickenpox. The medication works best if it is given within the first 24 hours after the rash starts.

Chapter 13

Chlamydia and Lymphogranuloma venereum *(LGV)*

Chlamydia

What Is Chlamydia?

Chlamydia is a common (sexually transmitted disease) STD that can infect both men and women. It can cause serious, permanent damage to a woman's reproductive system, making it difficult or impossible for her to get pregnant later on. Chlamydia can also cause a potentially fatal ectopic pregnancy (pregnancy that occurs outside the womb).

How Is Chlamydia Spread?

- You can get chlamydia by having vaginal, anal, or oral sex with someone who has chlamydia.

This chapter contains text excerpted from the following sources: Text beginning with the heading "Chlamydia" is excerpted from "Chlamydia," Centers for Disease Control and Prevention (CDC), January 23, 2014; Text under the heading "Chlamydial Infections in Adolescents and Adults" is excerpted from "2015–Sexually Transmitted Diseases Treatment Guidelines," Centers for Disease Control and Prevention (CDC), June 4, 2015.

101

- If your sex partner is male you can still get chlamydia even if he does not ejaculate (cum).

- If you've had chlamydia and were treated in the past, you can still get infected again if you have unprotected sex with someone who has chlamydia.

- If you are pregnant, you can give chlamydia to your baby during child birth.

How Can I Reduce My Risk of Getting Chlamydia?

The only way to avoid STDs is to not have vaginal, anal or oral sex. If you are sexually active, you can do the following things to lower your chances of getting chlamydia:

- Being in a long-term mutually monogamous relationship with a partner who has been tested and has negative STD test results.

- Using latex condoms the right way every time you have sex.

Am I at Risk for Chlamydia?

Anyone who has sex can get chlamydia through unprotected vaginal, anal, or oral sex. However, sexually active young people are at a higher risk of getting chlamydia. This is due to behaviors and biological factors common among young people. Gay, bisexual, and other men who have sex with men are also at risk since chlamydia can be spread through oral and anal sex.

Have an honest and open talk with your healthcare provider and ask whether you should be tested for chlamydia or other STDs. If you are a sexually active woman younger than 25 years, or an older woman with risk factors such as new or multiple sex partners, or a sex partner who has a sexually transmitted infection, you should get a test for chlamydia every year. Gay, bisexual, and men who have sex with men; as well as pregnant women should also be tested for chlamydia.

How Do I Know If I Have Chlamydia?

Most people who have chlamydia have no symptoms. If you do have symptoms, they may not appear until several weeks after you have sex with an infected partner. Even when chlamydia causes no symptoms, it can damage your reproductive system.

Women with symptoms may notice:

- An abnormal vaginal discharge
- A burning sensation when urinating

Symptoms in men can include:

- A discharge from their penis
- A burning sensation when urinating
- Pain and swelling in one or both testicles (although this is less common)

Men and women can also get infected with chlamydia in their rectum, either by having receptive anal sex, or by spread from another infected site (such as the vagina). While these infections often cause no symptoms, they can cause:

- Rectal pain
- Discharge
- Bleeding

You should be examined by your doctor if you notice any of these symptoms or if your partner has an STD or symptoms of an STD, such as an unusual sore, a smelly discharge, burning when urinating or bleeding between periods.

Chlamydial Infections in Adolescents and Adults

Chlamydial infection is the most frequently reported infectious disease in the United States, and prevalence is highest in persons aged ≤24 years. Several sequelae can result from *C. trachomatis* infection in women, the most serious of which include PID, ectopic pregnancy, and infertility. Some women who receive a diagnosis of uncomplicated cervical infection already have subclinical upper-reproductive-tract infection.

Asymptomatic infection is common among both men and women. To detect chlamydial infections, healthcare providers frequently rely on screening tests. Annual screening of all sexually active women aged <25 years is recommended, as is screening of older women at increased risk for infection (e.g., those who have a new sex partner, more than one sex partner, a sex partner with concurrent partners, or a sex partner who has a sexually transmitted infection. Although CT incidence might be higher in some women aged ≥25 years in some communities, overall the largest burden of infection is among women aged <25 years.

Chlamydia screening programs have been demonstrated to reduce the rates of PID in women. Although evidence is insufficient to recommend routine screening for *C. trachomatis* in sexually active young men because of several factors (e.g., feasibility, efficacy, and cost-effectiveness), the screening of sexually active young men should be considered in clinical settings with a high prevalence of chlamydia (e.g., adolescent clinics, correctional facilities, and STD clinics) or in populations with high burden of infection (e.g., MSM). Among women, the primary focus of chlamydia screening efforts should be to detect chlamydia, prevent complications, and test and treat their partners, whereas targeted chlamydia screening in men should only be considered when resources permit, prevalence is high, and such screening does not hinder chlamydia screening efforts in women. More frequent screening for some women (e.g., adolescents) or certain men (e.g., MSM) might be indicated.

Treatment

Treating persons infected with *C. trachomatis* prevents adverse reproductive health complications and continued sexual transmission, and treating their sex partners can prevent reinfection and infection of other partners. Treating pregnant women usually prevents transmission of *C. trachomatis* to neonates during birth. Chlamydia treatment should be provided promptly for all persons testing positive for infection; treatment delays have been associated with complications (e.g., PID) in a limited proportion of women.

A meta-analysis of 12 randomized clinical trials of azithromycin versus doxycycline for the treatment of urogenital chlamydial infection demonstrated that the treatments were equally efficacious, with microbial cure rates of 97% and 98%, respectively. These studies were conducted primarily in populations with urethral and cervical infection in which follow-up was encouraged, adherence to a 7-day regimen was effective, and culture or EIA (rather than the more sensitive NAAT) was used for determining microbiological outcome. More recent retrospective studies have raised concern about the efficacy of azithromycin for rectal *C. trachomatis* infection, however, these studies have limitations, and prospective clinical trials comparing azithromycin versus doxycycline regimens for rectal *C. trachomatis* infection are needed.

Although the clinical significance of oropharyngeal *C. trachomatis* infection is unclear and routine oropharyngeal screening for CT is not recommended, available evidence suggests oropharyngeal *C. trachomatis* can be sexually transmitted to genital sites; therefore, detection of *C. trachomatis* from an oropharyngeal specimen should be treated with azithromycin or doxycycline. The efficacy of alternative antimicrobial regimens in resolving oropharyngeal chlamydia remains unknown.

In a double-blinded randomized control trial, a doxycycline delayed-release 200 mg tablet administered daily for 7 days was as effective as generic doxycycline 100 mg twice daily for 7 days for treatment of urogenital *C. trachomatis* infection in men and women and had a lower frequency of gastrointestinal side effects. However, this regimen is more costly than those that involve multiple daily doses. Delayed-release doxycycline (Doryx) 200 mg daily for 7 days might be an alternative regimen to the doxycycline 100 mg twice daily for 7 days for treatment of urogenital *C. trachomatis* infection. Erythromycin might be less efficacious than either azithromycin or doxycycline, mainly because of the frequent occurrence of gastrointestinal side effects that can lead to nonadherence with treatment. Levofloxacin and ofloxacin are effective treatment alternatives, but they are more expensive and offer no advantage in the dosage regimen. Other quinolones either are not reliably effective against chlamydial infection or have not been evaluated adequately.

Lymphogranuloma venereum *(LGV)*

What Is LGV?

Lymphogranuloma venereum (LGV) is caused by *C. trachomatis* serovars L1, L2 or L3. The most common clinical manifestation of LGV among heterosexuals is tender inguinal and/or femoral lymphadenopathy that is typically unilateral. A self-limited genital ulcer or papule sometimes occurs at the site of inoculation. However, by the time patients seek care, the lesions have often disappeared. Rectal exposure in women or MSM can result in proctocolitis mimicking inflammatory bowel disease, and clinical findings may include mucoid and/or hemorrhagic rectal discharge, anal pain, constipation, fever, and/or tenesmus. Outbreaks of LGV protocolitis have been reported among MSM. LGV can be an invasive, systemic infection, and if it is not treated early, LGV proctocolitis can lead to chronic colorectal fistulas and strictures; reactive arthropathy has also been reported. However, reports indicate that rectal LGV can be asymptomatic. Persons with

105

genital and colorectal LGV lesions can also develop secondary bacterial infection or can be coinfected with other sexually and nonsexually transmitted pathogens.

Diagnostic Considerations

Diagnosis is based on clinical suspicion, epidemiologic information, and the exclusion of other etiologies for proctocolitis, inguinal lymphadenopathy or genital or rectal ulcers. Genital lesions, rectal specimens, and lymph node specimens (i.e., lesion swab or bubo aspirate) can be tested for *C. trachomatis* by culture, direct immunofluorescence or nucleic acid detection. NAATs for *C. trachomatis* perform well on rectal specimens, but are not FDA-cleared for this purpose. Many laboratories have performed the CLIA validation studies needed to provide results from rectal specimens for clinical management. MSM presenting with protocolitis should be tested for chlamydia; NAAT performed on rectal specimens is the preferred approach to testing.

Additional molecular procedures (e.g., PCR-based genotyping) can be used to differentiate LGV from non-LGV *C. trachomatis* in rectal specimens. However, they are not widely available, and results are not available in a timeframe that would influence clinical management.

Chlamydia serology (complement fixation titers >1:64 or microimmunofluorescence titers >1:256) might support the diagnosis of LGV in the appropriate clinical context. Comparative data between types of serologic tests are lacking, and the diagnostic utility of these older serologic methods has not been established. Serologic test interpretation for LGV is not standardized, tests have not been validated for clinical proctitis presentations, and *C. trachomatis* serovar-specific serologic tests are not widely available.

Treatment

At the time of the initial visit (before diagnostic tests for chlamydia are available), persons with a clinical syndrome consistent with LGV, including proctocolitis or genital ulcer disease with lymphadenopathy, should be presumptively treated for LGV. As required by state law, these cases should be reported to the health department.

Treatment cures infection and prevents ongoing tissue damage, although tissue reaction to the infection can result in scarring. Buboes might require aspiration through intact skin or incision and drainage to prevent the formation of inguinal/femoral ulcerations.

Although clinical data are lacking, azithromycin 1 g orally once weekly for 3 weeks is probably effective based on its chlamydial antimicrobial activity. Fluoroquinolone-based treatments also might be effective, but the optimal duration of treatment has not been evaluated.

Other Management Considerations

Patients should be followed clinically until signs and symptoms have resolved. Persons who receive an LGV diagnosis should be tested for other STDs, especially HIV, gonorrhea, and syphilis. Those who test positive for another infection should be referred for or provided with appropriate care and treatment.

Follow-up

Patients should be followed clinically until signs and symptoms resolve.

Management of Sex Partners

Persons who have had sexual contact with a patient who has LGV within the 60 days before onset of the patient's symptoms should be examined and tested for urethral, cervical, or rectal chlamydial infection depending on anatomic site of exposure. They should be presumptively treated with a chlamydia regimen (azithromycin 1 g orally single dose or doxycycline 100 mg orally twice a day for 7 days).

Special Considerations

Pregnancy

Pregnant and lactating women should be treated with erythromycin. Doxycycline should be avoided in the second and third trimester of pregnancy because of risk for discoloration of teeth and bones, but is compatible with breastfeeding. Azithromycin might prove useful for treatment of LGV in pregnancy, but no published data are available regarding an effective dose and duration of treatment.

HIV Infection

Persons with both LGV and HIV infection should receive the same regimens as those who are HIV negative. Prolonged therapy might be required, and delay in resolution of symptoms might occur.

Chapter 14

Cholera

What Is Cholera?

Cholera is an acute, diarrheal illness caused by infection of the intestine with the bacterium *Vibrio cholerae*. An estimated 3–5 million cases and over 100,000 deaths occur each year around the world. The infection is often mild or without symptoms, but can sometimes be severe. Approximately one in 10 (5–10%) infected persons will have severe disease characterized by profuse watery diarrhea, vomiting, and leg cramps. In these people, rapid loss of body fluids leads to dehydration and shock. Without treatment, death can occur within hours.

Where Is Cholera Found?

The cholera bacterium is usually found in water or food sources that have been contaminated by feces (poop) from a person infected with cholera. Cholera is most likely to be found and spread in places with inadequate water treatment, poor sanitation, and inadequate hygiene. The cholera bacterium may also live in the environment in brackish rivers and coastal waters. Shellfish eaten raw have been a source of cholera, and a few persons in the United States have contracted cholera after eating raw or undercooked shellfish from the Gulf of Mexico.

This chapter includes text excerpted from "Cholera-*Vibrio cholera* Infection," Centers for Disease Control and Prevention (CDC), November 6, 2014.

How Does a Person Get Cholera?

A person can get cholera by drinking water or eating food contaminated with the cholera bacterium. In an epidemic, the source of the contamination is usually the feces of an infected person that contaminates water and/or food. The disease can spread rapidly in areas with inadequate treatment of sewage and drinking water. The disease is not likely to spread directly from one person to another; therefore, casual contact with an infected person is not a risk for becoming ill.

What Are the Symptoms of Cholera?

Cholera infection is often mild or without symptoms, but can sometimes be severe. Approximately one in ten (5–10%) infected persons will have severe disease characterized by profuse watery diarrhea, vomiting, and leg cramps. In these people, rapid loss of body fluids leads to dehydration and shock. Without treatment, death can occur within hours.

How Long after Infection Do the Symptoms Appear?

It can take anywhere from a few hours to 5 days for symptoms to appear after infection. Symptoms typically appear in 2–3 days.

Who Is Most Likely to Get Cholera?

Individuals living in places with inadequate water treatment, poor sanitation, and inadequate hygiene are at a greater risk for cholera.

What Should I Do If I Think a Family Member or I Have Cholera?

If you think you or a member of your family may have cholera, seek medical attention immediately. Dehydration can be rapid so fluid replacement is essential. If you have oral rehydration solution (ORS), the ill person should start taking it now; it can save a life. He or she should continue to drink ORS at home and during travel to get treatment. If you have an infant who has watery diarrhea, continue to breastfeed.

How Is Cholera Diagnosed?

To test for cholera, doctors must take a stool sample or a rectal swab and send it to a laboratory to look for the cholera bacterium.

What Is the Treatment for Cholera?

Cholera can be simply and successfully treated by immediate replacement of the fluid and salts lost through diarrhea. Patients can be treated with oral rehydration solution, a prepackaged mixture of sugar and salts to be mixed with water and drunk in large amounts. This solution is used throughout the world to treat diarrhea. Severe cases also require intravenous fluid replacement. With prompt rehydration, fewer than 1% of cholera patients die. Antibiotics shorten the course and diminish the severity of the illness, but they are not as important as receiving rehydration. Persons who develop severe diarrhea and vomiting in countries where cholera occurs should seek medical attention promptly.

How Can I Avoid Getting Cholera?

The risk for cholera is very low for people visiting areas with epidemic cholera. When simple precautions are observed, contracting the disease is unlikely.

All people (visitors or residents) in areas where cholera is occurring or has occurred should observe the following recommendations:

- Drink only bottled, boiled, or chemically treated water and bottled or canned carbonated beverages. When using bottled drinks, make sure that the seal has not been broken.
  - To disinfect your own water: boil for 1 minute or filter the water and add 2 drops of household bleach or ½ an iodine tablet per liter of water.
  - Avoid tap water, fountain drinks, and ice cubes.
- Wash your hands often with soap and clean water.
- If no water and soap are available, use an alcohol-based hand cleaner (with at least 60% alcohol).
  - Clean your hands especially before you eat or prepare food and after using the bathroom.
- Use bottled, boiled, or chemically treated water to wash dishes, brush your teeth, wash and prepare food or make ice.
- Eat foods that are packaged or that are freshly cooked and served hot.
  - Do not eat raw and undercooked meats and seafood or unpeeled fruits and vegetables.

- Dispose of feces in a sanitary manner to prevent contamination of water and food sources.

Is a Vaccine Available to Prevent Cholera?

Two oral cholera vaccines are available: Dukoral® and ShanChol®, which are World Health Organization (WHO) prequalified. Cholera vaccines are not yet available in the United States and should not replace standard prevention and control measures.

What Is the Risk for Cholera in the United States?

In the United States, cholera was prevalent in the 1800s but water-related spread has been eliminated by modern water and sewage treatment systems. However, United States travelers to areas with epidemic cholera (for example, parts of Africa, Asia, or Latin America) may be exposed to the cholera bacterium. In addition, travelers may bring contaminated seafood back to the United States; foodborne outbreaks of cholera have been caused by contaminated seafood brought into the United States by travelers.

Where Can a Traveler Get Information about Cholera?

The global picture of cholera changes periodically, so travelers should seek updated information on countries of interest.

What Is the U.S. Government Doing to Combat Cholera?

United States and international public health authorities are working to enhance surveillance for cholera, investigate cholera outbreaks, and design and implement preventive measures across the globe. The Centers for Disease Control and Prevention (CDC) investigates epidemic cholera wherever it occurs at the invitation of the affected country and trains laboratory workers in proper techniques for identification of *Vibrio cholerae*. In addition, CDC provides information on diagnosis, treatment, and prevention of cholera to public health officials and educates the public about effective preventive measures.

The U.S. Agency for International Development sponsors some of the international U.S. government activities and provides medical supplies, and water, sanitation and hygiene supplies to affected countries.

The U.S. Food and Drug Administration (FDA) tests imported and domestic shellfish for *V. cholerae* and monitors the safety of U.S. shellfish beds through the shellfish sanitation program.

With cooperation at the state and local, national, and international levels, assistance will be provided to countries where cholera is present. The risk to U.S. residents remains small.

Chapter 15

Clostridium difficile
Infection

Clostridium difficile (C. difficile) is a bacterium that causes inflammation of the colon, known as colitis. People who have other illnesses or conditions requiring prolonged use of antibiotics, and the elderly, are at greater risk of acquiring this disease. The bacteria are found in the feces. People can become infected if they touch items or surfaces that are contaminated with feces and then touch their mouth or mucous membranes. Healthcare workers can spread the bacteria to patients or contaminate surfaces through hand contact.

Symptoms

Symptoms include:

- Watery diarrhea (at least three bowel movements per day for two or more days)
- Fever
- Loss of appetite
- Nausea
- Abdominal pain/tenderness

This chapter includes text excerpted from "*Clostridium difficile* Infection Information for Patients," Centers for Disease Control and Prevention (CDC), February 24, 2015.

Transmission

Clostridium difficile is shed in feces. Any surface, device, or material (e.g., toilets, bathing tubs, and electronic rectal thermometers) that becomes contaminated with feces may serve as a reservoir for the *Clostridium difficile* spores. *Clostridium difficile* spores are transferred to patients mainly via the hands of healthcare personnel who have touched a contaminated surface or item. *Clostridium difficile* can live for long periods on surfaces.

Treatment

Whenever possible, other antibiotics should be discontinued; in a small number of patients, diarrhea may go away when other antibiotics are stopped. Treatment of primary infection caused by *C. difficile* is an antibiotic such as metronidazole, vancomycin, or fidaxomicin. While metronidazole is not approved for treating *C. difficile* infections by the U.S. Food and Drug Administration (FDA), it has been commonly recommended and used for mild *C. difficile* infections; however, it should not be used for severe C. difficile infections. Whenever possible, treatment should be given by mouth and continued for a minimum of 10 days.

One problem with antibiotics used to treat primary *C. difficile* infection is that the infection returns in about 20 percent of patients. In a small number of these patients, the infection returns over and over and can be quite debilitating. While a first return of a *C. difficile* infection is usually treated with the same antibiotic used for primary infection, all future infections should be managed with oral vancomycin or fidaxomicin.

Transplanting stool from a healthy person to the colon of a patient with repeat *C. difficile* infections has been shown to successfully treat *C. difficile*. These "fecal transplants" appear to be the most effective method for helping patients with repeat *C. difficile* infections. This procedure may not be widely available and its long term safety has not been established.

Chapter 16

Common Cold

Common colds are the main reason that children miss school and adults miss work. Each year in the United States, there are millions of cases of the common cold. Adults have an average of 2–3 colds per year, and children have even more.

Most people get colds in the winter and spring, but it is possible to get a cold any time of the year. Symptoms usually include sore throat, runny nose, coughing, sneezing, watery eyes, headaches, and body aches. Most people recover within about 7–10 days. However, people with weakened immune systems, asthma, or respiratory conditions may develop serious illness, such as pneumonia.

Causes of the Common Cold

Many different viruses can cause the common cold, but rhinoviruses are the most common. Rhinoviruses can also trigger asthma attacks and have been linked to sinus and ear infections. Other viruses that can cause colds include respiratory syncytial virus, human parainfluenza viruses, and human metapneumovirus.

Viruses that cause colds can spread from infected people to others through the air and close personal contact. You can also get infected through contact with stool (poop) or respiratory secretions from an infected person. This can happen when you shake hands with someone

This chapter includes text excerpted from "Common Colds: Protect Yourself and Others," Centers for Disease Control and Prevention (CDC), February 8, 2016.

who has a cold, or touch a doorknob that has viruses on it, then touch your eyes, mouth or nose.

How to Protect Yourself and Others

You can help reduce your risk of getting a cold:

- **Wash your hands often with soap and water**

  Wash them for 20 seconds, and help young children do the same. If soap and water are not available, use an alcohol-based hand sanitizer. Viruses that cause colds can live on your hands, and regular handwashing can help protect you from getting sick.

- **Avoid touching your eyes, nose, and mouth with unwashed hands**

  Viruses that cause colds can enter your body this way and make you sick.

- **Stay away from people who are sick**

  Sick people can spread viruses that cause the common cold through close contact with others.

If you have a cold, you should follow these tips to prevent spreading it to other people:

- Stay at home while you are sick.
- Avoid close contact with others, such as hugging, kissing or shaking hands.
- Move away from people before coughing or sneezing.
- Cough and sneeze into a tissue then throw it away or cough and sneeze into your upper shirt sleeve, completely covering your mouth and nose.
- Wash your hands after coughing, sneezing or blowing your nose.
- Disinfect frequently touched surfaces, and objects such as toys and doorknobs.

There is no vaccine to protect you against the common cold.

How to Feel Better

There is no cure for a cold. To feel better, you should get lots of rest and drink plenty of fluids. Over-the-counter medicines may help ease symptoms but will not make your cold go away any faster. Always read the label and use medications as directed. Talk to your doctor before giving your child nonprescription cold medicines, since some medicines contain ingredients that are not recommended for children.

Antibiotics will not help you recover from a cold. They do not work against viruses, and they may make it harder for your body to fight future bacterial infections if you take them unnecessarily.

When to See a Doctor

You should call your doctor if you or your child has one or more of these conditions:

- a temperature higher than 100.4°F

- symptoms that last more than 10 days

- symptoms that are severe or unusual

If your child is younger than three months of age and has a fever, you should always call your doctor right away. Your doctor can determine if you or your child has a cold and can recommend therapy to help with symptoms.

Chapter 17

Conjunctivitis (Pinkeye)

Conjunctivitis, commonly called pinkeye, is an inflammation of the conjunctiva, the clear membrane that covers the white part of the eye and the inner surface of the eyelids.

Pinkeye can be alarming because it may make the eyes extremely red and can spread quickly. But it's fairly common and usually causes no long-term eye or vision damage.

Still, if your child has symptoms of pinkeye, it's important to see a doctor. Some kinds of pinkeye go away on their own, but others need treatment.

Causes

Pinkeye can be caused by many of the bacteria and viruses responsible for colds and other infections,—including ear infections, sinus infections, and sore throats—and by the same types of bacteria that cause chlamydia and gonorrhea, two sexually transmitted diseases (STDs). Pinkeye also can be caused by allergies. These cases tend to happen more often in kids who also have other allergic conditions, such as hay fever. Triggers of allergic conjunctivitis include grass, ragweed pollen, animal dander, and dust mites.

This chapter contains text excerpted from the following sources: Text in this chapter begins with excerpts from "Pinkeye (Conjunctivitis)" © 1995–2016. The Nemours Foundation/KidsHealth®. Reprinted with permission; Text under the heading "Preventing the Spread of Conjunctivitis" is excerpted from "Conjunctivitis (Pink Eye)," Centers for Disease Control and Prevention (CDC), January 9, 2014.

Sometimes a substance in the environment can irritate the eyes and cause pinkeye, such as chemicals (chlorine, soaps, etc.) or air pollutants (smoke and fumes).

Pinkeye in Newborns

Newborns are particularly at risk for pinkeye and can develop serious health complications if it's not treated.

If a baby is born to a mother who has an STD, during delivery the bacteria or virus can pass from the birth canal into the baby's eyes, causing pinkeye. To prevent this, doctors give antibiotic ointment or eye drops to all babies immediately after birth. Occasionally, this treatment causes a mild chemical conjunctivitis, which usually clears up on its own. Doctors also can screen pregnant women for STDs and treat them during pregnancy to prevent spreading the infection to the baby.

Symptoms

The different types of pinkeye can have different symptoms, which can vary from child to child. One of the most common symptoms is discomfort in the eye. A child may say that it feels like there's sand in the eye. Many kids have redness of the eye and inner eyelid, which is why conjunctivitis is often called pinkeye. It can also cause discharge from the eyes, which may cause the eyelids to stick together when a child wakes up. Some kids have swollen eyelids or sensitivity to bright light.

In cases of allergic conjunctivitis, itchiness and tearing are common symptoms.

Contagiousness

Pinkeye caused by bacteria and viruses is contagious; cases caused by allergies or environmental irritants are not. A child can get pinkeye by touching an infected person or something an infected person has touched, such as a used tissue. In the summertime, pinkeye can spread when kids swim in contaminated water or share contaminated towels. It also can spread through coughing and sneezing.

Doctors usually recommend keeping kids diagnosed with contagious conjunctivitis out of school, childcare or summer camp for a short time. Also, someone who has pinkeye in one eye can spread it to the other eye by rubbing or touching the infected eye, then touching the other eye.

Treatment

Pinkeye caused by a virus usually goes away without any treatment. If a doctor thinks that the pinkeye is due to a bacterial infection, antibiotic eye drops or ointment will be prescribed.

Sometimes it can be a challenge to get kids to tolerate eye drops several times a day. If you're having trouble, put the drops on the inner corner of your child's closed eye—when the child opens the eye, the medicine will flow into it. If you continue to have trouble with drops, ask the doctor about antibiotic ointment. It can be applied in a thin layer where the eyelids meet, and will melt and enter the eye.

If your child has allergic conjunctivitis, your doctor may prescribe anti-allergy medicine, which comes in the form of pills, liquid, or eye drops.

Using cool or warm compresses on the eyes and giving acetaminophen or ibuprofen may make your child more comfortable. Clean the edges of the infected eye carefully with warm water and gauze or cotton balls. This can also remove the crusts of dried discharge that may cause the eyelids to stick together first thing in the morning.

If your child wears contact lenses and has conjunctivitis, your doctor or eye doctor may recommend that the contact lenses not be worn until the infection is gone. After the infection is gone, clean the lenses carefully. Be sure to disinfect the lenses and their storage case at least twice before letting your child wear them again. If your child wears disposable contact lenses, throw away the current pair and use a new pair.

When to Call the Doctor

If you think your child has pinkeye, it's important to contact your doctor to learn what's causing it and how to treat it. Other serious eye conditions can have similar symptoms, so a child who complains of severe pain, changes in eyesight, swelling around the eyes, or sensitivity to light should be examined. If the pinkeye does not improve after 2 to 3 days of treatment, or after a week when left untreated, call your doctor.

If your child has pinkeye and starts to develop increased swelling, redness, and tenderness in the eyelids and around the eye, along with a fever, call your doctor. Those symptoms may mean the infection has started to spread beyond the conjunctiva and will need further treatment.

Preventing the Spread of Conjunctivitis

Viral and bacterial conjunctivitis (pinkeye) are very contagious. They can spread easily from person to person. You can greatly reduce the risk of getting conjunctivitis or spreading it to someone else by following some simple good-hygiene steps.

If You Have Conjunctivitis

If you have infectious (viral or bacterial) conjunctivitis, you can help limit its spread to other people by following these steps:

- Wash your hands often with soap and warm water. If soap and water are not available, use an alcohol-based hand sanitizer that contains at least 60 percent alcohol.

- Avoid touching or rubbing your eyes.

- Wash any discharge from around the eyes several times a day. Hands should be washed first and then a clean washcloth or fresh cotton ball or tissue can be used to cleanse the eye area. Throw away cotton balls or tissues after use; if a washcloth is used, it should be washed with hot water and detergent. Wash your hands with soap and warm water when done.

- Wash hands after applying eye drops or ointment.

- Do not use the same eye drop dispenser/bottle for infected and non-infected eyes—even for the same person.

- Wash pillowcases, sheets, washcloths, and towels in hot water and detergent; hands should be washed after handling such items.

- Avoid sharing articles like towels, blankets, and pillowcases.

- Clean eyeglasses, being careful not to contaminate items (like towels) that might be shared by other people.

- Do not share eye makeup, face make-up, make-up brushes, contact lenses and containers or eyeglasses.

- Do not use swimming pools.

If You Are around Someone with Conjunctivitis

If you are around someone with infectious (viral or bacterial) conjunctivitis, you can reduce your risk of infection by following these steps:

- Wash your hands often with soap and warm water. If soap and warm water are not available, use an alcohol-based hand rub.

- Wash your hands after contact with an infected person or items he or she uses; for example, wash your hands after applying eye drops or ointment to an infected person's eye(s) or after putting their bed linens in the washing machine.

- Avoid touching or rubbing your eyes.

- Do not share items used by an infected person; for example, do not share pillows, washcloths, towels, eye drops, eye or face makeup, makeup brushes, contact lenses, contact lens containers, or eyeglasses.

Avoid Getting Sick Again

In addition, if you have infectious conjunctivitis, the following steps can be taken to avoid re-infection, once the infection goes away.

- Throw away and replace any eye or face makeup you used while infected.

- Throw away contact lens solutions that you used while your eyes were infected.

- Throw away disposable contact lenses and cases that were used while your eyes were infected.

- Clean extended wear lenses as directed.

- Clean eyeglasses and cases that were used while infected.

There is no vaccine that prevents all types of conjunctivitis. However, there are vaccines to protect against some viral and bacterial diseases that are associated with conjunctivitis.

- rubella

- measles

- chickenpox

- shingles

- pneumococcal

- *Haemophilus influenzae* type b (Hib)

Conjunctivitis caused by allergens or irritants is not contagious unless a secondary viral or bacterial infection develops.

Chapter 18

Coxsackievirus Infections

Coxsackieviruses are part of the enterovirus family of viruses (which also includes polioviruses and hepatitis A virus) that live in the human digestive tract. They can spread from person to person, usually on unwashed hands and surfaces contaminated by feces, where they can live for several days. In cooler climates, outbreaks of coxsackievirus infections most often occur in the summer and fall, though they cause infections year-round in tropical parts of the world.

In most cases, coxsackieviruses cause mild flu-like symptoms and go away without treatment. But in some cases, they can lead to more serious infections.

Signs and Symptoms

Coxsackievirus can produce a wide variety of symptoms. About half of all kids infected with coxsackievirus have no symptoms. Others suddenly develop high fever, headache, and muscle aches, and some also develop a sore throat, abdominal discomfort, or nausea. A child with a coxsackievirus infection may simply feel hot but have no other symptoms. In most kids, the fever lasts about 3 days, then disappears.

Coxsackieviruses can also cause several different symptoms that affect different body parts, including:

- **Hand, foot, and mouth disease**, a type of coxsackievirus syndrome, causes painful red blisters in the throat and on the

This chapter includes excerpted from "Coxsackievirus Infections," © 1995–2016. The Nemours Foundation/KidsHealth®. Reprinted with permission.

tongue, gums, hard palate, inside of the cheeks, and the palms of hands and soles of the feet.

- **Herpangina**, an infection of the throat which causes red-ringed blisters and ulcers on the tonsils and soft palate, the fleshy back portion of the roof of the mouth.

- **Hemorrhagic conjunctivitis**, an infection that affects the whites of the eyes. Hemorrhagic conjunctivitis usually begins as eye pain, followed quickly by red, watery eyes with swelling, light sensitivity, and blurred vision.

Occasionally, coxsackieviruses can cause more serious infections that may need to be treated in a hospital, including:

- viral meningitis, an infection of the meninges (the three membranes that envelop the brain and spinal cord)

- encephalitis, a brain infection

- myocarditis, an infection of the heart muscle

Newborns can be infected from their mothers during or shortly after birth and are more at risk for developing serious infection, including myocarditis, hepatitis, and meningoencephalitis (an inflammation of the brain and meninges). In newborns, symptoms can develop within 2 weeks after birth.

Contagiousness

Coxsackieviruses are very contagious. They can be passed from person to person on unwashed hands and surfaces contaminated by feces. They also can be spread through droplets of fluid sprayed into the air when someone sneezes or coughs.

When an outbreak affects a community, risk for coxsackievirus infection is highest among infants and kids younger than five. The virus spreads easily in group settings like schools, childcare centers, and summer camps. People who are infected with a coxsackievirus are most contagious the first week they're sick.

Prevention

There is no vaccine to prevent coxsackievirus infection. Hand washing is the best protection. Remind everyone in your family to wash their hands frequently, particularly after using the toilet (especially those in public places), after changing a diaper, before meals, and before preparing food. Shared toys in childcare centers should be routinely cleaned with a disinfectant because the virus can live on these objects for days. Kids who are sick with a coxsackievirus infection should be kept out of school or childcare for a few days to avoid spreading the infection.

The duration of an infection varies widely. For fever without other symptoms, a child's temperature may return to normal within 24 hours, although the average fever lasts 3 to 4 days. Hand, foot, and mouth disease usually lasts for 2 or 3 days; viral meningitis can take 3 to 7 days to clear up.

Treating Coxsackievirus Infections

Depending on the type of infection and symptoms, the doctor may prescribe medications to make your child feel more comfortable. However, because antibiotics only work against bacteria, they can't be used to fight a coxsackievirus infection.

Acetaminophen may be given to relieve any minor aches and pains. If the fever lasts for more than 24 hours or if your child has any symptoms of a more serious coxsackievirus infection, call your doctor. Most kids with a simple coxsackievirus infection recover completely after a few days without needing any treatment. A child who has a fever without any other symptoms should rest in bed or play quietly indoors. Offer plenty of fluids to prevent dehydration.

When to Call the Doctor

Call the doctor immediately if your child develops any of the following symptoms:

- fever higher than 100.4°F (38°C) for infants younger than 6 months and higher than 102°F (38.8°C) for older kids

- poor appetite

- trouble feeding

- vomiting

- diarrhea

- difficulty breathing

- convulsions

- unusual sleepiness

- pain in the chest or abdomen
- sores on the skin or inside the mouth
- severe sore throat
- severe headache, especially with vomiting, confusion, or unusual sleepiness
- neck stiffness
- red, swollen, and watery eyes
- pain in one or both testicles

Chapter 19

Cryptosporidiosis

What Is Cryptosporidiosis?

Cryptosporidiosis is a disease that causes watery diarrhea. It is caused by microscopic germs—parasites called *Cryptosporidium*. *Cryptosporidium*, or "Crypto" for short, can be found in water, food, soil or on surfaces or dirty hands that have been contaminated with the feces of humans or animals infected with the parasite. During 2001–2010, Crypto was the leading cause of waterborne disease outbreaks, linked to recreational water in the United States. The parasite is found in every region of the United States and throughout the world.

How Is Cryptosporidiosis Spread?

Crypto lives in the gut of infected humans or animals. An infected person or animal sheds Crypto parasites in their poop. An infected person can shed 10,000,000 to 100,000,000 Crypto germs in a single bowel movement. Shedding of Crypto in poop begins when symptoms like diarrhea begin and can last for weeks after symptoms stop. Swallowing as few as 10 Crypto germs can cause infection.

Crypto can be spread by:

- Swallowing recreational water (for example, the water in swimming pools, fountains, lakes, rivers) contaminated with Crypto.

This chapter includes text excerpted from "Parasites-Cryptosporidium (Also Known As "Crypto")," Centers for Disease Control and Prevention (CDC), April 20, 2015.

- Crypto's high tolerance to chlorine enables the parasite to survive for long periods of time in chlorinated drinking and swimming pool water.

- Drinking untreated water from a lake or river that is contaminated with Crypto.

- Swallowing water, ice, or beverages contaminated with poop from infected humans or animals.

- Eating undercooked food or drinking unpasteurized/raw apple cider or milk that gets contaminated with Crypto.

- Touching your mouth with contaminated hands.

- Hands can become contaminated through a variety of activities, such as touching surfaces or objects (e.g., toys, bathroom fixtures, changing tables, diaper pails) that have been contaminated by poop from an infected person, changing diapers, caring for an infected person, and touching an infected animal.

- Exposure to poop from an infected person through oral-anal sexual contact.

Crypto is not spread through contact with blood.

What Are the Symptoms of Cryptosporidiosis, When Do They Begin, and How Long Do They Last?

Symptoms of Crypto generally begin 2 to 10 days (average 7 days) after becoming infected with the parasite. Symptoms include:

- Watery diarrhea

- Stomach cramps or pain

- Dehydration

- Nausea

- Vomiting

- Fever

- Weight loss

Symptoms usually last about 1 to 2 weeks (with a range of a few days to 4 or more weeks) in people with healthy immune systems. The most common symptom of cryptosporidiosis is watery diarrhea. Some people with Crypto will have no symptoms at all.

Who Is Most at Risk for Cryptosporidiosis?

People who are most likely to become infected with *Cryptosporidium* include:

- Children who attend childcare centers, including diaper-aged children
- Childcare workers
- Parents of infected children
- People who take care of other people with Crypto
- International travelers
- Backpackers, hikers, and campers who drink unfiltered, untreated water
- People who drink from untreated shallow, unprotected wells
- People, including swimmers, who swallow water from contaminated sources
- People who handle infected calves or other ruminants like sheep
- People exposed to human poop through sexual contact

Contaminated water might include water that has not been boiled or filtered, as well as contaminated recreational water sources (e.g., swimming pools, lakes, rivers, ponds, and streams). Several community-wide outbreaks have been linked to drinking tap water or recreational water contaminated with *Cryptosporidium*. Crypto's high tolerance to chlorine enables the parasite to survive for long periods of time in chlorinated drinking and swimming pool water. This means anyone swallowing contaminated water could get ill.

Although Crypto can infect all people, some groups are likely to develop more serious illness.

- **Young children and pregnant women** may be more likely to get dehydrated because of their diarrhea so they should drink plenty of fluids while ill.

- People with **severely weakened immune systems** are at risk for more serious disease. Symptoms may be more severe and could lead to serious or life-threatening illness. Examples of people with weakened immune systems include those with AIDS; those with inherited diseases that affect the immune system; and cancer and transplant patients who are taking certain immunosuppressive drugs.

What Should I Do If I Think I Might Have Cryptosporidiosis?

For diarrhea whose cause has not been determined, the following actions may help relieve symptoms:

- Drink plenty of fluids to remain well hydrated and avoid dehydration. Serious health problems can occur if the body does not maintain proper fluid levels. For some people, diarrhea can be severe resulting in hospitalization due to dehydration.

- Maintain a well-balanced diet. Doing so may help speed recovery.

- Avoid beverages that contain caffeine, such as tea, coffee, and many soft drinks.

- Avoid alcohol, as it can lead to dehydration.

Contact your healthcare provider if you suspect that you have cryptosporidiosis.

How Is Cryptosporidiosis Diagnosed?

Cryptosporidiosis is a diarrheal disease that is spread through contact with the stool of an infected person or animal. The disease is diagnosed by examining stool samples. People infected with Crypto can shed the parasite irregularly in their poop (for example, one day they shed parasite, the next day they don't, the third day they do) so patients may need to give three samples collected on three different days to help make sure that a negative test result is accurate and really means they do not have Crypto. Healthcare providers should specifically request testing for Crypto. Routine ova and parasite testing does not normally include Crypto testing.

What Is the Treatment for Cryptosporidiosis?

Most people with healthy immune systems will recover from cryptosporidiosis without treatment. Individuals who have health concerns should talk to their healthcare provider.

Over-the-counter anti-diarrheal medicine might help slow down diarrhea, but a healthcare provider should be consulted before such medicine is taken. A drug called nitazoxanide has been U.S. Food and Drug Administration (FDA)-approved for treatment of diarrhea caused by *Cryptosporidium* in people with healthy immune systems and is available by prescription.

Consult with your healthcare provider for more information about potential advantages and disadvantages of taking nitazoxanide. Infants, young children, and pregnant women may be more likely than others to suffer from dehydration. Losing a lot of fluids from diarrhea can be dangerous—and especially life-threatening in infants. These people should drink extra fluids when they are sick. Severe dehydration may require hospitalization for treatment with fluids given through your vein (intravenous or IV fluids).

If you are pregnant or a parent and you suspect you or your child is severely dehydrated, contact a healthcare provider about fluid replacement options.

How Should I Clean My House to Help Prevent the Spread of Cryptosporidiosis?

No cleaning method is guaranteed to be completely effective against Crypto. However, you can lower the chance of spreading Crypto by taking the following precautions:

- **Wash linens, clothing, dishwasher- or dryer-safe soft toys, etc. soiled with poop or vomit as soon as possible.**
- Flush excess vomit or poop on clothes or objects down the toilet.
- Use laundry detergent, and wash in hot water: 113°F or hotter for at least 20 minutes or at 122°F or hotter for at least 5 minutes.
- Machine dry on the highest heat setting.
- For other household object and surfaces (for example, diaper-change areas):
- Remove all visible poop.
- Clean with soap and water.
- Let dry completely for at least 4 hours.
- If possible, expose to direct sunlight during the 4 hours.
- Wash your hands with soap and water after cleaning objects or surfaces that could be contaminated with Crypto.

The best way to prevent the spread of *Cryptosporidium* in the home is by practicing good hygiene. Wash your hands frequently with soap and water, especially after using the toilet, after changing diapers, and before eating or preparing food. Alcohol-based hand sanitizers are not effective against Crypto.

Chapter 20

Diphtheria

Diphtheria once was a major cause of illness and death among children. The United States recorded 206,000 cases of diphtheria in 1921 and 15,520 deaths. Before there was treatment for diphtheria, up to half of the people who got the disease died from it.

Starting in the 1920s, diphtheria rates dropped quickly in the United States and other countries with the widespread use of vaccines. In the past decade, there were less than five cases of diphtheria in the United States reported to Centers for Disease Control and Prevention (CDC). However, the disease continues to cause illness globally. In 2014, 7,321 cases of diphtheria were reported to the World Health Organization (WHO), but there are likely many more cases.

Causes and Transmission

Diphtheria is an infection caused by the *Corynebacterium diphtheriae* bacterium.

Diphtheria is spread (transmitted) from person to person, usually through respiratory droplets, like from coughing or sneezing. Rarely, people can get sick from touching open sores (skin lesions) or clothes that touched open sores of someone sick with diphtheria. A person also can get diphtheria by coming in contact with an object, like a toy, that has the bacteria that cause diphtheria on it.

This chapter includes text excerpted from "Diphtheria," Centers for Disease Control and Prevention (CDC), January 15, 2016.

Symptoms

When the bacteria that cause diphtheria get into and attach to the lining of the respiratory system, which includes parts of the body that help you breathe, they produce a poison (toxin) that can cause:

- Weakness

- Sore throat

- Fever

- Swollen glands in the neck

The poison destroys healthy tissues in the respiratory system. Within two to three days, the dead tissue forms a thick, gray coating that can build up in the throat or nose. This thick gray coating is called a "pseudomembrane." It can cover tissues in the nose, tonsils, voice box, and throat, making it very hard to breathe and swallow.

The poison may also get into the bloodstream and cause damage to the heart, kidneys, and nerves.

Diagnosis

Doctors usually decide if a person has diphtheria by looking for common signs and symptoms. They can use a swab from the back of the throat and test it for the bacteria that cause diphtheria. A doctor can also take a sample from a skin lesion (like a sore) and try and grow the bacteria to be sure a patient has diphtheria.

Treatment

It is important to start treatment right away if a doctor suspects diphtheria and not to wait for laboratory confirmation. In the United States, before there was treatment for diphtheria, up to half of the people who got the disease died from it. Diphtheria treatment today involves:

- Using diphtheria antitoxin to stop the poison (toxin) produced by the bacteria from damaging the body.

- Using medicines (called antibiotics) to kill and get rid of the bacteria.

Diphtheria patients are usually kept in isolation, until they are no longer contagious—this usually takes about 48 hours after starting antibiotics. After the patient finishes taking the antibiotic, the doctor will run tests to make sure the bacteria are not in the patient's body anymore.

Prevention

The best way to prevent diphtheria is to get vaccinated. In the United States, there are four vaccines used to prevent diphtheria: DTaP, Tdap, DT, and Td. Each of these vaccines prevents diphtheria and tetanus; DTaP and Tdap also help prevent pertussis (whooping cough). DTaP and DT are given to children younger than seven years old, while Tdap and Td are given to older children, teens, and adults.

Babies and Children

The current childhood immunization schedule for diphtheria includes five doses of DTaP for children younger than seven years old.

Preteens and Teens

The adolescent immunization schedule recommends that preteens get a booster dose of Tdap at 11 or 12 years old. Teens who did not get Tdap when they were 11 or 12 years old should get a dose the next time they see their doctor.

Adults

Adults should get a dose of Td every 10 years according to the adult immunization schedule. For added protection against whooping cough, any adult who never received a dose of Tdap should get one as soon as possible. The dose of Tdap takes the place of one of the Td shots.

Chapter 21

Ebola

Ebola, previously known as Ebola hemorrhagic fever, is a rare and deadly disease caused by infection with one of the Ebola virus species. Ebola can cause disease in humans and nonhuman primates (monkeys, gorillas, and chimpanzees).

Ebola viruses are found in several African countries. Ebola was first discovered in 1976 near the Ebola River in what is now the Democratic Republic of the Congo. Since then, outbreaks have appeared sporadically in Africa.

The natural reservoir host of Ebola virus remains unknown. However, on the basis of evidence and the nature of similar viruses, researchers believe that the virus is animal-borne and that bats are the most likely reservoir. Four of the five virus strains occur in an animal host native to Africa.

Signs and Symptoms

Symptoms of Ebola include:

- Fever

- Severe headache

- Muscle pain

- Weakness

This chapter includes text excerpted from "Ebola (Ebola Virus Disease)," Centers for Disease Control and Prevention (CDC), February 18, 2016.

- Fatigue

- Diarrhea

- Vomiting

- Abdominal (stomach) pain

- Unexplained hemorrhage (bleeding or bruising)

Symptoms may appear anywhere from 2 to 21 days after exposure to Ebola, but the average is 8 to 10 days. Recovery from Ebola depends on good supportive clinical care and the patient's immune response. People who recover from Ebola infection develop antibodies that last for at least 10 years.

Transmission

Because the natural reservoir host of Ebola viruses has not yet been identified, the way in which the virus first appears in a human at the start of an outbreak is unknown. However, scientists believe that the first patient becomes infected through contact with an infected animal, such as a fruit bat or primate (apes and monkeys), which is called a spillover event. Person-to-person transmission follows and can lead to large numbers of affected people. In some past Ebola outbreaks, primates were also affected by Ebola and multiple spillover events occurred when people touched or ate infected primates.

When an infection occurs in humans, the virus can be spread to others through direct contact (through broken skin or mucous membranes in, for example, the eyes, nose, or mouth) with

- blood or body fluids (including but not limited to urine, saliva, sweat, feces, vomit, breast milk, and semen) of a person who is sick with or has died from Ebola,

- objects (like needles and syringes) that have been contaminated with body fluids from a person who is sick with Ebola or the body of a person who has died from Ebola,

- infected fruit bats or primates (apes and monkeys), and

- possibly from contact with semen from a man who has recovered from Ebola (for example, by having oral, vaginal, or anal sex).

Ebola is not spread through the air, by water, or in general, by food. However, in Africa, Ebola may be spread as a result of handling bushmeat (wild animals hunted for food) and contact with infected bats. There is no evidence that mosquitoes or other insects can transmit Ebola virus. Only a few species of mammals (e.g., humans, bats, monkeys, and apes) have shown the ability to become infected with and spread Ebola virus.

Healthcare providers caring for Ebola patients and family and friends in close contact with Ebola patients are at the highest risk of getting sick because they may come in contact with infected blood or body fluids.

During outbreaks of Ebola, the disease can spread quickly within healthcare settings (such as a clinic or hospital). Exposure to Ebola can occur in healthcare settings where hospital staff are not wearing appropriate personal protective equipment.

Dedicated medical equipment (preferably disposable, when possible) should be used by healthcare personnel providing patient care. Proper cleaning and disposal of instruments, such as needles and syringes, also are important. If instruments are not disposable, they must be sterilized before being used again. Without adequate sterilization of instruments, virus transmission can continue and amplify an outbreak.

Ebola virus has been found in the semen of some men who have recovered from Ebola. It is possible that Ebola could be spread through sex or other contact with semen. It is not known how long Ebola might be found in the semen of male Ebola survivors. The time it takes for Ebola to leave the semen is different for each man. Based on the results from limited studies conducted to date, it appears that the amount of virus decreases over time and eventually leaves the semen. Until more information is known, avoid contact with semen from a man who has had Ebola. It is not known if Ebola can be spread through sex or other contact with vaginal fluids from a woman who has had Ebola.

Prevention

If you travel to or are in an area affected by an Ebola outbreak, make sure to do the following:

- Practice careful hygiene. For example, wash your hands with soap and water or an alcohol-based hand sanitizer and avoid contact with blood and body fluids (such as urine, feces, saliva, sweat, urine, vomit, breast milk, semen, and vaginal fluids).

- Do not handle items that may have come in contact with an infected person's blood or body fluids (such as clothes, bedding, needles, and medical equipment).

- Avoid funeral or burial rituals that require handling the body of someone who has died from Ebola.

- Avoid contact with bats and nonhuman primates or blood, fluids, and raw meat prepared from these animals.

- Avoid facilities in West Africa where Ebola patients are being treated. The U.S. embassy or consulate is often able to provide advice on facilities.

- Avoid contact with semen from a man who has had Ebola until you know Ebola is gone from his semen.

- After you return, monitor your health for 21 days and seek medical care immediately if you develop symptoms of Ebola.

Healthcare workers who may be exposed to people with Ebola should follow these steps:

- Wear appropriate personal protective equipment (PPE).

- Practice proper infection control and sterilization measures.

- Isolate patients with Ebola from other patients.

- Avoid direct, unprotected contact with the bodies of people who have died from Ebola.

- Notify health officials if you have had direct contact with the blood or body fluids, such as but not limited to, feces, saliva, urine, vomit, and semen of a person who is sick with Ebola. The virus can enter the body through broken skin or unprotected mucous membranes in, for example, the eyes, nose or mouth.

Diagnosis

Diagnosing Ebola in a person who has been infected for only a few days is difficult because the early symptoms, such as fever, are non-specific to Ebola infection and often are seen in patients with more common diseases, such as malaria and typhoid fever.

However, a person should be isolated and public health authorities notified if they have the early symptoms of Ebola and have had contact with:

- blood or body fluids from a person sick with or who has died from Ebola

- objects that have been contaminated with the blood or body fluids of a person sick with or who has died from Ebola

- infected fruit bats and primates (apes and monkeys)

- semen from a man who has recovered from Ebola

Samples from the patient can then be collected and tested to confirm infection.

Ebola virus is detected in blood only after onset of symptoms, most notably fever, which accompany the rise in circulating virus within the patient's body. It may take up to three days after symptoms start for the virus to reach detectable levels. Laboratory tests used in diagnosis include:

Table 21.1. Infections and Diagnostic Tests

Timeline of Infection	Diagnostic Tests Available
Within a few days after symptoms begin	• Antigen-capture enzyme-linked immunosorbent assay (ELISA) testing • IgM ELISA • Polymerase chain reaction (PCR) • Virus isolation
Later in disease course or after recovery	• IgM and IgG antibodies
Retrospectively in deceased patients	• Immunohistochemistry testing • PCR • Virus isolation

Treatment

No FDA-approved vaccine or medicine (e.g., antiviral drug) is available for Ebola.

Symptoms of Ebola and complications are treated as they appear. The following basic interventions, when used early, can significantly improve the chances of survival:

- Providing intravenous fluids (IV) and balancing electrolytes (body salts)

- Maintaining oxygen status and blood pressure

- Treating other infections if they occur

Experimental vaccines and treatments for Ebola are under development, but they have not yet been fully tested for safety or effectiveness.

Recovery from Ebola depends on good supportive care and the patient's immune response. People who recover from Ebola infection develop antibodies that last for at least 10 years, possibly longer. It is not known if people who recover are immune for life or if they can become infected with a different species of Ebola. Some people who have recovered from Ebola have developed long-term complications, such as joint and vision problems.

Even after recovery, Ebola might be found in some body fluids, including semen. The time it takes for Ebola to leave the semen is different for each man. For some men who survived Ebola, the virus left their semen in three months. For other men, the virus did not leave their semen for more than nine months. Based on the results from limited studies conducted to date, it appears that the amount of virus decreases over time and eventually leaves the semen.

Chapter 22

Epstein-Barr Virus and Infectious Mononucleosis

Epstein-Barr Virus (EBV)

Epstein-Barr virus (EBV), also known as human herpesvirus 4, is a member of the herpesvirus family. It is one of the most common human viruses. EBV is found all over the world. Most people get infected with EBV at some point in their lives. EBV spreads most commonly through bodily fluids, primarily saliva. EBV can cause infectious mononucleosis, also called mono, and other illnesses.

Symptoms

Symptoms of EBV infection can include:

- fatigue
- fever
- inflamed throat
- swollen lymph nodes in the neck
- enlarged spleen

This chapter includes text excerpted from "Epstein-Barr Virus and Infectious Mononucleosis," Centers for Disease Control and Prevention (CDC), January 7, 2014.

- swollen liver

- rash

Many people become infected with EBV in childhood. EBV infections in children usually do not cause symptoms, or the symptoms are not distinguishable from other mild, brief childhood illnesses. People who get symptoms from EBV infection, usually teenagers or adults, get better in 2 to 4 weeks. However, some people may feel fatigued for several weeks or even months.

After you get an EBV infection, the virus becomes latent (inactive) in your body. In some cases, the virus may reactivate. This does not always cause symptoms, but people with compromised immune systems are more likely to develop symptoms if EBV reactivates.

Transmission

EBV spreads most commonly through bodily fluids, especially saliva. However, EBV can also spread through blood and semen during sexual contact, blood transfusions, and organ transplantations. EBV can be spread by using objects, such as a toothbrush or drinking glass, that an infected person recently used. The virus probably survives on an object at least as long as the object remains moist. There is no evidence that disinfecting the objects will prevent EBV from spreading.

The first time you get infected with EBV (primary EBV infection) you can spread the virus for weeks and even before you have symptoms. Once the virus is in your body, it stays there in a latent (inactive) state. If the virus reactivates, you can potentially spread EBV to others no matter how much time has passed since the initial infection.

Diagnosis

Diagnosing EBV infection can be challenging since symptoms are similar to other illnesses. EBV infection can be confirmed with a blood test that detects antibodies. About 90% of adults have antibodies that show that they have a current or past EBV infection.

Prevention and Treatment

There is no vaccine to protect against EBV infection. You can help protect yourself by not kissing or sharing drinks, food, or personal items, like toothbrushes, with people who have EBV infection.

There is no specific treatment for EBV. However, some things can be done to help relieve symptoms including:

- drinking fluids to stay hydrated
- getting plenty of rest

Infectious Mononucleosis

Infectious mononucleosis, also called "mono," is a contagious disease. Epstein-Barr virus (EBV) is the most common cause of infectious mononucleosis, but other viruses can also cause this disease. It is common among teenagers and young adults, especially college students. At least 25% of teenagers and young adults who get infected with EBV will develop infectious mononucleosis.

Symptoms

Typical symptoms of infectious mononucleosis usually appear 4 to 6 weeks after you get infected with EBV. Symptoms may develop slowly and may not all occur at the same time.

These symptoms include:

- extreme fatigue
- fever
- sore throat
- head and body aches
- swollen lymph nodes in the neck and armpits
- swollen liver or spleen or both
- rash

Enlarged spleen and a swollen liver are less common symptoms. For some people, their liver or spleen or both may remain enlarged even after their fatigue ends. Most people get better in 2 to 4 weeks; however, some people may feel fatigued for several more weeks. Occasionally, the symptoms of infectious mononucleosis can last for 6 months or longer.

Transmission

EBV is the most common cause of infectious mononucleosis, but other viruses can cause this disease. Typically, these viruses spread most commonly through bodily fluids, especially saliva. However, these viruses can also spread through blood and semen during sexual contact, blood transfusions, and organ transplantations.

Prevention and Treatment

There is no vaccine to protect against infectious mononucleosis. You can help protect yourself by not kissing or sharing drinks, food, or personal items, like toothbrushes, with people who have infectious mononucleosis.

You can help relieve symptoms of infectious mononucleosis by:

- drinking fluids to stay hydrated

- getting plenty of rest

- taking over-the-counter medications for pain and fever

If you have infectious mononucleosis, you should not take ampicillin or amoxicillin. Based on the severity of the symptoms, a healthcare provider may recommend treatment of specific organ systems affected by infectious mononucleosis. Because your spleen may become enlarged as a result of infectious mononucleosis, you should avoid contact sports until you fully recover. Participating in contact sports can be strenuous and may cause the spleen to rupture.

Diagnosing Infectious Mononucleosis

Healthcare providers typically diagnose infectious mononucleosis based on symptoms. Laboratory tests are not usually needed to diagnose infectious mononucleosis. However, specific antibody tests may be needed to identify the cause of illness in people who do not have a typical case of infectious mononucleosis.

The blood work of patients who have infectious mononucleosis due to EBV infection may show:

- more white blood cells (lymphocytes) than normal

- unusual looking white blood cells (atypical lymphocytes)

- fewer than normal neutrophils or platelets

- abnormal liver function

Chapter 23

Fifth Disease (Parvovirus B19)

Fifth disease is a mild rash illness caused by parvovirus B19. This disease, also called erythema infectiosum, got its name because it was fifth in a list of historical classifications of common skin rash illnesses in children. It is more common in children than adults. A person usually gets sick with fifth disease within 4 to 14 days after getting infected with parvovirus B19.

Signs and Symptoms

The first symptoms of fifth disease are usually mild and may include:

- fever

- runny nose

- headache

Then you can get a rash on your face and body. After several days, you may get a red rash on your face called "slapped cheek" rash. This rash is the most recognized feature of fifth disease. It is more common in children than adults. Some people may get a second rash

---

This chapter includes text excerpted from "Parvovirus B19 and Fifth Disease," Centers for Disease Control and Prevention (CDC), November 2, 2015.

a few days later on their chest, back, buttocks, or arms and legs. The rash may be itchy, especially on the soles of the feet. It can vary in intensity and usually goes away in 7 to 10 days, but it can come and go for several weeks. As it starts to go away, it may look lacy.

You may also have painful or swollen joints. People with fifth disease can also develop pain and swelling in their joints (polyarthropathy syndrome). This is more common in adults, especially women. Some adults with fifth disease may only have painful joints, usually in the hands, feet or knees, and no other symptoms. The joint pain usually lasts 1 to 3 weeks, but it can last for months or longer. It usually goes away without any long-term problems.

Complications

Fifth disease is usually mild for children and adults who are otherwise healthy. But for some people fifth disease cause serious health complications. People with weakened immune systems caused by leukemia, cancer, organ transplants or HIV infection are at risk for serious complications from fifth disease. It can cause chronic anemia that requires medical treatment.

Transmission

Parvovirus B19—which causes fifth disease—spreads through respiratory secretions (such as saliva, sputum, or nasal mucus) when an infected person coughs or sneezes. You are most contagious when it seems like you have "just a cold" and before you get the rash or joint pain and swelling. After you get the rash you are not likely to be contagious, so then it is usually safe for you or your child to go back to work or school.

People with fifth disease who have weakened immune systems may be contagious for a longer amount of time. Parvovirus B19 can also spread through blood or blood products. A pregnant woman who is infected with parvovirus B19 can pass the virus to her baby. Once you recover from fifth disease, you develop immunity that generally protects you from parvovirus B19 infection in the future.

Diagnosis

Healthcare providers can often diagnose fifth disease just by seeing "slapped cheek" rash on a patient's face. A blood test can also be done to determine if you are susceptible or immune to parvovirus

B19 infection or if you were recently infected. The blood test may be particularly helpful for pregnant women who may have been exposed to parvovirus B19 and are suspected to have fifth disease.

Prevention

There is no vaccine or medicine that can prevent parvovirus B19 infection. You can reduce your chance of being infected or infecting others by:

- washing your hands often with soap and water
- covering your mouth and nose when you cough or sneeze
- not touching your eyes, nose, or mouth
- avoiding close contact with people who are sick
- staying home when you are sick

After you get the rash, you are probably not contagious. So it is usually then safe for you to go back to work or for your child to return to school or a child care center. Healthcare providers who are pregnant should know about potential risks to their baby and discuss this with their doctor. All healthcare providers and patients should follow strict infection control practices to prevent parvovirus B19 from spreading.

Treatment

Fifth disease is usually mild and will go away on its own. Children and adults who are otherwise healthy usually recover completely. Treatment usually involves relieving symptoms, such as fever, itching, and joint pain and swelling. People who have complications from fifth disease should see their healthcare provider for medical treatment.

Chapter 24

Genital Herpes

Herpes is a common sexually transmitted disease (STD) that any sexually active person can get. Most people with the virus don't have symptoms. It is important to know that even without signs of the disease, it can still spread to sexual partners.

What Is Genital Herpes?

Genital herpes is an STD caused by two types of viruses. The viruses are called herpes simplex type 1 and herpes simplex type 2.

How Common Is Genital Herpes?

Genital herpes is common in the United States. In the United States, about one out of every six people aged 14 to 49 years have genital herpes.

How Is Genital Herpes Spread?

You can get herpes by having vaginal, anal, or oral sex with someone who has the disease.

Fluids found in a herpes sore carry the virus, and contact with those fluids can cause infection. You can also get herpes from an infected sex partner who does not have a visible sore or who may not know he

---

This chapter includes text excerpted from "Genital Herpes—CDC Fact Sheet," Centers for Disease Control and Prevention (CDC), January 23, 2014.

or she is infected because the virus can be released through your skin and spread the infection to your sex partner(s).

How Can I Reduce My Risk of Getting Herpes?

The only way to avoid STDs is to not have vaginal, anal, or oral sex.

If you are sexually active, you can do the following things to lower your chances of getting herpes:

- Being in a long-term mutually monogamous relationship with a partner who has been tested and has negative STD test results.

- Using latex condoms the right way every time you have sex.

Herpes symptoms can occur in both male and female genital areas that are covered by a latex condom. However, outbreaks can also occur in areas that are not covered by a condom so condoms may not fully protect you from getting herpes.

I'm Pregnant. How Could Genital Herpes Affect My Baby?

If you are pregnant and have genital herpes, it is even more important for you to go to prenatal care visits. You need to tell your doctor if you have ever had symptoms of, been exposed to, or been diagnosed with genital herpes. Sometimes genital herpes infection can lead to miscarriage. It can also make it more likely for you to deliver your baby too early. Herpes infection can be passed from you to your unborn child and cause a potentially deadly infection (neonatal herpes). It is important that you avoid getting herpes during pregnancy.

If you are pregnant and have genital herpes, you may be offered herpes medicine towards the end of your pregnancy to reduce the risk of having any symptoms and passing the disease to your baby. At the time of delivery your doctor should carefully examine you for symptoms. If you have herpes symptoms at delivery, a 'C-section' is usually performed.

Can Herpes Be Cured?

There is no cure for herpes. However, there are medicines that can prevent or shorten outbreaks. One of these herpes medicines can be taken daily, and makes it less likely that you will pass the infection onto your sex partner(s).

What Happens If I Don't Get Treated?

Genital herpes can cause painful genital sores and can be severe in people with suppressed immune systems. If you touch your sores or the fluids from the sores, you may transfer herpes to another part of your body, such as your eyes. Do not touch the sores or fluids to avoid spreading herpes to another part of your body. If you touch the sores or fluids, immediately wash your hands thoroughly to help avoid spreading your infection.

Some people who get genital herpes have concerns about how it will impact their overall health, sex life, and relationships. It is best for you to talk to a healthcare provider about those concerns, but it also is important to recognize that while herpes is not curable, it can be managed. Since a genital herpes diagnosis may affect how you will feel about current or future sexual relationships, it is important to understand how to talk to sexual partners about STDs.

Can I Still Have Sex If I Have Herpes?

If you have herpes, you should tell your sex partner(s) and let him or her know that you do and the risk involved. Using condoms may help lower this risk but it will not get rid of the risk completely. Having sores or other symptoms of herpes can increase your risk of spreading the disease. Even if you do not have any symptoms, you can still infect your sex partners.

What Is the Link between Genital Herpes and HIV?

Genital herpes can cause sores or breaks in the skin or lining of the mouth, vagina, and rectum. The genital sores caused by herpes can bleed easily. When the sores come into contact with the mouth, vagina, or rectum during sex, they increase the risk of giving or getting HIV if you or your partner has HIV.

What Is the Link between Genital Herpes and Oral Herpes (Cold Sores on the Mouth)?

Oral herpes (such as cold sores or fever blisters on or around the mouth) is usually caused by HSV-1. Most people are infected with

HSV-1 during childhood from non-sexual contact. For example, people can get infected from a kiss from a relative or friend with oral herpes. More than half of the population in the United States has HSV-1, even if they don't show any signs or symptoms. HSV-1 can also be spread from the mouth to the genitals through oral sex. This is why some cases of genital herpes are caused by HSV-1.

Chapter 25

Gonorrhea

What Is Gonorrhea?

Gonorrhea is a sexually transmitted disease (STD) caused by infection with the *Neisseria gonorrhoeae* bacterium. *N. gonorrhoeae* infects the mucous membranes of the reproductive tract, including the cervix, uterus, and fallopian tubes in women, and the urethra in women and men. *N. gonorrhoeae* can also infect the mucous membranes of the mouth, throat, eyes, and rectum.

How Common Is Gonorrhea?

Gonorrhea is a very common infectious disease. Centers for Disease Control and Prevention (CDC) estimates that approximately 820,000 new gonorrheal infections occur in the United States each year, and that less than half of these infections are detected and reported to CDC. CDC estimates that 570,000 of them were among young people 15–24 years of age. In 2014, 350,062 cases of gonorrhea were reported to CDC.

How Do People Get Gonorrhea?

Gonorrhea is transmitted through sexual contact with the penis, vagina, mouth or anus of an infected partner. Ejaculation does not

This chapter includes text excerpted from "Gonorrhea—CDC Fact Sheet (Detailed Version)," Centers for Disease Control and Prevention (CDC), August 27, 2015.

have to occur for gonorrhea to be transmitted or acquired. Gonorrhea can also be spread perinatally from mother to baby during childbirth.

People who have had gonorrhea and received treatment may be reinfected if they have sexual contact with a person infected with gonorrhea.

Who Is at Risk for Gonorrhea?

Any sexually active person can be infected with gonorrhea. In the United States, the highest reported rates of infection are among sexually active teenagers, young adults, and African Americans.

What Are the Signs and Symptoms of Gonorrhea?

Many men with gonorrhea are asymptomatic. When present, signs and symptoms of urethral infection in men include dysuria or a white, yellow, or green urethral discharge that usually appears one to fourteen days after infection. In cases where urethral infection is complicated by epididymitis, men with gonorrhea may also complain of testicular or scrotal pain.

Most women with gonorrhea are asymptomatic. Even when a woman has symptoms, they are often so mild and nonspecific that they are mistaken for a bladder or vaginal infection. The initial symptoms and signs in women include dysuria, increased vaginal discharge, or vaginal bleeding between periods. Women with gonorrhea are at risk of developing serious complications from the infection, regardless of the presence or severity of symptoms.

Symptoms of rectal infection in both men and women may include discharge, anal itching, soreness, bleeding, or painful bowel movements. Rectal infection also may be asymptomatic. Pharyngeal infection may cause a sore throat, but usually is asymptomatic.

What Are the Complications of Gonorrhea?

Untreated gonorrhea can cause serious and permanent health problems in both women and men.

In women, gonorrhea can spread into the uterus or fallopian tubes and cause pelvic inflammatory disease (PID). The symptoms may be quite mild or can be very severe and can include abdominal pain and fever. PID can lead to internal abscesses and chronic pelvic pain. PID can also damage the fallopian tubes enough to cause infertility or increase the risk of ectopic pregnancy.

In men, gonorrhea may be complicated by epididymitis. In rare cases, this may lead to infertility.

If left untreated, gonorrhea can also spread to the blood and cause disseminated gonococcal infection (DGI). DGI is usually characterized by arthritis, tenosynovitis, and/or dermatitis. This condition can be life threatening.

What about Gonorrhea and HIV?

Untreated gonorrhea can increase a person's risk of acquiring or transmitting HIV, the virus that causes AIDS.

How Does Gonorrhea Affect a Pregnant Woman and Her Baby?

If a pregnant woman has gonorrhea, she may give the infection to her baby as the baby passes through the birth canal during delivery. This can cause blindness, joint infection, or a life-threatening blood infection in the baby. Treatment of gonorrhea as soon as it is detected in pregnant women will reduce the risk of these complications. Pregnant women should consult a healthcare provider for appropriate examination, testing, and treatment, as necessary.

Who Should Be Tested for Gonorrhea?

Any sexually active person can be infected with gonorrhea. Anyone with genital symptoms such as discharge, burning during urination, unusual sores, or rash should stop having sex and see a healthcare provider immediately.

Also, anyone with an oral, anal, or vaginal sex partner who has been recently diagnosed with an STD should see a healthcare provider for evaluation.

Some people should be tested (screened) for gonorrhea even if they do not have symptoms or know of a sex partner who has gonorrhea. Anyone who is sexually active should discuss his or her risk factors with a healthcare provider and ask whether he or she should be tested for gonorrhea or other STDs.

CDC recommends yearly gonorrhea screening for all sexually active women younger than 25 years, as well as older women with risk factors such as new or multiple sex partners, or a sex partner who has a sexually transmitted infection.

People who have gonorrhea should also be tested for other STDs.

How Is Gonorrhea Diagnosed?

Urogenital gonorrhea can be diagnosed by testing urine, urethral (for men), or endocervical or vaginal (for women) specimens using nucleic acid amplification testing (NAAT). It can also be diagnosed using gonorrhea culture, which requires endocervical or urethral swab specimens.

If a person has had oral and/or anal sex, pharyngeal and/or rectal swab specimens should be collected either for culture or for NAAT (if the local laboratory has validated the use of NAAT for extra-genital specimens).

What Is the Treatment for Gonorrhea?

Gonorrhea can be cured with the right treatment. CDC now recommends dual therapy (i.e., using two drugs) for the treatment of gonorrhea. It is important to take all of the medication prescribed to cure gonorrhea. Medication for gonorrhea should not be shared with anyone. Although medication will stop the infection, it will not repair any permanent damage done by the disease. Antimicrobial resistance in gonorrhea is of increasing concern, and successful treatment of gonorrhea is becoming more difficult. If a person's symptoms continue for more than a few days after receiving treatment, he or she should return to a healthcare provider to be reevaluated.

What about Partners

If a person has been diagnosed and treated for gonorrhea, he or she should tell all recent anal, vaginal, or oral sex partners (all sex partners within 60 days before the onset of symptoms or diagnosis) so they can see a health provider and be treated. This will reduce the risk that the sex partners will develop serious complications from gonorrhea and will also reduce the person's risk of becoming reinfected. A person with gonorrhea and all of his or her sex partners must avoid having sex until they have completed their treatment for gonorrhea and until they no longer have symptoms.

How Can Gonorrhea Be Prevented?

Latex condoms, when used consistently and correctly, can reduce the risk of transmission of gonorrhea. The surest way to avoid transmission of gonorrhea or other STDs is to abstain from vaginal, anal, and oral sex, or to be in a long-term mutually monogamous relationship with a partner who has been tested and is known to be uninfected.

Chapter 26

Hand, Foot, and Mouth Disease

Hand, foot, and mouth disease is common in infants and young children. It usually causes fever, painful sores in the mouth, and a rash on the hands and feet. Most infected people recover in a week or two. Wash your hands often and practice good hygiene to reduce your risk of infection.

Hand, foot, and mouth disease (HFMD) is a contagious illness that is caused by different viruses. It is common in infants and children younger than five years old, because they do not yet have immunity (protection) to the viruses that cause HFMD. However, older children and adults can also get HFMD. In the United States, it is more common for people to get HFMD during spring, summer, and fall.

What Are the Symptoms of HFMD?

Symptoms of hand, foot, and mouth disease often include the following:

- Fever

- Reduced appetite

- Sore throat

This chapter includes text excerpted from "Hand, Foot, and Mouth Disease," Centers for Disease Control and Prevention (CDC), July 5, 2016.

- A feeling of being unwell

- Painful sores in the mouth that usually begin as flat red spots

- A rash of flat red spots that may blister on the palms of the hands, soles of the feet, and sometimes the knees, elbows, buttocks, and/or genital area.

These symptoms usually appear in stages, not all at once. Also, not everyone will get all of these symptoms. Some people may show no symptoms at all, but they can still pass the virus to others.

Is HFMD Serious?

HFMD is usually not serious. The illness is typically mild, and nearly all people recover in 7 to 10 days without medical treatment. Complications are uncommon.

Rarely, an infected person can develop viral meningitis (characterized by fever, headache, stiff neck, lack of energy, sleepiness or trouble waking up from sleep) and may need to be hospitalized for a few days. Other even more rare complications can include polio-like paralysis, or encephalitis (brain inflammation) which can be fatal.

Is HFMD Contagious?

Yes. The viruses that cause HFMD can be found in an infected person's:

- Nose and throat secretions (such as saliva, sputum, or nasal mucus)

- Blister fluid

- Feces (poop)

HFMD spreads from an infected person to others through:

- Close contact, such as kissing, hugging, or sharing cups and eating utensils

- Coughing and sneezing

- Contact with feces, for example when changing a diaper

- Contact with blister fluid

- Touching objects or surfaces that have the virus on them

People with HFMD are most contagious during the first week of their illness. However, they may sometimes remain contagious for weeks after symptoms go away. Some people, especially adults, may not develop any symptoms, but they can still spread the viruses to others. This is why you should always try to maintain good hygiene, like washing hands often with soap and water, so you can minimize your chance of getting and spreading infections.

Who Is at Risk for HFMD?

HFMD mostly affects infants and children younger than 5 years old. However, older children and adults can get it, too. When someone gets HFMD, they develop immunity to the specific virus that caused their infection. However, because HFMD is caused by several different viruses, people can get the disease again.

Can HFMD Be Treated?

There is no specific treatment for HFMD. Fever and pain can be managed with over-the-counter fever reducers and pain relievers, such as acetaminophen or ibuprofen. It is important for people with HFMD to drink enough fluids to prevent dehydration (loss of body fluids).

Can HFMD Be Prevented?

There is no vaccine to protect against HFMD. However, you can reduce the risk of getting infected with the viruses that cause HFMD by following a few simple steps:

- Wash your hands often with soap and water for 20 seconds, especially after changing diapers, and help young children do the same.

- Avoid touching your eyes, nose and mouth with unwashed hands.

- Avoid close contact such as kissing, hugging, and sharing cups and eating utensils with people who have HFMD.

- Disinfect frequently touched surfaces and objects, such as toys and doorknobs, especially if someone is sick.

Is HFMD the Same as Foot-And-Mouth Disease?

No. HFMD is often confused with foot-and-mouth disease (also called hoof-and-mouth disease), which affects cattle, sheep, and swine. Humans do not get the animal disease, and animals do not get the human disease.

Chapter 27

Hepatitis: A through E and Beyond

What Is Viral Hepatitis?

Viral hepatitis is inflammation of the liver caused by a virus. Several different viruses, named the hepatitis A, B, C, D, and E viruses, cause viral hepatitis.

All of these viruses cause acute, or short-term, viral hepatitis. The hepatitis B, C, and D viruses can also cause chronic hepatitis, in which the infection is prolonged, sometimes lifelong. Chronic hepatitis can lead to cirrhosis, liver failure, and liver cancer.

Researchers are looking for other viruses that may cause hepatitis, but none have been identified with certainty. Other viruses that less often affect the liver include cytomegalovirus; Epstein-Barr virus, also called infectious mononucleosis; herpesvirus; parvovirus; and adenovirus.

What Are the Symptoms of Viral Hepatitis?

Symptoms include:

- jaundice, which causes a yellowing of the skin and eyes

This chapter includes text excerpted from "Viral Hepatitis: A through E and Beyond," National Institute of Diabetes and Digestive and Kidney Diseases (NIDDK), April 2012. Reviewed August 2016.

- fatigue
- abdominal pain
- loss of appetite
- nausea
- vomiting
- diarrhea
- low grade fever
- headache

However, some people do not have symptoms.

Hepatitis A

How Is Hepatitis A Spread?

Hepatitis A is spread primarily through food or water contaminated by feces from an infected person. Rarely, it spreads through contact with infected blood.

Who Is at Risk for Hepatitis A?

People most likely to get hepatitis A are:

- international travelers, particularly those traveling to developing countries
- people who live with or have sex with an infected person
- people living in areas where children are not routinely vaccinated against hepatitis A, where outbreaks are more likely
- day care children and employees, during outbreaks
- men who have sex with men
- users of illicit drugs

How Can Hepatitis A Be Prevented?

The hepatitis A vaccine offers immunity to adults and children older than age 1. The Centers for Disease Control and Prevention recommends routine hepatitis A vaccination for children aged 12 to 23 months and for adults who are at high risk for infection. Treatment with immune globulin can provide short-term immunity to hepatitis A when given before exposure or within 2 weeks of exposure to the virus. Avoiding tap water when traveling internationally and practicing good hygiene and sanitation also help prevent hepatitis A.

What Is the Treatment for Hepatitis A?

Hepatitis A usually resolves on its own over several weeks.

Hepatitis B

How Is Hepatitis B Spread?

Hepatitis B is spread through contact with infected blood, through sex with an infected person, and from mother to child during childbirth, whether the delivery is vaginal or via cesarean section.

Who Is at Risk for Hepatitis B?

People most likely to get hepatitis B are:

- people who live with or have sexual contact with an infected person
- men who have sex with men
- people who have multiple sex partners
- injection drug users
- immigrants and children of immigrants from areas with high rates of hepatitis B
- infants born to infected mothers
- healthcare workers
- hemodialysis patients
- people who received a transfusion of blood or blood products before 1987, when better tests to screen blood donors were developed
- international travelers

How Can Hepatitis B Be Prevented?

The hepatitis B vaccine offers the best protection. All infants and unvaccinated children, adolescents, and at-risk adults should be vaccinated. For people who have not been vaccinated, reducing exposure to the virus can help prevent hepatitis B. Reducing exposure means using latex condoms, which may lower the risk of transmission; not sharing drug needles; and not sharing personal items such as toothbrushes, razors, and nail clippers with an infected person.

What Is the Treatment for Hepatitis B?

Drugs approved for the treatment of chronic hepatitis B include alpha interferon and peginterferon, which slow the replication of the virus in the body and also boost the immune system, and the antiviral drugs lamivudine, adefovir dipivoxil, entecavir, and telbivudine. Other drugs are also being evaluated. Infants born to infected mothers should receive hepatitis B immune globulin and the hepatitis B vaccine within 12 hours of birth to help prevent infection.

People who develop acute hepatitis B are generally not treated with antiviral drugs because, depending on their age at infection, the disease often resolves on its own. Infected newborns are most likely to progress to chronic hepatitis B, but by young adulthood, most people with acute infection recover spontaneously. Severe acute hepatitis B can be treated with an antiviral drug such as lamivudine.

Hepatitis C

How Is Hepatitis C Spread?

Hepatitis C is spread primarily through contact with infected blood. Less commonly, it can spread through sexual contact and childbirth.

Who Is at Risk for Hepatitis C?

People most likely to be exposed to the hepatitis C virus are:

- injection drug users
- people who have sex with an infected person
- people who have multiple sex partners
- healthcare workers
- infants born to infected women
- hemodialysis patients
- people who received a transfusion of blood or blood products before July 1992, when sensitive tests to screen blood donors for hepatitis C were introduced

- people who received clotting factors made before 1987, when methods to manufacture these products were improved

How Can Hepatitis C Be Prevented?

There is no vaccine for hepatitis C. The only way to prevent the disease is to reduce the risk of exposure to the virus. Reducing exposure means avoiding behaviors like sharing drug needles or personal items such as toothbrushes, razors, and nail clippers with an infected person.

What Is the Treatment for Hepatitis C?

Chronic hepatitis C is treated with peginterferon together with the antiviral drug ribavirin.

If acute hepatitis C does not resolve on its own within 2 to 3 months, drug treatment is recommended.

Hepatitis D

How Is Hepatitis D Spread?

Hepatitis D is spread through contact with infected blood. This disease only occurs at the same time as infection with hepatitis B or in people who are already infected with hepatitis B.

Who Is at Risk for Hepatitis D?

Anyone infected with hepatitis B is at risk for hepatitis D. Injection drug users have the highest risk. Others at risk include:

- people who live with or have sex with a person infected with hepatitis D

- people who received a transfusion of blood or blood products before 1987

How Can Hepatitis D Be Prevented?

People not already infected with hepatitis B should receive the hepatitis B vaccine. Other preventive measures include avoiding exposure to infected blood, contaminated needles, and an infected person's personal items such as toothbrushes, razors, and nail clippers.

What Is the Treatment for Hepatitis D?

Chronic hepatitis D is usually treated with pegylated interferon, although other potential treatments are under study.

Hepatitis E

How Is Hepatitis E Spread?

Hepatitis E is spread through food or water contaminated by feces from an infected person. This disease is uncommon in the United States.

Who Is at Risk for Hepatitis E?

People most likely to be exposed to the hepatitis E virus are:

- international travelers, particularly those traveling to developing countries

- people living in areas where hepatitis E outbreaks are common

- people who live with or have sex with an infected person

How Can Hepatitis E Be Prevented?

There is no U.S. Food and Drug Administration (FDA)-approved vaccine for hepatitis E. The only way to prevent the disease is to reduce the risk of exposure to the virus. Reducing risk of exposure means avoiding tap water when traveling internationally and practicing good hygiene and sanitation.

What Is the Treatment for Hepatitis E?

Hepatitis E usually resolves on its own over several weeks to months.

What Else Causes Viral Hepatitis?

Some cases of viral hepatitis cannot be attributed to the hepatitis A, B, C, D, or E viruses, or even the less common viruses that can infect the liver, such as cytomegalovirus, Epstein-Barr virus, herpesvirus, parvovirus, and adenovirus. These cases are called non-A–E hepatitis. Scientists continue to study the causes of non-A–E hepatitis.

Chapter 28

Hib Disease

What Is Hib Disease?

Hib disease is a serious illness caused by the bacteria *Haemophilus influenzae* type b. Babies and children younger than 5 years old are most at risk for Hib disease. It can cause lifelong disability and be deadly.

What Are the Symptoms of Hib Disease?

Hib disease causes different symptoms depending on which part of the body it affects.

The most common type of Hib disease is meningitis. This is an infection of the covering of the brain and spinal cord. It causes the following:

- Fever and headache

- Confusion

- Stiff neck

- Pain from bright lights

- Poor eating and drinking, low alertness, and vomiting (in babies)

This chapter includes text excerpted from "Hib Disease and the Vaccine (Shot) to Prevent It," Centers for Disease Control and Prevention (CDC), November 10, 2014.

Hib disease can also cause the following:

- Throat swelling that makes it hard to breathe
- Joint infection
- Skin infection
- Pneumonia (lung infection)
- Bone infection

How Serious Is It?

Hib disease is very serious. Most children with Hib disease need care in the hospital. Even with treatment, as many as 1 out of 20 children with Hib meningitis dies. As many as 1 out of 5 children who survive Hib meningitis will have brain damage or become deaf.

How Does Hib Spread?

Hib spreads when an infected person coughs or sneezes. Usually, the Hib bacteria stay in a person's nose and throat and do not cause illness. But if the bacteria spread into the lungs or blood, the person will get very sick. Spread of Hib is common among family members and in childcare centers.

Why Should My Child Get the Hib Vaccine?

The Hib vaccine:

- Protects your child from Hib disease, which can cause lifelong disability and be deadly.
- Protects your child from the most common type of Hib disease, meningitis (an infection of the covering of the brain and spinal cord).
- Keeps your child from missing school or childcare (and keeps you from missing work to care for your sick child).

Is It Safe?

The Hib vaccine is very safe, and it is effective at preventing Hib disease. Vaccines, like any medicine, can have side effects. Most children who get the Hib shot have no side effects.

What Are the Side Effects?

The most common side effects are usually mild and last 2 or 3 days. They include the following:

- Redness, swelling, and warmth where the child got the shot

- Fever

Chapter 29

Human Immunodeficiency Virus (HIV) and Acquired Immunodeficiency Syndrome (AIDS)

What Is Human Immunodeficiency Virus (HIV)?

HIV stands for human immunodeficiency virus. If left untreated, HIV can lead to the disease AIDS (acquired immunodeficiency syndrome). Unlike some other viruses, the human body can't get rid of HIV completely. So once you have HIV, you have it for life.

HIV attacks the body's immune system, specifically the CD4 cells (T cells), which help the immune system fight off infections. If left untreated, HIV reduces the number of CD4 cells (T cells) in the body, making the person more likely to get infections or infection-related cancers. Over time, HIV can destroy so many of these cells that the

This chapter contains text excerpted from the following sources: Text beginning with the heading "What Is Human Immunodeficiency Virus (HIV)?" is excerpted from "What Is HIV/AIDS?" AIDS.gov, U.S. Department of Health and Human Services (HHS), July 14, 2016; Text beginning with the heading "How Is HIV Spread?" is excerpted from "How Do You Get HIV or AIDS?" AIDS.gov, U.S. Department of Health and Human Services (HHS), December 31, 2015; Text beginning with the heading "How Is HIV Passed from One Person to Another?" is excerpted from "HIV Transmission," Centers for Disease Control and Prevention (CDC), July 12, 2016.

body can't fight off infections and disease. These opportunistic infections or cancers take advantage of a very weak immune system and signal that the person has AIDS, the last state of HIV infection.

What Is Acquired Immunodeficiency Syndrome (AIDS)?

AIDS stands for acquired immunodeficiency syndrome. AIDS is the final stage of HIV infection, and not everyone who has HIV advances to this stage.

AIDS is the stage of infection that occurs when your immune system is badly damaged and you become vulnerable to *opportunistic infections*. When the number of your CD4 cells falls below 200 cells per cubic millimeter of blood (200 cells/mm^3), you are considered to have progressed to AIDS. (The CD4 count of an uninfected adult/adolescent who is generally in good health ranges from 500 cells/mm^3 to 1,600 cells/mm^3.) You can also be diagnosed with AIDS if you develop one or more opportunistic infections, regardless of your CD4 count.

Without treatment, people who are diagnosed with AIDS typically survive about three years. Once someone has a dangerous opportunistic illness, life expectancy without treatment falls to about one year. People with AIDS need medical treatment to prevent death.

How Is HIV Spread?

You can get or transmit human immunodeficiency virus (HIV) only through specific activities. Most commonly, people get or transmit HIV through sexual behaviors and needle or syringe use.

HIV is not spread easily. Only certain body fluids from a person who has HIV can transmit HIV:

- Blood
- Semen (cum)
- Pre-seminal fluid (pre-cum)
- Rectal fluids
- Vaginal fluids
- Breast milk

These body fluids must come into contact with a mucous membrane or damaged tissue or be directly injected into your bloodstream (by a needle or syringe) for transmission to occur. Mucous membranes are found inside the rectum, vagina, penis, and mouth.

If you think you may have been exposed to HIV, get tested. You can get tested at your healthcare provider's office, a clinic, and other locations. You can also get a HIV home test kit from your local pharmacy.

Ways HIV Is Transmitted

In the United States, HIV is spread mainly by:

- Having anal or vaginal sex with someone who has HIV without using a condom or taking medicines to prevent or treat HIV.

  - Anal sex is the highest-risk sexual behavior. For the HIV-negative partner, receptive anal sex ("bottoming") is riskier than insertive anal sex ("topping").

  - Vaginal sex is the second highest-risk sexual behavior.

- Sharing needles or syringes, rinse water, or other equipment ("works") used to prepare injection drugs with someone who has HIV. HIV can live in a used needle up to 42 days depending on temperature and other factors.

Less commonly, HIV may be spread:

- From mother to child during pregnancy, birth or breastfeeding. Although the risk can be high if a mother is living with HIV and not taking medicine, recommendations to test all pregnant women for HIV and start HIV treatment immediately have lowered the number of babies who are born with HIV.

- By being stuck with an HIV-contaminated needle or other sharp object. This is a risk mainly for healthcare workers.

In extremely rare cases, HIV has been transmitted by:

- Oral sex—putting the mouth on the penis (fellatio), vagina (cunnilingus), or anus (rimming). In general, there is little to no risk of getting HIV from oral sex. But transmission of HIV, though extremely rare, is theoretically possible if an HIV-positive man ejaculates in his partner's mouth during oral sex.

- Receiving blood transfusions, blood products, or organ/tissue transplants that are contaminated with HIV. This was more common in the early years of HIV, but now the risk is extremely small because of rigorous testing of the U.S. blood supply and donated organs and tissues.

- Eating food that has been pre-chewed by an HIV-infected person. The contamination occurs when infected blood from a caregiver's mouth mixes with food while chewing. The only known cases are among infants.

- Being bitten by a person with HIV. Each of the very small number of documented cases has involved severe trauma with extensive tissue damage and the presence of blood. There is no risk of transmission if the skin is not broken.

- Contact between broken skin, wounds, or mucous membranes and HIV-infected blood or blood-contaminated body fluids.

- Deep, open-mouth kissing if the person with HIV has sores or bleeding gums and blood from the HIV-positive partner gets into the bloodstream of the HIV-negative partner. HIV is not spread through saliva.

HIV Is Not Spread by...

HIV does not survive long outside the human body (such as on surfaces) and it cannot reproduce outside a human host. It is not spread by:

- Air or water

- Mosquitoes, ticks or other insects

- Saliva, tears, or sweat that is not mixed with the blood of an HIV-positive person

- Shaking hands, hugging, sharing toilets, sharing dishes/drinking glasses, or closed-mouth or "social" kissing with someone who is HIV-positive

- Drinking fountains

- Other sexual activities that don't involve the exchange of body fluids (for example, touching)

HIV Treatment Reduces Transmission Risk

People with HIV who are using antiretroviral therapy (ART) consistently and who have achieved viral suppression (having the virus reduced to an undetectable level in the body) are very unlikely to transmit the virus to their uninfected partners. However, there is still some risk of transmission, so even with an undetectable viral load, people with HIV and their partners should continue to take steps to reduce the risk of HIV transmission.

I Have HIV, Does That Mean I Have Aids?

No. The terms "HIV" and "acquired immune deficiency syndrome (AIDS)" can be confusing because both terms refer to the same disease. However, "HIV" refers to the virus itself, and "AIDS" refers to the late stage of HIV infection, when an HIV-infected person's immune system is severely damaged and has difficulty fighting diseases and certain cancers. Before the development of certain medications, people with HIV could progress to AIDS in just a few years. But today, most people who are HIV-positive do not progress to AIDS. That's because if you have HIV and you take ART consistently, you can keep the level of HIV in your body low. This will help keep your body strong and healthy and reduce the likelihood that you will ever progress to AIDS. It will also help lower your risk of transmitting HIV to others.

How Is HIV Passed from One Person to Another?

You can get or transmit HIV only through specific activities. Most commonly, people get or transmit HIV through sexual behaviors and needle or syringe use.

Only certain body fluids—blood, semen (cum), pre-seminal fluid (pre-cum), rectal fluids, vaginal fluids, and breast milk—from a person who has HIV can transmit HIV. These fluids must come in contact with a mucous membrane or damaged tissue or be directly injected into the bloodstream (from a needle or syringe) for transmission to occur. Mucous membranes are found inside the rectum, vagina, penis, and mouth.

In the United States, HIV is spread mainly by:

- Having anal or vaginal sex with someone who has HIV without using a condom or taking medicines to prevent or treat HIV.

  - Anal sex is the highest-risk sexual behavior. For the HIV-negative partner, receptive anal sex (bottoming) is riskier than insertive anal sex (topping).

  - Vaginal sex is the second-highest-risk sexual behavior.

- Sharing needles or syringes, rinse water, or other equipment (works) used to prepare drugs for injection with someone who has HIV. HIV can live in a used needle up to 42 days depending on temperature and other factors.

Less commonly, HIV may be spread:

- From mother to child during pregnancy, birth, or breastfeeding. Although the risk can be high if a mother is living with HIV and not taking medicine, recommendations to test all pregnant women for HIV and start HIV treatment immediately have lowered the number of babies who are born with HIV.

- By being stuck with an HIV-contaminated needle or other sharp object. This is a risk mainly for healthcare workers.

How Well Does HIV Survive outside the Body?

HIV does not survive long outside the human body (such as on surfaces), and it cannot reproduce outside a human host. It is not spread by:

- Mosquitoes, ticks or other insects.

- Saliva, tears, or sweat that is not mixed with the blood of an HIV-positive person.

- Hugging, shaking hands, sharing toilets, sharing dishes or closed-mouth or "social" kissing with someone who is HIV-positive.

- Other sexual activities that don't involve the exchange of body fluids (for example, touching).

Can I Get HIV from Anal Sex?

Yes. In fact, having anal sex is the riskiest type of sex for getting or spreading HIV.

HIV can be found in the blood, semen (*cum*), preseminal fluid (*pre-cum*), or rectal fluid of a person infected with the virus. The *bottom* is at greater risk of getting HIV because the lining of the rectum is thin and may allow HIV to enter the body during anal sex, but the top is also at risk because HIV can enter through the opening of the penis or through small cuts, abrasions or open sores on the penis.

Can I Get HIV from Vaginal Sex?

Yes. Vaginal sex is the sexual behavior with the second-highest risk for getting or transmitting HIV.

It is possible for either partner to get HIV from vaginal sex.

When a woman has vaginal sex with a partner who's HIV-positive, HIV can enter her body through the mucous membranes that line the vagina and cervix. Most women who get HIV get it from vaginal sex.

Men can also get HIV from having vaginal sex with a woman who's HIV-positive. This is because vaginal fluid and blood can carry HIV. Men get HIV through the opening at the tip of the penis (or urethra); the foreskin if they're not circumcised; or small cuts, scratches or open sores anywhere on the penis.

Can I Get HIV from Oral Sex?

The chance that an HIV-negative person will get HIV from oral sex with an HIV-positive partner is extremely low.

Oral sex involves putting the mouth on the penis (fellatio), vagina (cunnilingus), or anus (anilingus). In general, there's little to no risk of getting or transmitting HIV through oral sex.

Factors that may increase the risk of transmitting HIV through oral sex are ejaculation in the mouth with oral ulcers, bleeding gums, genital sores, and the presence of other sexually transmitted diseases (STDs), which may or may not be visible.

You can get other STDs from oral sex. And, if you get feces in your mouth during anilingus, you can get hepatitis A and B, parasites like *Giardia*, and bacteria like *Shigella*, *Salmonella*, *Campylobacter*, and *E. coli*.

Is There a Connection between HIV and Other Sexually Transmitted Infections?

Yes. Having another sexually transmitted disease (STD) can increase the risk of getting or transmitting HIV.

If you have another STD, you're more likely to get or transmit HIV to others. Some of the most common STDs include gonorrhea, chlamydia, syphilis, trichomoniasis, human papillomavirus (HPV), genital herpes, and hepatitis. The only way to know for sure if you have an STD is to get tested. If you're sexually active, you and your partners should get tested for STDs (including HIV if you're HIV-negative) regularly, even if you don't have symptoms.

If you are HIV-negative but have an STD, you are about 3 times as likely to get HIV if you have unprotected sex with someone who has HIV. There are two ways that having an STD can increase the likelihood of getting HIV. If the STD causes irritation of the skin (for example, from syphilis, herpes, or human papillomavirus), breaks or sores may make it easier for HIV to enter the body during sexual contact. Even STDs that cause no breaks or open sores (for example, chlamydia, gonorrhea, trichomoniasis) can increase your risk by causing inflammation that increases the number of cells that can serve as targets for HIV.

If you are HIV-positive and also infected with another STD, you are about 3 times as likely as other HIV-infected people to spread HIV through sexual contact. This appears to happen because there is an increased concentration of HIV in the semen and genital fluids of HIV-positive people who also are infected with another STD.

Does My HIV-Positive Partner's Viral Load Affect My Risk of Getting HIV?

Yes, as an HIV-positive person's viral load goes down, the chance of transmitting HIV goes down.

Viral load is the amount of HIV in the blood of someone who is HIV-positive. When the viral load is very low, it is called viral suppression. Undetectable viral load is when the amount of HIV in the blood is so low that it can't be measured.

In general, the higher someone's viral load, the more likely that person is to transmit HIV. People who have HIV but are in care, taking HIV medicines, and have a very low or undetectable viral load are much less likely to transmit HIV than people who have HIV and do not have a low viral load.

However, a person with HIV can still potentially transmit HIV to a partner even if they have an undetectable viral load, because:

- HIV may still be found in genital fluids (semen, vaginal fluids). The viral load test only measures virus in blood.

- A person's viral load may go up between tests. When this happens, they may be more likely to transmit HIV to partners.

- Sexually transmitted diseases increase viral load in genital fluids.

If you're HIV-positive, getting into care and taking HIV medicines (called antiretroviral therapy or ART) the right way, every day will give you the greatest chance to get and stay virally suppressed, live a longer, healthier life, and reduce the chance of transmitting HIV to your partners.

If you're HIV-negative and have an HIV-positive partner, encourage your partner to get into care and take HIV treatment medicines.

Taking other actions, like using a condom the right way every time you have sex or taking daily medicine to prevent HIV (called pre-exposure prophylaxis or PrEP) if you're HIV-negative, can lower your chances of transmitting or getting HIV even more.

Can I Get HIV from Injecting Drugs?

Yes. Your risk for getting HIV is very high if you use needles or works (such as cookers, cotton, or water) after someone with HIV has used them.

People who inject drugs, hormones, steroids, or silicone can get HIV by sharing needles or syringes and other injection equipment. The needles and equipment may have someone else's blood in them, and blood can transmit HIV. Likewise, you're at risk for getting hepatitis B and C if you share needles and works because these infections are also transmitted through blood.

Another reason people who inject drugs can get HIV (and other sexually transmitted diseases) is that when people are high, they're more likely to have risky sex.

Stopping injection and other drug use can lower your chances of getting HIV a lot. You may need help to stop or cut down using drugs, but many resources are available. To find a substance abuse treatment center near you, check out the locator tools on SAMHSA.gov or AIDS. gov, or call 1-800-662-HELP (1-800-662-4357).

If you keep injecting drugs, you can lower your risk for getting HIV by using only new, sterile needles and works each time you inject. Never share needles or works.

Can I Get HIV from Using Other Kinds of Drugs?

When you're drunk or high, you're more likely to make decisions that put you at risk for HIV, such as having sex without a condom.

Drinking alcohol, particularly binge drinking, and using "club drugs" like Ecstasy, ketamine, GHB, and poppers can alter your judgment, lower your inhibitions, and impair your decisions about sex or other drug use. You may be more likely to have unplanned and unprotected sex, have a harder time using a condom the right way every time you have sex, have more sexual partners, or use other drugs, including injection drugs or meth. Those behaviors can increase your risk of exposure to HIV. If you have HIV, they can also increase your risk of spreading HIV to others. Being drunk or high affects your ability to make safe choices.

If you're going to a party or another place where you know you'll be drinking or using drugs, you can bring a condom so that you can reduce your risk if you have vaginal or anal sex.

Therapy, medicines, and other methods are available to help you stop or cut down on drinking or using drugs. Talk with a counselor, doctor, or other healthcare provider about options that might be right for you. To find a substance abuse treatment center near you, check out the locator tools on SAMHSA.gov or AIDS.gov, or call 1-800-662-HELP (4357).

If I Already Have HIV, Can I Get Another Kind of HIV?

Yes. This is called HIV superinfection.

HIV superinfection is when a person with HIV gets infected with another strain of the virus. The new strain of HIV can replace the original strain or remain along with the original strain.

The effects of superinfection differ from person to person. Superinfection may cause some people to get sicker faster because they become infected with a new strain of the virus that is resistant to the medicine (antiretroviral therapy or ART) they're taking to treat their original infection.

Research suggests that a hard-to-treat superinfection is rare. Taking medicine to treat HIV (ART) may reduce someone's chance of getting a superinfection.

Are Healthcare Workers at Risk of Getting HIV on the Job?

The risk of healthcare workers being exposed to HIV on the job (occupational exposure) is very low, especially if they use protective practices and personal protective equipment to prevent HIV and other blood-borne infections. For healthcare workers on the job, the main risk of HIV transmission is from being stuck with an HIV-contaminated needle or other sharp object. However, even this risk is small. Scientists estimate that the risk of HIV infection from being stuck with a needle used on an HIV-infected person is less than 1%.

Can I Get HIV from Receiving Medical Care?

When you're drunk or high, you're more likely to make decisions that put you at risk for HIV, such as having sex without a condom.

Drinking alcohol, particularly binge drinking, and using "club drugs" like Ecstasy, ketamine, GHB, and poppers can alter your judgment, lower your inhibitions, and impair your decisions about sex or other drug use. You may be more likely to have unplanned and unprotected sex, have a harder time using a condom the right way every time you have sex, have more sexual partners, or use other drugs, including injection drugs or meth. Those behaviors can increase your risk of exposure to HIV. If you have HIV, they can also increase your risk of spreading HIV to others. Being drunk or high affects your ability to make safe choices.

If you're going to a party or another place where you know you'll be drinking or using drugs, you can bring a condom so that you can reduce your risk if you have vaginal or anal sex.

Therapy, medicines, and other methods are available to help you stop or cut down on drinking or using drugs. Talk with a counselor, doctor, or other healthcare provider about options that might be right for you. To find a substance abuse treatment center near you, check out the locator tools on SAMHSA.gov or AIDS.gov, or call 1-800-662-HELP (1-800-662-4357).

Can I Get HIV from Casual Contact ("Social Kissing," Shaking Hands, Hugging, Using a Toilet, Drinking from the Same Glass, or the Sneezing and Coughing of an Infected Person)?

No. HIV isn't transmitted

- By hugging, shaking hands, sharing toilets, sharing dishes, or closed-mouth or "social" kissing with someone who is HIV-positive.

- Through saliva, tears, or sweat that is not mixed with the blood of an HIV-positive person.

- By mosquitoes, ticks or other blood-sucking insects.

- Through the air.

Only certain body fluids—blood, semen (*cum*), pre-seminal fluid (*pre-cum*), rectal fluids, vaginal fluids, and breast milk—from an HIV-infected person can transmit HIV. Most commonly, people get or transmit HIV through sexual behaviors and needle or syringe use. Babies can also get HIV from an HIV-positive mother during pregnancy, birth, or breastfeeding.

Can I Get HIV from a Tattoo or a Body Piercing?

There are no known cases in the United States of anyone getting HIV this way. However, it is possible to get HIV from a reused or not properly sterilized tattoo or piercing needle or other equipment, or from contaminated ink.

It's possible to get HIV from tattooing or body piercing if the equipment used for these procedures has someone else's blood in it or if the ink is shared. The risk of getting HIV this way is very low, but the risk increases when the person doing the procedure is unlicensed, because of the potential for unsanitary practices such as sharing needles or ink. If you get a tattoo or a body piercing, be sure that the person doing the procedure is properly licensed and that they use only new or sterilized needles, ink, and other supplies.

Can I Get HIV from Being Spit on or Scratched by an HIV-Infected Person?

No. HIV isn't spread through saliva, and there is no risk of transmission from scratching because no body fluids are transferred between people.

Can I Get HIV from Mosquitoes?

No. HIV is not transmitted by mosquitoes, ticks or any other insects.

Can I Get HIV from Food?

You can't get HIV from consuming food handled by an HIV-infected person. Even if the food contained small amounts of HIV-infected blood or semen, exposure to the air, heat from cooking, and stomach acid would destroy the virus.

Though it is very rare, HIV can be spread by eating food that has been pre-chewed by an HIV-infected person. The contamination occurs when infected blood from a caregiver's mouth mixes with food while chewing. The only known cases are among infants.

Are Lesbians or Other Women Who Have Sex with Women at Risk for HIV?

Case reports of female-to-female transmission of HIV are rare. The well-documented risk of female-to-male transmission shows that vaginal fluids and menstrual blood may contain the virus and that exposure to these fluids through mucous membranes (in the vagina or mouth) could potentially lead to HIV infection.

Is the Risk of HIV Different for Different People?

Some groups of people in the United States are more likely to get HIV than others because of many factors, including the status of their sex partners, their risk behaviors, and where they live.

When you live in a community where many people have HIV infection, the chances of having sex or sharing needles or other injection equipment with someone who has HIV are higher. You can use CDC's HIV, STD, hepatitis, and tuberculosis atlas to see the percentage of people with HIV ("prevalence") in different US communities. Within any community, the prevalence of HIV can vary among different populations.

Gay and bisexual men have the largest number of new diagnoses in the United States. Blacks/African Americans and Hispanics/Latinos are disproportionately affected by HIV compared to other racial and ethnic groups. Also, transgender women who have sex with men are among the groups at highest risk for HIV infection, and injection drug users remain at significant risk for getting HIV.

Risky behaviors, like having anal or vaginal sex without using a condom or taking medicines to prevent or treat HIV, and sharing needles or syringes play a big role in HIV transmission. Anal sex is the highest-risk sexual behavior. If you don't have HIV, being a receptive partner (or bottom) for anal sex is the highest-risk sexual activity for getting HIV. If you do have HIV, being the insertive partner (or top) for anal sex is the highest-risk sexual activity for transmitting HIV.

But there are more tools available today to prevent HIV than ever before. Choosing less risky sexual behaviors, taking medicines to prevent and treat HIV, and using condoms with lubricants are all highly effective ways to reduce the risk of getting or transmitting HIV.

Chapter 30

Human Papillomavirus (HPV)

Human papillomavirus (HPV) is a sexually transmitted virus. It is passed on through genital contact (such as vaginal and anal sex). It is also passed on by skin-to-skin contact. At least 50% of people who have had sex will have HPV at some time in their lives. HPV is not a new virus. **But many people don't know about it. Most people don't have any signs. HPV may go away on its own**—without causing any health problems.

Who Can Get HPV?

Anyone who has ever had genital contact with another person may have HPV. Both men and women may get it—and pass it on—without knowing it. Since there might not be any signs, a person may have HPV even if years have passed since he or she had sex.

You are more likely to get HPV if you have:

- sex at an early age

- many sex partners

- a sex partner who has had many partners

This chapter includes text excerpted from "HPV (Human Papillomavirus)," U.S. Food and Drug Administration (FDA), May 23, 2016.

If There Are No Signs, Why Do I Need to Worry about HPV?

There are over 100 different kinds of HPV and not all of them cause health problems. Some kinds of HPV may cause problems like genital warts. Some kinds of HPV can also cause cancer of the cervix, vagina, vulva or anus. Most of these problems are caused by types 6, 11, 16 or 18.

Is There a Test for HPV?

Yes. It tests for the kinds of HPV that may lead to cervical cancer. The U.S. Food and Drug Administration (FDA) approved the HPV test to be used for women over 30 years old. It may find HPV even before there are changes to the cervix. Women who have the HPV test still need to get the Pap test.

Can I Prevent HPV?

FDA has approved vaccines that prevent certain diseases, including cervical cancer, caused by some types of HPV. Ask your doctor if you should get the HPV vaccine.

What Else Can I Do to Lower My Chances of Getting HPV?

- You can choose not to have sex (abstinence).
- If you have sex, you can limit the number of partners you have.
- Choose a partner who has had no or few sex partners. The fewer partners your partner has had—the less likely he or she is to have HPV.
- It is not known how much condoms protect against HPV. Areas not covered by a condom can be exposed to the virus.

Is There a Cure for HPV?

There is no cure for the virus (HPV) itself. There are treatments for the health problems that HPV can cause, such as genital warts, cervical changes, and cervical cancer.

What Should I Know about Genital Warts?

There are many treatment choices for genital warts. But even after the warts are treated, the virus might still be there and may be passed on to others. If genital warts are not treated they may go away, stay the same or increase in size or number, but they will not turn into cancer.

HPV and Cancer

What Should I Know about Cervical Cancer?

All women should get regular Pap tests. The Pap test looks for cell changes caused by HPV. The test finds cell changes early—so the cervix can be treated before the cells turn into cancer. This test can also find cancer in its early stages so it can be treated before it becomes too serious. It is rare to die from cervical cancer if the disease is caught early.

What Should I Know about Vaginal or Vulvar Cancer?

Vaginal cancer is cancer of the vagina (birth canal). Vulvar cancer is cancer of the clitoris, vaginal lips, and opening to the vagina. Both of these kinds of cancer are very rare. Not all vaginal or vulvar cancer is caused by HPV.

What Should I Know about Anal Cancer?

Anal cancer is cancer that forms in tissues of the anus. The anus is the opening of the rectum (last part of the large intestine) to the outside of the body.

Chapter 31

Impetigo

Impetigo is an infection of the top layers of the skin and is most common among children ages 2 to 6 years. It usually starts when bacteria get into a cut, scratch or insect bite.

Cause

Impetigo is usually caused by *staphylococcus* (staph) bacteria, but it also can be caused by group A *streptococcus* bacteria. Skin infections are usually caused by different types (strains) of strep bacteria than those that cause strep throat. Therefore, the types of strep germs that cause impetigo are usually different from those that cause strep throat.

Transmission

The infection is spread by direct contact with lesions (wounds or sores) or nasal discharge from an infected person. Scratching may spread the lesions. It usually takes 1 to 3 days from the time of infection until you show symptoms. If your skin doesn't have breaks in it, you can't be infected by dried strep bacteria in the air.

Symptoms

Symptoms start with red or pimple-like lesions surrounded by reddened skin. These sores can be anywhere on your body, but mostly on

This chapter includes text excerpted from "Impetigo," National Institute of Allergy and Infectious Diseases (NIAID), October 22, 2013.

195

your face, arms, and legs. The sores fill with pus, then break open after a few days and form a thick crust. Itching is common.

Diagnosis

Your healthcare provider can diagnose the infection by looking at the skin lesions.

Treatment

If your impetigo is caused by strep bacteria, your healthcare provider will prescribe oral antibiotics, as with strep throat. This treatment may also include an antibiotic ointment to be used on your skin.

Chapter 32

Influenza

Chapter Contents

197

Section 32.1

Seasonal Flu

This section contains text excerpted from the following sources: Text beginning with the heading "What Is Influenza (Also Called Flu)?" is excerpted from "Key Facts about Influenza (Flu)," Centers for Disease Control and Prevention (CDC), May 6, 2016; Text beginning with the heading "When Is the Flu Season in the United States?" is excerpted from "Seasonal Influenza, More Information," Centers for Disease Control and Prevention (CDC), May 4, 2016.

What Is Influenza (Also Called Flu)?

The flu is a contagious respiratory illness caused by influenza viruses that infect the nose, throat, and lungs. It can cause mild to severe illness, and at times can lead to death. The best way to prevent the flu is by getting a flu vaccine each year.

Signs and Symptoms of Flu

People who have the flu often feel some or all of these signs and symptoms:

- Fever* or feeling feverish/chills

- Cough

- Sore throat

- Runny or stuffy nose

- Muscle or body aches

- Headaches

- Fatigue (very tired)

- Some people may have vomiting and diarrhea, though this is more common in children than adults.

It's important to note that not everyone with flu will have a fever.

198

How Flu Spreads

Most experts believe that flu viruses spread mainly by droplets made when people with flu cough, sneeze or talk. These droplets can land in the mouths or noses of people who are nearby. Less often, a person might also get flu by touching a surface or object that has flu virus on it and then touching their own mouth, eyes or possibly their nose.

Period of Contagiousness

You may be able to pass on the flu to someone else before you know you are sick, as well as while you are sick. Most healthy adults may be able to infect others beginning 1 day **before** symptoms develop and up to 5 to 7 days **after** becoming sick. Some people, especially young children and people with weakened immune systems, might be able to infect others for an even longer time.

Onset of Symptoms

The time from when a person is exposed to flu virus to when symptoms begin is about 1 to 4 days, with an average of about 2 days.

Complications of Flu

Complications of flu can include bacterial pneumonia, ear infections, sinus infections, dehydration, and worsening of chronic medical conditions, such as congestive heart failure, asthma or diabetes.

People at High Risk from Flu

Anyone can get the flu (even healthy people), and serious problems related to the flu can happen at any age, but some people are at high risk of developing serious flu-related complications if they get sick. This includes people 65 years and older, people of any age with certain chronic medical conditions (such as asthma, diabetes or heart disease), pregnant women, and young children.

Preventing Flu

The first and most important step in preventing flu is to get a flu vaccination each year. Centers for Disease Control and Prevention (CDC) also recommends everyday preventive actions (like staying away from people who are sick, covering coughs and sneezes and frequent handwashing) to help slow the spread of germs that cause respiratory (nose, throat, and lungs) illnesses, like flu.

Diagnosing Flu

It is very difficult to distinguish the flu from other viral or bacterial causes of respiratory illnesses on the basis of symptoms alone. There are tests available to diagnose flu.

Treating

There are influenza antiviral drugs that can be used to treat flu illness.

When Is the Flu Season in the United States?

In the United States, flu season occurs in the fall and winter. The peak of flu season has occurred anywhere from late November through March. The overall health impact (e.g., infections, hospitalizations, and deaths) of a flu season varies from year to year. CDC monitors circulating flu viruses and their related disease activity and provides influenza reports (called " FluView") each week from October through May.

How Does CDC Monitor the Progress of the Flu Season?

CDC collects data year-round and reports on influenza (flu) activity in the United States each week from October through May. The U.S. influenza surveillance system consists of five separate categories.

1. Laboratory-based viral surveillance, which tracks the number and percentage of influenza-positive tests from laboratories across the country, and monitors for human infections with influenza A viruses that are different from currently circulating human influenza H1 and H3 viruses.

2. Outpatient physician surveillance for influenza-like illness (ILI), which tracks the percentage of doctor visits for flu-like symptoms.

3. Mortality surveillance as reported through the 122 Cities Mortality Reporting System, which tracks the percentage of deaths reported to be caused by pneumonia and influenza in 122 cities in the United States; and influenza-associated pediatric

mortality as reported through the Nationally Notifiable Disease Surveillance System, which tracks the number of deaths in children with laboratory confirmed influenza infection.

4. Hospitalization surveillance, which tracks laboratory confirmed influenza-associated hospitalizations in children and adults through the Influenza Hospitalization Network (Flu-Surv-NET) and Aggregate Hospitalization and Death Reporting Activity (AHDRA).

5. State and territorial epidemiologist reports of influenza activity, which indicates the number of states affected by flu and the degree to which they are affected.

These surveillance components allow CDC to determine when and where influenza activity is occurring, determine what types of influenza viruses are circulating, detect changes in the influenza viruses collected and analyzed, track patterns of influenza-related illness, and measure the impact of influenza in the United States. All influenza activity reporting by states, laboratories, and healthcare providers is voluntary.

Why Is There a Week-Long Lag between the Data and When It's Reported?

The influenza surveillance system is one of the largest and most timely surveillance systems at CDC. The system consists of 5 complementary surveillance categories. These categories include reports from more than 145 laboratories, about 3,000 outpatient healthcare providers, vital statistics offices in 122 cities, research and healthcare personnel at the Emerging Infections Program (EIP) sites, and influenza surveillance coordinators and state epidemiologists from all 50 state health departments and the New York City and District of Columbia health departments. Influenza surveillance data collection is based on a reporting week that starts on Sunday and ends on Saturday of each week. Each surveillance participant is requested to summarize weekly data and submit it to CDC by Tuesday afternoon of the following week. The data are then downloaded, compiled, and analyzed at CDC each Wednesday. The compiled data are interpreted and checked for anomalies which are resolved before the report is written and submitted for clearance at CDC. On Friday the report is approved, distributed, and posted on the Internet.

How Many People Get Sick or Die from the Flu Every Year?

Flu seasons vary in severity depending on a number of factors including the characteristics of circulating viruses, the timing of the season, how well the vaccine is protecting against influenza infection, and how many people got vaccinated. While the numbers vary, in the United States, millions of people are sickened, hundreds of thousands are hospitalized and thousands or tens of thousands of people die from flu every year.

Is The "Stomach Flu" Really the Flu?

Many people use the term "stomach flu" to describe illnesses with nausea, vomiting or diarrhea. These symptoms can be caused by many different viruses, bacteria or even parasites. While vomiting, diarrhea, and being nauseous or "sick to your stomach" can sometimes be related to the flu—more commonly in children than adults—these problems are rarely the main symptoms of influenza. The flu is a respiratory disease and not a stomach or intestinal disease.

Do Other Respiratory Viruses Circulate during the Flu Season?

In addition to the flu virus, several other respiratory viruses also can circulate during the flu season and can cause symptoms and illness similar to those seen with flu infection. These non-flu viruses include rhinovirus (one cause of the "common cold") and respiratory syncytial virus (RSV), which is the most common cause of severe respiratory illness in young children as well as a leading cause of death from respiratory illness in those aged 65 years and older.

Section 32.2

Pandemic Flu

This section includes text excerpted from "About Pandemics,"
Flu.gov, U.S. Department of Health and Human Services (HHS),
February 10, 2012. Reviewed August 2016.

About Pandemics

A pandemic is a global disease outbreak. It is determined by how the disease spreads, not how many deaths it causes.

When a new influenza A virus emerges, a flu pandemic can occur. Because the virus is new, the human population has little to no immunity against it. The virus spreads quickly from person-to-person worldwide.

Characteristics and Challenges of a Flu Pandemic

1. Rapid worldwide spread.

    •   When a pandemic flu virus emerges, expect it to spread around the world.

    •   You should prepare for a pandemic flu as if the entire world population is susceptible.

    •   Countries may try to delay the pandemic flu's arrival through border closings and travel restrictions, but they cannot stop it.

2. Overloaded healthcare systems.

    •   Most people have little or no immunity to a pandemic virus. Infection and illness rates soar. A substantial percentage of the world's population will require some form of medical care.

    •   Nations are unlikely to have the staff, facilities, equipment, and hospital beds needed to cope with the number of people who get the pandemic flu.

- Death rates may be high. Four factors largely determine the death toll:

  - The number of people who become infected.

  - The strength of the virus.

  - The underlying characteristics and vulnerability of affected populations.

  - The effectiveness of preventive measures.

- Past pandemics spread globally in two or sometimes three waves.

3. Inadequate medical supplies.

   - The need for vaccines is likely to be larger than the supply. Those at highest risk will likely get the vaccine first.

   - Early in a pandemic, the need for antiviral medications is likely to be larger than the supply. Those at highest risk will likely get antiviral medications first.

4. A pandemic can create a shortage of hospital beds, ventilators, and other supplies. Alternative sites, such as schools, may serve as medical facilities.

5. Disrupted economy and society.

   - Travel bans, event cancellations, and school and business closings could have a major impact on communities and citizens.

   - Caring for sick family members and fear of exposure could result in significant employee absenteeism.

Seasonal Flu versus Pandemic Flu

Table 32.1. Seasonal Flu versus Pandemic Flu

Pandemic Flu	Seasonal Flu
Rarely happens (three times in 20th century)	Happens annually and usually peaks in January or February
People have little or no immunity because they have no previous exposure to the virus	Usually some immunity built up from previous exposure

Table 32.1. Continued

Pandemic Flu	Seasonal Flu
Healthy people may be at increased risk for serious complications	Usually only people at high risk, not healthy adults, are at risk of serious complications
Healthcare providers and hospitals may be overwhelmed	Healthcare providers and hospitals can usually meet public and patient needs
Vaccine probably would not be available in the early stages of a pandemic	Vaccine available for annual flu season
Effective antivirals may be in limited supply	Adequate supplies of antivirals are usually available
Number of deaths could be high (The U.S. death toll during the 1918 pandemic was approximately 675,000)	Seasonal flu-associated deaths in the United States over 30 years ending in 2007 have ranged from about 3,000 per season to about 49,000 per season.
Symptoms may be more severe	Symptoms include fever, cough, runny nose, and muscle pain
May cause major impact on the general public, such as widespread travel restrictions and school or business closings	Usually causes minor impact on the general public, some schools may close and sick people are encouraged to stay home
Potential for severe impact on domestic and world economy	Manageable impact on domestic and world economy

Section 32.3

Avian Flu

This section includes text excerpted from "Avian Influenza A
Virus Infections in Humans," Centers for Disease Control and
Prevention (CDC), May 25, 2016.

Avian Influenza A Virus Infections in Humans

Although avian influenza A viruses usually do not infect humans,
rare cases of human infection with these viruses have been reported.

Infected birds shed avian influenza virus in their saliva, mucous and feces. Human infections with bird flu viruses can happen when enough virus gets into a person's eyes, nose or mouth, or is inhaled. This can happen when virus is in the air (in droplets or possibly dust) and a person breathes it in, or when a person touches something that has virus on it then touches their mouth, eyes or nose. Rare human infections with some avian viruses have occurred most often after unprotected contact with infected birds or surfaces contaminated with avian influenza viruses. However, some infections have been identified where direct contact was not known to have occurred. Illness in humans has ranged from mild to severe.

Signs and Symptoms of Avian Influenza A Virus Infections in Humans

The reported signs and symptoms of low pathogenic avian influenza (LPAI) A virus infections in humans have ranged from conjunctivitis to influenza-like illness (e.g., fever, cough, sore throat, muscle aches) to lower respiratory disease (pneumonia) requiring hospitalization. Highly pathogenic avian influenza (HPAI) A virus infections in people have been associated with a wide range of illness from conjunctivitis only, to influenza-like illness, to severe respiratory illness (e.g., shortness of breath, difficulty breathing, pneumonia, acute respiratory distress, viral pneumonia, respiratory failure) with multi-organ disease, sometimes accompanied by nausea, abdominal pain, diarrhea, vomiting and sometimes neurologic changes (altered mental status, seizures). LPAI H7N9 and HPAI Asian H5N1 have been responsible for most human illness worldwide to date, including the most serious illnesses and deaths.

Detecting Avian Influenza A Virus Infection in Humans

Avian influenza A virus infection in humans cannot be diagnosed by clinical signs and symptoms alone; laboratory testing is required. Avian influenza A virus infection is usually diagnosed by collecting a swab from the nose or throat of the sick person during the first few days of illness. This specimen is sent to a lab; the laboratory looks for avian influenza A virus either by using a molecular test, by trying to grow the virus, or both. (Growing avian influenza A viruses should only be done in laboratories with high levels of protection).

For critically ill patients, collection and testing of lower respiratory tract specimens may lead to diagnosis of avian influenza virus infection.

For some patients who are no longer very sick or who have fully recovered, it may be difficult to find the avian influenza A virus in the specimen, using these methods. Sometimes it may still be possible to diagnose avian influenza A virus infection by looking for evidence of the body's immune response to the virus infection by detecting specific antibodies the body has produced in response to the virus. This is not always an option because it requires two blood specimens (one taken during the first week of illness and another taken 3–4 weeks later). Also, it can take several weeks to verify the results, and testing must be performed in a special laboratory, such as at Centers for Disease Control and Prevention (CDC).

Treating Avian Influenza A Virus Infections in Humans

CDC recommends oseltamivir, peramivir, or zanamivir for treatment of human infection with avian influenza A viruses. Analyses of available avian influenza viruses circulating worldwide suggest that most viruses are susceptible to oseltamivir, peramivir, and zanamivir. However, some evidence of antiviral resistance has been reported in HPAI Asian H5N1 viruses and influenza A H7N9 viruses isolated from some human cases. Monitoring for antiviral resistance among avian influenza A viruses is crucial and ongoing. These data directly inform CDC and WHO antiviral treatment recommendations.

Preventing Human Infection with Avian Influenza A Viruses

The best way to prevent infection with avian influenza A viruses is to avoid sources of exposure. Most human infections with avian influenza A viruses have occurred following direct or close contact with infected poultry.

People who have had contact with infected birds may be given influenza antiviral drugs preventatively. While antiviral drugs are most often used to treat flu, they also can be used to prevent infection in someone who has been exposed to influenza viruses. When used to prevent seasonal influenza, antiviral drugs are 70% to 90% effective.

Seasonal influenza vaccination will not prevent infection with avian influenza A viruses, but can reduce the risk of co-infection with human and avian influenza A viruses. It's also possible to make a vaccine that can protect people against avian influenza viruses. For example, the United States government maintains a stockpile of vaccine to protect against avian influenza A H5N1 vaccine. The stockpiled vaccine could be used if a similar H5N1 virus were to begin transmitting easily from person to person. Creating a candidate vaccine virus is the first step in producing a vaccine.

Section 32.4

H1N1 Flu (Swine Flu)

This section includes text excerpted from "Key Facts about Human Infections with Variant Viruses (Swine Origin Influenza Viruses in Humans)," Centers for Disease Control and Prevention (CDC), August 19, 2014.

What Is Swine Influenza?

Swine influenza (swine flu) is a respiratory disease of pigs caused by type A influenza viruses that regularly cause outbreaks of influenza in pigs. Swine flu viruses can cause high levels of illness in swine herds, but usually cause few deaths. Common signs in sick pigs include fever, depression, coughing (barking), discharge from the nose or eyes, sneezing, breathing difficulties, eye redness or inflammation, and going off feed. However, influenza-infected pigs also may not appear ill or be only mildly ill. Swine influenza viruses may circulate among swine throughout the year, but most outbreaks occur during the late fall and winter months similar to outbreaks of seasonal influenza in humans.

What Is a Variant Influenza Virus?

When an influenza virus that normally circulates in swine (but not people) is detected in a person, it is called a "variant influenza virus." For example, if a swine origin influenza A H3N2 virus is detected in a person, that virus will be called an "H3N2 variant" virus or "H3N2v" virus.

Can Humans Be Infected with Swine Influenza Viruses?

Yes. Swine flu viruses do not normally infect humans, however, sporadic human infections with influenza viruses that normally infect swine have occurred. When this happens, these viruses are called "variant viruses." Most commonly, human infections with variant viruses have occurred in people exposed to infected pigs (e.g., children near pigs at a fair or workers in the swine industry). In addition, there have been documented cases of multiple persons becoming sick after exposure to one or more sick pigs. Also cases of limited person-to-person spread of variant viruses have occurred.

How Common Is It for Humans to Be Infected with Influenza Viruses That Normally Infect Swine?

In the past, Centers for Disease Control and Prevention (CDC) received reports of approximately one human infected with influenza viruses that usually are found in swine every one to two years, but over the last few years, these cases have been detected more frequently. The increased detection and reporting of these cases could be occurring for a number of reasons, including one or more of the following factors: First, pandemic preparedness efforts have improved state level surveillance and laboratory capacity to detect novel viruses in the United States. Second, in 2007, novel influenza virus infections were made domestically and internationally reportable. And three, it's also possible that there is a true increase in the number of these cases, possibly occurring from exposure to infected swine or through subsequent, limited human-to-human transmission.

Why Are Human Infections with Variant Viruses of Concern?

Influenza viruses that infect pigs may be different from human influenza viruses. Thus, influenza vaccines made against human influenza viruses are generally not expected to protect people from influenza viruses that normally circulate in pigs. In addition, because pigs are susceptible to avian, human and swine influenza viruses, they potentially may be infected with influenza viruses from different species (e.g., ducks and humans) at the same time. If this happens, it is possible for the genes of these viruses to mix and create a new virus that could spread easily from person-to-person. This type of major change in the influenza A viruses is known as antigenic shift. Antigenic shift results when a new influenza A virus to which most people have little or no immune protection infects humans. If this new virus causes illness in people and can be transmitted easily from person-to-person, an influenza pandemic can occur. This is what happened in 2009 when an influenza A H1N1 virus with swine, avian and human genes emerged in the spring of 2009 and caused the first pandemic in more than 40 years.

What Symptoms Do People Have When They Are Infected with Variant Viruses?

People who have been infected with variant viruses have had symptoms similar to the symptoms of regular human seasonal influenza. These include fever, lethargy, lack of appetite and coughing. Some people also have reported runny nose, sore throat, eye irritation, nausea, vomiting, and diarrhea.

Can People Catch Swine Flu/Variant Flu from Eating Pork?

Swine influenza has not been shown to be transmissible to people through eating properly handled and prepared pork (pig meat) or other products derived from pigs.

How Are Variant Influenza Viruses Spread?

Influenza viruses can be directly transmitted from pigs to people and from people to pigs. When a human is infected with a flu virus that normally circulates in pigs, this virus is called a "variant virus" because it is different from seasonal influenza viruses. These infections have been most likely to occur when people are in close proximity to infected pigs, such as in pig barns and livestock exhibits housing pigs at fairs. This is thought to happen mainly when an infected pig coughs or sneezes and droplets with influenza virus in them spread through the air. If these droplets land in your nose or mouth, or are inhaled, you can be infected. There also is some evidence that you might get infected by touching something that has virus on it and then touching your own mouth or nose. A third way to possibly get infected is to inhale dust containing influenza virus. Scientists aren't really sure which of these ways of spread is the most common.

Human-to-human transmission of variant flu viruses also has occurred, though this method of spread has been limited. This kind of transmission is thought to occur in the same way that seasonal flu transmits in people, which is mainly through coughing or sneezing by people who are infected. People also may become infected by touching something with flu viruses on it and then touching their mouth or nose. It's important to note that in most cases, variant flu viruses have not shown the ability to spread easily and sustainably from person to person.

How Can Human Infections with Variant Influenza Viruses Be Diagnosed?

To diagnose variant influenza A virus infection, a respiratory specimen would generally need to be collected within the first 4 to 5 days of illness (when an infected person is most likely to be shedding virus). However, some persons, especially children, may shed virus for 10 days or longer. Since the 2009 H1N1 pandemic, state health departments have the ability to test for novel (non-human) influenza viruses. However, if a variant influenza virus is suspected, it is sent to CDC for further testing.

What Medications Are Available to Treat Variant Flu Infections in Humans?

There are four different antiviral drugs that are licensed for use in the United States for the treatment of influenza:

1. Amantadine
2. Rimantadine
3. Oseltamivir
4. Zanamivir

In the past, most variant influenza viruses had been susceptible to all four drugs, however the most recent variant influenza viruses isolated from humans are resistant to amantadine and rimantadine. At this time, CDC recommends the use of oseltamivir or zanamivir for the treatment of infection with these variant influenza viruses.

Chapter 33

Lice

Chapter Contents

Section 33.1

Body Lice

This section includes text excerpted from
"Parasites-Lice-Body Lice," Centers for Disease
Control and Prevention (CDC), September 24, 2013.

What Are Body Lice?

Body lice are parasitic insects that live on clothing and bedding used by infested persons. Body lice frequently lay their eggs on or near the seams of clothing. Body lice must feed on blood and usually only move to the skin to feed. Body lice exist worldwide and infest people of all races. Body lice infestations can spread rapidly under crowded living conditions where hygiene is poor (the homeless, refugees, victims of war or natural disasters).

In the United States, body lice infestations are found only in homeless transient populations who do not have access to bathing and regular changes of clean clothes. Infestation is unlikely to persist on anyone who bathes regularly and who has at least weekly access to freshly laundered clothing and bedding.

What Do Body Lice Look Like?

Body lice have three forms: the egg (also called a nit), the nymph, and the adult.

Nit: Nits are lice eggs. They are generally easy to see in the seams of an infested person's clothing, particularly around the waistline and under armpits. Body lice nits occasionally also may be attached to body hair. They are oval and usually yellow to white in color. Body lice nits may take 1–2 weeks to hatch.

Nymph: A nymph is an immature louse that hatches from the nit (egg). A nymph looks like an adult body louse, but is smaller. Nymphs mature into adults about 9–12 days after hatching. To live, the nymph must feed on blood.

214

Adult: The adult body louse is about the size of a sesame seed, has 6 legs, and is tan to greyish-white. Females lay eggs. To live, lice must feed on blood. If a louse falls off of a person, it dies within about 5–7 days at room temperature.

Where Are Body Lice Found?

Body lice generally are found on clothing and bedding used by infested people. Sometimes body lice are seen on the body when they feed. Body lice eggs usually are seen in the seams of clothing or on bedding. Occasionally eggs are attached to body hair.

Lice found on the head and scalp are not body lice; they are head lice.

What Are the Signs and Symptoms of Body Lice?

Intense itching ("pruritus") and rash caused by an allergic reaction to the louse bites are common symptoms of body lice infestation. When body lice infestation has been present for a long time, heavily bitten areas of the skin can become thickened and discolored, particularly around the midsection of the body (waist, groin, upper thighs); this condition is called "vagabond's disease." As with other lice infestations, intense itching can lead to scratching which can cause sores on the body; these sores sometimes can become infected with bacteria or fungi.

Can Body Lice Transmit Disease?

Yes. Body lice can spread epidemic typhus, trench fever, and louse-borne relapsing fever. Although louse-borne (epidemic) typhus is no longer widespread, outbreaks of this disease still occur during times of war, civil unrest, natural or man-made disasters, and in prisons where people live together in unsanitary conditions. Louse-borne typhus still exists in places where climate, chronic poverty, and social customs or war and social upheaval prevent regular changes and laundering of clothing.

How Are Body Lice Spread?

Body lice are spread through direct physical contact with a person who has body lice or through contact with articles such as clothing, beds, bed linens or towels that have been in contact with an infested person. In the United States, actual infestation with body lice tends to occur only in persons, such as homeless, transient persons, who do not have access to regular (at least weekly) bathing and changes of clean clothes, such as homeless, transient persons.

How Are Body Lice Infestations Diagnosed?

Body lice infestation is diagnosed by finding eggs and crawling lice in the seams of clothing. Sometimes a body louse can be seen on the skin crawling or feeding. Although body lice and nits can be large enough to be seen with the naked eye, sometimes a magnifying lens may be necessary to find lice or nits diagnosis should be made by a healthcare provider if you are unsure about an infestation.

Section 33.2

Head Lice

This section includes text excerpted from
"Parasites-Lice-Head Lice," Centers for Disease Control
and Prevention (CDC), September 2, 2015.

What Are Head Lice?

The head louse, or *Pediculus humanus capitis*, is a parasitic insect that can be found on the head, eyebrows, and eyelashes of people. Head lice feed on human blood several times a day and live close to the human scalp. Head lice are not known to spread disease.

Who Is at Risk for Getting Head Lice?

Head lice are found worldwide. In the United States, infestation with head lice is most common among pre-school children attending child care, elementary schoolchildren, and the household members of infested children. Although reliable data on how many people in the United States get head lice each year are not available, an estimated 6 million to 12 million infestations occur each year in the United States among children 3 to 11 years of age.

216

In the United States, infestation with head lice is much less common among African-Americans than among persons of other races, possibly because the claws of the of the head louse found most frequently in the United States are better adapted for grasping the shape and width of the hair shaft of other races. Head lice move by crawling; they cannot hop or fly. Head lice are spread by direct contact with the hair of an infested person. Anyone who comes in head-to-head contact with someone who already has head lice is at greatest risk. Spread by contact with clothing (such as hats, scarves, coats) or other personal items (such as combs, brushes or towels) used by an infested person is uncommon. Personal hygiene or cleanliness in the home or school has nothing to do with getting head lice.

What Do Head Lice Look Like?

Head lice have three forms: the egg (also called a nit), the nymph, and the adult.

Egg/Nit: Nits are lice eggs laid by the adult female head louse at the base of the hair shaft nearest the scalp. Nits are firmly attached to the hair shaft and are oval-shaped and very small (about the size of a knot in thread) and hard to see. Nits often appear yellow or white although live nits sometimes appear to be the same color as the hair of the infested person. Nits are often confused with dandruff, scabs, or hair spray droplets. Head lice nits usually take about 8–9 days to hatch. Eggs that are likely to hatch are usually located no more than 1/4 inch from the base of the hair shaft. Nits located further than 1/4 inch from the base of hair shaft may very well be already hatched, non-viable nits, or empty nits or casings. This is difficult to distinguish with the naked eye.

Nymph: A nymph is an immature louse that hatches from the nit. A nymph looks like an adult head louse, but is smaller. To live, a nymph must feed on blood. Nymphs mature into adults about 9–12 days after hatching from the nit.

Adult: The fully grown and developed adult louse is about the size of a sesame seed, has six legs, and is tan to grayish-white in color. Adult head lice may look darker in persons with dark hair than in persons with light hair. To survive, adult head lice must feed on blood. An adult head louse can live about 30 days on a person's head but will die within one or two days if it falls off a person. Adult female head lice are usually larger than males and can lay about six eggs each day.

Where Are Head Lice Most Commonly Found?

Head lice and head lice nits are found almost exclusively on the scalp, particularly around and behind the ears and near the neckline at the back of the head. Head lice or head lice nits sometimes are found on the eyelashes or eyebrows but this is uncommon. Head lice hold tightly to hair with hook-like claws at the end of each of their six legs. Head lice nits are cemented firmly to the hair shaft and can be difficult to remove even after the nymphs hatch and empty casings remain.

What Are the Signs and Symptoms of Head Lice Infestation?

- Tickling feeling of something moving in the hair.
- Itching, caused by an allergic reaction to the bites of the head louse.
- Irritability and difficulty sleeping; head lice are most active in the dark.
- Sores on the head caused by scratching. These sores can sometimes become infected with bacteria found on the person's skin.

How Did My Child Get Head Lice?

Head-to-head contact with an already infested person is the most common way to get head lice. Head-to-head contact is common during play at school, at home, and elsewhere (sports activities, playground, slumber parties, camp).

Although uncommon, head lice can be spread by sharing clothing or belongings. This happens when lice crawl or nits attached to shed hair hatch, and get on the shared clothing or belongings. Examples include:

- sharing clothing (hats, scarves, coats, sports uniforms) or articles (hair ribbons, barrettes, combs, brushes, towels, stuffed animals) recently worn or used by an infested person;
- or lying on a bed, couch, pillow or carpet that has recently been in contact with an infested person.

Dogs, cats, and other pets do not play a role in the spread of head lice.

How Is Head Lice Infestation Diagnosed?

The diagnosis of a head lice infestation is best made by finding a live nymph or adult louse on the scalp or hair of a person. Because nymphs and adult lice are very small, move quickly, and avoid light, they can be difficult to find. Use of a magnifying lens and a fine-toothed comb may be helpful to find live lice. If crawling lice are not seen, finding nits firmly attached within a 1/4 inch of base of the hair shafts strongly suggests, but does not confirm, that a person is infested and should be treated. Nits that are attached more than 1/4 inch from the base of the hair shaft are almost always dead or already hatched. Nits are often confused with other things found in the hair such as dandruff, hair spray droplets, and dirt particles. If no live nymphs or adult lice are seen, and the only nits found are more than 1/4-inch from the scalp, the infestation is probably old and no longer active and does not need to be treated.

If you are not sure if a person has head lice, the diagnosis should be made by their healthcare provider, local health department, or other person trained to identify live head lice.

Is Infestation with Head Lice Reportable to Health Departments?

Most health departments do not require reporting of head lice infestation. However, it may be beneficial for the sake of others to share information with school nurses, parents of classmates, and others about contact with head lice.

I Don't Like My School's "No-Nit" Policy; Can CDC Do Something?

No. Centers for Disease Control and Prevention (CDC) is not a regulatory agency. School head lice policies often are determined by local school boards. Local health departments may have guidelines that address school head lice policies; check with your local and state health departments to see if they have such recommendations.

Do Head Lice Spread Disease?

Head lice should not be considered as a medical or public health hazard. Head lice are not known to spread disease. Head lice can be an annoyance because their presence may cause itching and loss of sleep. Sometimes the itching can lead to excessive scratching that can sometimes increase the chance of a secondary skin infection.

219

Can Head Lice Be Spread by Sharing Sports Helmets or Headphones?

Head lice are spread most commonly by direct contact with the hair of an infested person. Spread by contact with inanimate objects and personal belongings may occur but is very uncommon. Head lice feet are specially adapted for holding onto human hair. Head lice would have difficulty attaching firmly to smooth or slippery surfaces like plastic, metal, polished synthetic leathers, and other similar materials.

Can Wigs or Hair Pieces Spread Lice?

Head lice and their eggs (nits) soon perish if separated from their human host. Adult head lice can live only a day or so off the human head without blood for feeding. Nymphs (young head lice) can live only for several hours without feeding on a human. Nits (head lice eggs) generally die within a week away from their human host and cannot hatch at a temperature lower than that close to the human scalp. For these reasons, the risk of transmission of head lice from a wig or other hairpiece is extremely small, particularly if the wig or hairpiece has not been worn within the preceding 48 hours by someone who is actively infested with live head lice.

Can Swimming Spread Lice?

Data show that head lice can survive under water for several hours but are unlikely to be spread by the water in a swimming pool. Head lice have been seen to hold tightly to human hair and not let go when submerged under water. Chlorine levels found in pool water do not kill head lice.

Head lice may be spread by sharing towels or other items that have been in contact with an infested person's hair, although such spread is uncommon. Children should be taught not to share towels, hair brushes, and similar items either at poolside or in the changing room.

Swimming or washing the hair within 1–2 days after treatment with some head lice medicines might make some treatments less effective. Seek the advice of your healthcare provider or health department if you have questions.

Section 33.3

Pubic Lice

This section contains text excerpted from the following sources: Text beginning with the heading "What Are Pubic Lice?" is excerpted from "Parasites-Lice-Pubic "Crab" Lice," Centers for Disease Control and Prevention (CDC), September 24, 2013; Text under with the heading "Prevention and Control" is excerpted from "Parasites-Lice-Pubic "Crab" Lice," Centers for Disease Control and Prevention (CDC), September 24, 2013.

What Are Pubic Lice?

Also called crab lice or "crabs," pubic lice are parasitic insects found primarily in the pubic or genital area of humans. Pubic lice infestation is found worldwide and occurs in all races, ethnic groups, and levels of society.

What Do Pubic Lice Look Like?

Pubic lice have three forms: the egg (also called a nit), the nymph, and the adult.

Nit: Nits are lice eggs. They can be hard to see and are found firmly attached to the hair shaft. They are oval and usually yellow to white. Pubic lice nits take about 6–10 days to hatch.

Nymph: The nymph is an immature louse that hatches from the nit (egg). A nymph looks like an adult pubic louse but it is smaller. Pubic lice nymphs take about 2–3 weeks after hatching to mature into adults capable of reproducing. To live, a nymph must feed on blood.

Adult: The adult pubic louse resembles a miniature crab when viewed through a strong magnifying glass. Pubic lice have six legs; their two front legs are very large and look like the pincher claws of a crab. This is how they got the nickname "crabs." Pubic lice are tan to grayish-white in color. Females lay nits and are usually larger than males. To live, lice must feed on blood. If the louse falls off a person, it dies within 1–2 days.

Where Are Pubic Lice Found?

Pubic lice usually are found in the genital area on pubic hair; but they may occasionally be found on other coarse body hair, such as hair on the legs, armpits, mustache, beard, eyebrows or eyelashes. Pubic lice on the eyebrows or eyelashes of children may be a sign of sexual exposure or abuse. Lice found on the head generally are head lice, not pubic lice. Animals do not get or spread pubic lice.

What Are the Signs and Symptoms of Pubic Lice?

Signs and symptoms of pubic lice include:

• Itching in the genital area

• Visible nits (lice eggs) or crawling lice

How Did I Get Pubic Lice?

Pubic lice usually are spread through sexual contact and are most common in adults. Pubic lice found on children may be a sign of sexual exposure or abuse. Occasionally, pubic lice may be spread by close personal contact or contact with articles such as clothing, bed linens, or towels that have been used by an infested person. A common misconception is that pubic lice are spread easily by sitting on a toilet seat. This would be extremely rare because lice cannot live long away from a warm human body and they do not have feet designed to hold onto or walk on smooth surfaces such as toilet seats.

Persons infested with pubic lice should be examined for the presence of other sexually transmitted diseases (STDs).

How Is a Pubic Lice Infestation Diagnosed?

A pubic lice infestation is diagnosed by finding a "crab" louse or egg (nit) on hair in the pubic region or, less commonly, elsewhere on the body (eyebrows, eyelashes, beard, mustache, armpit, perianal area, groin, trunk, scalp). Pubic lice may be difficult to find because there may be only a few. Pubic lice often attach themselves to more than one hair and generally do not crawl as quickly as head and body lice. If crawling lice are not seen, finding nits in the pubic area strongly suggests that a person is infested and should be treated. If you are unsure about infestation or if treatment is not successful, see a health-care provider for a diagnosis. Persons infested with pubic lice should be investigated for the presence of other sexually transmitted diseases.

Although pubic lice and nits can be large enough to be seen with the naked eye, a magnifying lens may be necessary to find lice or eggs.

Prevention and Control

Pubic ("crab") lice most commonly are spread directly from person to person by sexual contact. Pubic lice very rarely may be spread by clothing, bedding or a toilet seat. The following are steps that can be taken to help prevent and control the spread of pubic ("crab") lice:

- All sexual contacts of the infested person should be examined. All those who are infested should be treated.

- Sexual contact between the infested person(s)and their sexual partner(s) should be avoided until all have been examined, treated as necessary, and reevaluated to rule out persistent infestation.

- Machine wash and dry clothing worn and bedding used by the infested person in the hot water (at least 130°F) laundry cycle and the high heat drying cycle. Clothing and items that are not washable can be dry-cleaned OR sealed in a plastic bag and stored for 2 weeks.

- Do not share clothing, bedding, and towels used by an infested person.

- Do not use fumigant sprays or fogs; they are not necessary to control pubic ("crab") lice and can be toxic if inhaled or absorbed through the skin. Persons with pubic lice should be examined and treated for any other sexually transmitted diseases (STDs) that may be present.

Chapter 34

Measles

Measles History

Pre-Vaccine Era

In the 9th century, a Persian doctor published one of the first written accounts of measles disease.

Francis Home, a Scottish physician, demonstrated in 1757 that measles is caused by an infectious agent in the blood of patients.

In 1912, measles became a nationally notifiable disease in the United States, requiring U.S. healthcare providers and laboratories to report all diagnosed cases. In the first decade of reporting, an average of 6,000 measles-related deaths were reported each year.

In the decade before 1963 when a vaccine became available, nearly all children got measles by the time they were 15 years of age. It is estimated 3 to 4 million people in the United States were infected each year. Also each year an estimated 400 to 500 people died, 48,000 were hospitalized, and 4,000 suffered encephalitis (swelling of the brain) from measles.

Vaccine Development

In 1954, John F. Enders and Dr. Thomas C. Peebles collected blood samples from several ill students during a measles outbreak in Boston,

---

About This chapter includes text excerpted from "Measles (Rubeola)," Centers for Disease Control and Prevention (CDC), November 3, 2014.

Massachusetts. They wanted to isolate the measles virus in the student's blood and create a measles vaccine. They succeeded in isolating measles in 13-year-old David Edmonston's blood.

In 1963, John Enders and colleagues transformed their Edmonston-B strain of measles virus into a vaccine and licensed it in the United States. In 1968, an improved and even weaker measles vaccine, developed by Maurice Hilleman and colleagues, began to be distributed. This vaccine, called the Edmonston-Enders (formerly "Moraten") strain has been the only measles vaccine used in the United States since 1968. Measles vaccine is usually combined with mumps and rubella (MMR), or combined with mumps, rubella and varicella (MMRV).

Measles Elimination

In 1978, Centers for Disease Control and Prevention (CDC) set a goal to eliminate measles from the United States by 1982. Although this goal was not met, widespread use of measles vaccine drastically reduced the disease rates. By 1981, the number of reported measles cases was 80% less compared with the previous year. However, a 1989 measles outbreaks among vaccinated school-aged children prompted the Advisory Committee on Immunization Practices (ACIP), the American Academy of Pediatrics (AAP), and the American Academy of Family Physicians (AAFP) to recommend a second dose of MMR vaccine for all children. Following widespread implementation of this recommendation and improvements in first-dose MMR vaccine coverage, reported measles cases declined even more.

Measles was declared eliminated (absence of continuous disease transmission for greater than 12 months) from the United States in 2000. This was possible thanks to a highly effective vaccination program and better measles control in the Americas region.

Signs and Symptoms

The symptoms of measles generally appear about 7 to 14 days after a person is infected.

Measles typically begins with:

- high fever
- cough
- runny nose (coryza)
- red, watery eyes (conjunctivitis)

Two or three days after symptoms begin, tiny white spots (Koplik spots) may appear inside the mouth.

Three to five days after symptoms begin, a rash breaks out. It usually begins as flat red spots that appear on the face at the hairline and spread downward to the neck, trunk, arms, legs, and feet. Small raised bumps may also appear on top of the flat red spots. The spots may become joined together as they spread from the head to the rest of the body. When the rash appears, a person's fever may spike to more than 104° Fahrenheit.

After a few days, the fever subsides and the rash fades.

Transmission of Measles

Measles is a highly contagious virus that lives in the nose and throat mucus of an infected person. It can spread to others through coughing and sneezing. Also, measles virus can live for up to two hours in an airspace where the infected person coughed or sneezed. If other people breathe the contaminated air or touch the infected surface, then touch their eyes, noses, or mouths, they can become infected. Measles is so contagious that if one person has it, 90% of the people close to that person who are not immune will also become infected.

Infected people can spread measles to others from four days before through four days after the rash appears.

Measles is a disease of humans; measles virus is not spread by any other animal species.

Top Four Things Parents Need to Know about Measles

1. Measles can be serious.

    Some people think of measles as just a little rash and fever that clears up in a few days, but measles can cause serious health complications, especially in children younger than 5 years of age. There is no way to tell in advance the severity of the symptoms your child will experience.

    - About 1 in 4 people in the U.S. who get measles will be hospitalized.

    - 1 out of every 1,000 people with measles will develop brain swelling, which could lead to brain damage.

- 1 or 2 out of 1,000 people with measles will die, even with the best care.

  Some of the more common measles symptoms include:

  - Fever

  - Rash

  - Runny nose

  - Red eyes

2. Measles is very contagious.

   Measles spreads through the air when an infected person coughs or sneezes. It is so contagious that if one person has it, 9 out of 10 people around him or her will also become infected if they are not protected. Your child can get measles just by being in a room where a person with measles has been, even up to two hours after that person has left. An infected person can spread measles to others even before knowing he/she has the disease—from four days before developing the measles rash through four days afterward.

3. Your child can still get measles in United States.

   Measles was declared eliminated from the United States in 2000 thanks to a highly effective vaccination program. Eliminated means that the disease is no longer constantly present in this country. However, measles is still common in many parts of the world, including some countries in Europe, Asia, the Pacific, and Africa. Worldwide, an estimated 20 million people get measles and 146,000 people, mostly children, die from the disease each year.

   Even if your family does not travel internationally, you could come into contact with measles anywhere in your community. Every year, measles is brought into the United States by unvaccinated travelers (Americans or foreign visitors) who get measles while they are in other countries. Anyone who is not protected against measles is at risk.

4. You have the power to protect your child against measles with a safe and effective vaccine.

   The best protection against measles is measles-mumps-rubella (MMR) vaccine. MMR vaccine provides long-lasting protection against all strains of measles. Your child needs two doses of MMR vaccine for best protection:

- The first dose at 12 through 15 months of age.

- The second dose 4 through 6 years of age.

If your family is traveling overseas, the vaccine recommendations are a little different:

- If your baby is 6 through 11 months old, he or she should receive 1 dose of MMR vaccine before leaving.

- If your child is 12 months of age or older, he or she will need 2 doses of MMR vaccine (separated by at least 28 days) before departure.

Measles Vaccination

Measles can be prevented with the MMR (measles, mumps, and rubella) vaccine. One dose of MMR vaccine is about 93% effective at preventing measles if exposed to the virus, and two doses are about 97% effective. In the United States, widespread use of measles vaccine has led to a greater than 99% reduction in measles cases compared with the pre-vaccine era. Since 2000, when measles was declared eliminated from the United States, the annual number of people reported to have measles ranged from a low of 37 people in 2004 to a high of 668 people in 2014. Most of these originated outside the country or were linked to a case that originated outside the country.

Measles is still common in other countries. The virus is highly contagious and can spread rapidly in areas where people are not vaccinated. Worldwide, an estimated 20 million people get measles and 146,000 people die from the disease each year—that equals about 400 deaths every day or about 17 deaths every hour.

Vaccine Recommendations

Children

CDC recommends all children get two doses of MMR vaccine, starting with the first dose at 12 through 15 months of age, and the second dose at 4 through 6 years of age. Children can receive the second dose earlier as long as it is at least 28 days after the first dose.

Students at Post-High School Educational Institutions

Students at post-high school educational institutions who do not have evidence of immunity against measles need two doses of MMR vaccine, separated by at least 28 days.

Adults

Adults who do not have evidence of immunity against measles should get at least one dose of MMR vaccine.

International Travelers

People 6 months of age and older who will be traveling internationally should be protected against measles. Before any international travel:

- Infants 6 through 11 months of age should receive one dose of MMR vaccine. Infants who get one dose of MMR vaccine before their first birthday should get two more doses (one dose at 12 through 15 months of age and another dose at least 28 days later).

- Children 12 months of age and older should receive two doses of MMR vaccine, separated by at least 28 days.

- Teenagers and adults who do not have evidence of immunity against measles should get two doses of MMR vaccine separated by at least 28 days.

Chapter 35

Meningitis

Meningitis is an inflammation of the meninges, the membranes that cover the brain and spinal cord. Most cases are caused by bacteria or viruses, but some can be due to certain medications or illnesses.

Bacterial meningitis is rare, but is usually serious and can be life threatening if not treated right away. **Viral meningitis** (also called **aseptic meningitis**) is relatively common and far less serious. It often remains undiagnosed because its symptoms can be similar to those of the common flu.

People of any age can get meningitis, but because it can be easily spread among those living in close quarters, teens, college students, and boarding-school students are at higher risk for infection.

If dealt with promptly, meningitis can be treated successfully. So it's important to get routine vaccinations, know the signs of meningitis, and if you suspect that your child has the illness, seek medical care right away.

Causes of Meningitis

Many of the bacteria and viruses that cause meningitis are fairly common and associated with other routine illnesses. Bacteria and viruses that infect the skin, urinary system, or gastrointestinal and respiratory tract can spread by the bloodstream to the meninges through cerebrospinal fluid, the fluid that circulates in and around the spinal cord.

In some cases of bacterial meningitis, the bacteria spread to the meninges from a severe head trauma or a severe local infection, such as a serious ear infection (otitis media) or nasal sinus infection (sinusitis).

Bacterial and Viral Types

Many different types of bacteria can cause bacterial meningitis. In newborns, the most common causes are Group B streptococcus, *Escherichia coli*, and less commonly, *Listeria monocytogenes*. In older kids, *Streptococcus pneumoniae* (pneumococcus) and *Neisseria meningitidis* (meningococcus) are more often the causes. Another bacteria, *Haemophilus influenza* type b (Hib), also can cause the illness but because of widespread childhood immunization, these cases are rarer.

Similarly, many different viruses can lead to viral meningitis, including enteroviruses (such as coxsackievirus and poliovirus) and the herpesvirus.

Symptoms of Meningitis

Meningitis symptoms vary, depending both on the age of the patient and the cause of the infection. The first symptoms of bacterial or viral meningitis can come on quickly or surface several days after someone has had a cold, diarrhea and vomiting, or other signs of an infection.

Common symptoms include:

- fever
- lethargy (decreased consciousness)
- irritability
- headache
- photophobia (eye sensitivity to light)
- stiff neck
- skin rashes
- seizures

Meningitis in Infants

Infants with meningitis may not have common symptoms. They might simply have extreme irritability, lethargy or fever. They may be difficult to comfort, even when they are picked up and rocked.

Other symptoms of meningitis in infants can include:

- jaundice (a yellowish tint to the skin)
- stiffness of the body and neck
- fever or lower-than-normal temperature

- poor feeding

- a weak suck

- a high-pitched cry

- bulging fontanelles (the soft spot at the top/front of the baby's skull)

Viral meningitis tends to cause flu-like symptoms, such as fever and headache, and may be so mild that the illness goes undiagnosed. Most cases of viral meningitis resolve completely within 7 to 10 days, without any complications or need for treatment.

Treatment

Because bacterial meningitis can be so serious, if you think that your child has any form of meningitis, it's important to see the doctor right away.

If meningitis is suspected, the doctor will order laboratory tests to help make the diagnosis, probably including a lumbar puncture (spinal tap) to collect a sample of spinal fluid. This test will show any signs of inflammation and whether a virus or bacteria is causing the infection.

Someone with viral meningitis may be hospitalized, although some kids are allowed to recover at home if they are not too ill. Treatment aimed at relieving symptoms includes rest, fluids, and over-the-counter pain medication.

If bacterial meningitis is diagnosed—or even suspected—doctors will start intravenous (IV) antibiotics as soon as possible. Fluids may be given to replace those lost to fever, sweating, vomiting, and poor appetite.

Possible Complications

Complications of bacterial meningitis might require additional treatment. For example, anticonvulsants might be given for seizures. If someone develops shock or low blood pressure, additional IV fluids and certain medications might be given to increase blood pressure. Some kids may need supplemental oxygen or mechanical ventilation if they have difficulty breathing.

Bacterial meningitis complications can be severe and include neurological problems such as hearing loss, visual impairment, seizures, and learning disabilities. Because impaired hearing is a common complication, those who've had bacterial meningitis should have a hearing test following their recovery.

The heart, kidneys, and adrenal glands also might be affected, depending on the cause of the infection. Although some kids develop long-lasting neurological problems, most who receive prompt diagnosis and treatment recover fully.

Contagiousness

Most cases of meningitis—both viral and bacterial—are due to infections that are contagious, spread via tiny drops of fluid from the throat and nose of someone who is infected. The drops may become airborne when the person coughs, laughs, talks, or sneezes. They then can infect others when people breathe them in or touch the drops and then touch their own noses or mouths.

Sharing food, drinking glasses, eating utensils, tissues, or towels all can transmit infection as well. Some infectious organisms can spread through a person's stool (poop), and someone who comes in contact with the stool—such as kids in daycare—may develop the infection.

Infections most often spread between people who are in close contact, such as those who live together or people who are exposed by kissing or sharing eating utensils. Casual contact at school or work with someone who has one of these infections usually will not transmit the infectious agent.

Prevention

Routine immunization can go a long way toward preventing meningitis. The vaccines against Hib, measles, mumps, polio, meningococcus, and pneumococcus can protect against meningitis caused by these microorganisms.

Doctors now recommend that kids get vaccinated for meningococcal disease with a vaccine called MCV4 when they're 11 years old, with a booster shot at age 16. Kids who have not been vaccinated and are older than 11 also should be immunized, particularly if they're going to college, boarding school, camp, or other settings where they'll live in close quarters with others.

This vaccine also might be recommended for kids between 2 months and 10 years old who have certain high-risk medical problems, and for people traveling to countries where meningitis is more common.

A new type of meningococcal vaccine called MenB (which protects against a type of meningococcal bacterium not covered by the older vaccine) *may* be given to teens and young adults at the discretion of their doctor. For kids 10 and older who are at higher risk of developing meningococcal disease (those with immune system disorders, or those who live in or travel to countries where the disease is common), it is recommended that they receive the MenB vaccine in addition to the MCV4 vaccine.

Many of the bacteria and viruses responsible for meningitis are fairly common, so good hygiene is an important way to prevent infection. Encourage kids to wash their hands thoroughly and often, particularly before eating and after using the bathroom. Avoiding close contact with someone who is obviously ill and not sharing food, drinks, or eating utensils can help halt the spread of germs as well.

In certain cases, doctors may give antibiotics to anyone who has been in close contact with a person who has bacterial meningitis to help prevent additional infections.

When to Call the Doctor

Seek medical attention immediately if you suspect your child has meningitis or has symptoms such as vomiting, headache, lethargy or confusion, neck stiffness, rash, and fever. Infants who have fever, irritability, poor feeding, and lethargy should also be assessed by a doctor right away.

If your child has had contact with someone who has meningitis (for example, in a childcare center or a college dorm), call your doctor to ask whether preventive medication is recommended.

Chapter 36

Methicillin-Resistant Staphylococcus aureus *(MRSA)*

General Information about MRSA in the Community

Methicillin-resistant *Staphylococcus aureus* (MRSA) is a type of staph bacteria that is resistant to several antibiotics. In the general community, MRSA most often causes skin infections. In some cases, it causes pneumonia (lung infection) and other issues. If left untreated, MRSA infections can become severe and cause sepsis-a life-threatening reaction to severe infection in the body.

In a healthcare setting, such as a hospital or nursing home, MRSA can cause severe problems such as bloodstream infections, pneumonia, and surgical site infections.

Who Is at Risk, and How Is MRSA Spread in the Community?

Anyone can get MRSA on their body from contact with an infected wound or by sharing personal items, such as towels or razors, that

This chapter includes text excerpted from "Methicillin-Resistant *Staphylococcus aureus* (MRSA)," Centers for Disease Control and Prevention (CDC), February 9, 2016.

have touched infected skin. MRSA infection risk can be increased when a person is in activities or places that involve crowding, skin-to-skin contact, and shared equipment or supplies. People including athletes, daycare and school students, military personnel in barracks, and those who recently received inpatient medical care are at higher risk.

How Common Is MRSA?

Studies show that about one in three people carry staph in their nose, usually without any illness. 2 in 100 people carry MRSA. There are not data showing the total number of people who get MRSA skin infections in the community.

Can I Prevent MRSA? How?

There are the steps you can take to reduce your risk of MRSA infection:

- Maintain good hand and body hygiene. Wash hands often, and clean your body regularly, especially after exercise.
- Keep cuts, scrapes and wounds clean and covered until healed.
- Avoid sharing personal items such as towels and razors.
- Get care early if you think you might have an infection.

What Are MRSA Symptoms?

Sometimes, people with MRSA skin infections first think they have a spider bite. However, unless a spider is actually seen, the irritation is likely not a spider bite. Most staph skin infections, including MRSA, appear as a bump or infected area on the skin that might be:

- Red
- Swollen
- Painful
- Warm to the touch
- Full of pus or other drainage
- Accompanied by a fever

What Should I Do If I See These Symptoms?

If you or someone in your family experiences these signs and symptoms, cover the area with a bandage, wash your hands, and contact your doctor. It is especially important to contact your doctor if signs and symptoms of an MRSA skin infection are accompanied by a fever.

What Should I Do If I Think I Have a Skin Infection?

- You can't tell by looking at the skin if it is a staph infection (including MRSA).

- Contact your doctor if you think you have an infection. Finding infections early and getting care make it less likely that the infection will become severe.

- Do not try to treat the infection yourself by picking or popping the sore.

- Cover possible infections with clean, dry bandages until you can be seen by a doctor, nurse or other healthcare provider.

How to Prevent Spreading MRSA

- Cover your wounds. Keep wounds covered with clean, dry bandages until healed. Follow your doctor's instructions about proper care of the wound. Pus from infected wounds can contain MRSA so keeping the infection covered will help prevent the spread to others. Bandages and tape can be thrown away with the regular trash. Do not try to treat the infection yourself by picking or popping the sore.

- Clean your hands often. You, your family, and others in close contact should wash their hands often with soap and water or use an alcohol-based hand rub, especially after changing the bandage or touching the infected wound.

- Do not share personal items. Personal items include towels, washcloths, razors and clothing, including uniforms.

- Wash used sheets, towels, and clothes with water and laundry detergent. Use a dryer to dry them completely.

- Wash clothes according to manufacturer's instructions on the label. Clean your hands after touching dirty clothes.

239

Chapter 37

Mumps

Mumps is a contagious disease caused by a virus. It typically starts with a few days of fever, headache, muscle aches, tiredness, and loss of appetite, followed by swollen salivary glands. You can protect yourself and your family against mumps with vaccination.

Signs and Symptoms

Mumps is best known for the puffy cheeks and swollen jaw that it causes. This is a result of swollen salivary glands.

The most common symptoms include:

- Fever

- Headache

- Muscle aches

- Tiredness

- Loss of appetite

- Swollen and tender salivary glands under the ears on one or both sides (parotitis)

Symptoms typically appear 16–18 days after infection, but this period can range from 12–25 days after infection. Some people who get

This chapter includes text excerpted from "Mumps," Centers for Disease Control and Prevention (CDC), May 29, 2015.

mumps have very mild or no symptoms, and often they do not know they have the disease. Most people with mumps recover completely in a few weeks.

Transmission

Mumps is a contagious disease caused by a virus. It spreads through saliva or mucus from the mouth, nose or throat. An infected person can spread the virus by:

- coughing, sneezing or talking

- sharing items, such as cups or eating utensils, with others

- touching objects or surfaces with unwashed hands that are then touched by others

Mumps likely spreads before the salivary glands begin to swell and up to five days after the swelling begins.

Complications

Mumps can occasionally cause complications, especially in adults.

Complications include:

- inflammation of the testicles (orchitis) in males who have reached puberty; rarely does this lead to fertility problems

- inflammation of the brain (encephalitis)

- inflammation of the tissue covering the brain and spinal cord (meningitis)

- inflammation of the ovaries (oophoritis) and/or breasts (mastitis) in females who have reached puberty

- deafness

Mumps Vaccination

Mumps can be prevented with MMR (measles-mumps-rubella) vaccine. MMR vaccine prevents most, but not all, cases of mumps and complications caused by the disease. Two doses of the vaccine are 88% (range: 66–95%) effective at preventing mumps; one dose is 78% (range: 49%–92%) effective.

The first vaccine against mumps was licensed in the United States in 1967. By 2005, mumps rates declined by more than 99% thanks to high two-dose vaccination coverage among children.

Vaccination Recommendations

Children

Centers for Disease Control and Prevention (CDC) recommends that children routinely receive get two doses of MMR vaccine:

- the first dose at 12 through 15 months of age
- the second dose at 4 through 6 years of age

Children can receive the second dose earlier as long as it is at least 28 days after the first dose.

Students at Post-High School Educational Institutions

Students at post-high school educational institutions, such as college, trade schools, and training programs, who do not have evidence of immunity (protection) against mumps need two doses of MMR vaccine, separated by at least 28 days.

Adults

People who are born during or after 1957 who do not have evidence of immunity against mumps should get at least one dose of MMR vaccine.

International Travelers

- Children 12 months of age or older should have two doses of MMR vaccine, separated by at least 28 days.
- Teenagers and adults without evidence of immunity (protection) to mumps should have two doses of MMR vaccine, separated by at least 28 days.

Healthcare Personnel

Healthcare personnel should have documented evidence of immunity against mumps, according to the recommendations of the Advisory Committee on Immunization Practices

Acceptable presumptive evidence of immunity to mumps includes: documented administration of two doses of live mumps virus vaccine at least 28 days apart, on or after the first birthday; laboratory evidence of immunity; birth before 1957; or documentation of physician-diagnosed mumps.

Chapter 38

Non-Polio Enterovirus

Overview

Non-polio enteroviruses are very common viruses. They cause about 10 to 15 million infections in the United States each year. Tens of thousands of people are hospitalized each year for illnesses caused by enteroviruses.

Anyone can get infected with non-polio enteroviruses. But infants, children, and teenagers are more likely to get infected and become sick. That's because they do not yet have immunity (protection) from previous exposures to the viruses.

Most people who get infected with non-polio enteroviruses do not get sick. Or, they may have mild illness, like the common cold. But some people can get very sick and have infection of their heart or brain or even become paralyzed. Infants and people with weakened immune systems have a greater chance of having these complications.

You can get infected with non-polio enteroviruses by having close contact with an infected person. You can also get infected by touching objects or surfaces that have the virus on them then touching your mouth, nose or eyes.

In the United States, people are more likely to get infected with non-polio enteroviruses in the summer and fall.

This chapter includes text excerpted from "Non-Polio Enterovirus," Centers for Disease Control and Prevention (CDC), June 10, 2016.

Symptoms

Most people who are infected with non-polio enteroviruses do not get sick, or they only have mild illness, like the common cold. Infants, children, and teenagers are more likely than adults to get infected and become sick because they do not yet have immunity (protection) from previous exposures to the viruses. Adults can get infected too, but they are less likely to have symptoms, or their symptoms may be milder. Symptoms of mild illness may include:

• fever

• runny nose, sneezing, cough

• skin rash

• mouth blisters

• body and muscle aches

Some non-polio enterovirus infections can cause:

• viral conjunctivitis,

• hand, foot, and mouth disease

• viral meningitis (infection of the covering of the spinal cord and/ or brain)

• viral encephalitis (infection of the brain)

• myocarditis (infection of the heart)

• pericarditis (infection of the sac around the heart)

• acute flaccid paralysis (a sudden onset of weakness in one or more arms or legs)

• inflammatory muscle disease (slow, progressive muscle weakness)

Infants and people with weakened immune systems have a greater chance of having these complications.

People who develop myocarditis may have heart failure and require long term care. Some people who develop encephalitis or paralysis may not fully recover.

Newborns infected with a non-polio enterovirus may develop sepsis (the body's overwhelming response to infection which can lead to tissue damage, organ failure, and death). But this is very rare.

Non-polio enterovirus infections may play a role in the development of type 1 diabetes in children.

Transmission

Non-polio enteroviruses can be found in an infected person's:

- feces (stool)
- eyes, nose, and mouth secretions (such as saliva, nasal mucus, or sputum)
- blister fluid

You can get exposed to the virus by:

- having close contact, such as touching or shaking hands, with an infected person
- touching objects or surfaces that have the virus on them, then touching your eyes, nose or mouth before washing your hands
- changing diapers of an infected person, then touching your eyes, nose or mouth before washing your hands
- drinking water that has the virus in it

Pregnant women who are infected with a non-polio enterovirus shortly before delivery can pass the virus to their babies. Mothers who are breastfeeding should talk with their doctor if they are sick or think they may have an infection.

Non-polio enteroviruses can be shed (passed from a person's body into the environment) in your stool for several weeks or longer after you have been infected. The virus can be shed from your respiratory tract for 1 to 3 weeks or less. Infected people can shed the virus even if they don't have symptoms.

Prevention

Many people who are infected with non-polio enteroviruses do not have symptoms, but can still spread the virus to other people. This makes it is difficult to prevent them from spreading. But the best way to help protect yourself and others from non-polio enterovirus infections is to:

- Wash your hands often with soap and water, especially after using the toilet and changing diapers.

- Avoid close contact, such as touching and shaking hands, with people who are sick.

- Clean and disinfecting frequently touched surfaces.

There is no vaccine to protect you from non-polio enterovirus infection.

Treatment

There is no specific treatment for non-polio enterovirus infection. People with mild illness caused by non-polio enterovirus infection typically only need symptom treatment. They usually recover completely. However, some illnesses caused by non-polio enteroviruses can be severe enough to require hospitalization.

If you are concerned about your symptoms, you should contact your healthcare provider.

Chapter 39

Norovirus

Norovirus is a very contagious virus that can infect anyone. You can get it from an infected person, contaminated food or water or by touching contaminated surfaces.

Symptoms

Norovirus causes inflammation of the stomach or intestines or both. This is called acute gastroenteritis.

The most common symptoms:

- diarrhea
- throwing up
- nausea
- stomach pain

Other symptoms:

- fever
- headache
- body aches

A person usually develops symptoms 12 to 48 hours after being exposed to norovirus. Most people with norovirus illness get better within 1 to 3 days.

This chapter contains text excerpted from the following sources: Text in this chapter begins with excerpts from "Norovirus," Centers for Disease Control and Prevention (CDC), June 24, 2016; Text beginning with the heading "Prevent the Spread of Norovirus" is excerpted from "Diseases and Conditions," Centers for Disease Control and Prevention (CDC), December 21, 2015.

If you have norovirus illness, you can feel extremely ill and throw up or have diarrhea many times a day. This can lead to dehydration, especially in young children, older adults, and people with other illnesses.

Symptoms of dehydration:

- decrease in urination
- dry mouth and throat
- feeling dizzy when standing up

Children who are dehydrated may cry with few or no tears and be unusually sleepy or fussy.

Transmission

Norovirus is a highly contagious virus. Anyone can get infected with norovirus and get sick. Also, you can get norovirus illness many times in your life. One reason for this is that there are many different types of noroviruses. Being infected with one type of norovirus may not protect you against other types.

Norovirus can be found in your stool (feces) even before you start feeling sick. The virus can stay in your stool for 2 weeks or more after you feel better.

You are most contagious:

- when you are sick with norovirus illness
- during the first few days after you recover from norovirus illness

You can become infected with norovirus by accidentally getting stool or vomit from infected people in your mouth. This usually happens by:

- eating food or drinking liquids that are contaminated with norovirus
- touching surfaces or objects contaminated with norovirus then putting your fingers in your mouth
- having contact with someone who is infected with norovirus (for example, caring for or sharing food or eating utensils with someone with norovirus illness)

Norovirus can spread quickly in closed places like daycare centers, nursing homes, schools, and cruise ships. Most norovirus outbreaks happen from November to April in the United States.

Treatment

There is no specific medicine to treat people with norovirus illness. Norovirus infection cannot be treated with antibiotics because it is a viral (not a bacterial) infection.

If you have norovirus illness, you should drink plenty of liquids to replace fluid lost from throwing up and diarrhea. This will help prevent dehydration.

Sports drinks and other drinks without caffeine or alcohol can help with mild dehydration. But, these drinks may not replace important nutrients and minerals. Oral rehydration fluids that you can get over the counter are most helpful for mild dehydration.

Dehydration can lead to serious problems. Severe dehydration may require hospitalization for treatment with fluids given through your vein (intravenous or IV fluids). If you think you or someone you are caring for is severely dehydrated, call the doctor.

Prevent the Spread of Norovirus

Norovirus causes many people to become ill with vomiting and diarrhea each year. You can help protect yourself and others by washing your hands often and following simple tips to stay healthy.

Noroviruses are a group of related viruses that can cause gastro-enteritis, which is inflammation of the stomach and intestines. This leads to cramping, nausea, vomiting, and diarrhea.

Norovirus Is the Most Common Cause of Gastroenteritis in United States

Centers for Disease Control and Prevention (CDC) estimates that each year Norovirus causes 19 to 21 million illnesses, 56,000 to 71,000 hospitalizations and 570 to 800 deaths. Anyone can get infected with norovirus and you can get it more than once. It is estimated that a person will get norovirus about 5 times during their lifetime. Many people usually get sick with norovirus in cooler months, especially from November to April.

Norovirus spreads quickly. It is found in the vomit and stool of infected people. You can get it by:

- Eating food or drinking liquids that are contaminated with norovirus.

- Touching surfaces or objects with norovirus on them and then putting your hand or fingers in your mouth.

- Having direct contact with a person who is infected with noro-virus, for example, when caring for someone with norovirus or sharing foods or eating utensils with them.

People with norovirus illness are contagious from the moment they begin feeling sick and for the first few days after they recover. Some people may be contagious for even longer. There is no vaccine to prevent norovirus infection or drug to treat sick people. Learn how to protect yourself and others by following a few simple steps.

Norovirus and Food

Norovirus is the leading cause of illness and outbreaks from contaminated food in the United States. Most of these outbreaks occur in the food service settings like restaurants. Infected food workers are frequently the source of the outbreaks, often by touching ready-to-eat foods, such as raw fruits and vegetables, with their bare hands before serving them. However, any food served raw or handled after being cooked can get contaminated with norovirus.

Norovirus outbreaks can also occur from foods, such as oysters, fruits, and vegetables, that are contaminated at their source.

Protect Yourself and Others from Norovirus

- Practice proper hand hygiene. Wash your hands carefully with soap and water, especially after using the toilet and changing diapers and always before eating or preparing food. If soap and water aren't available, use an alcohol-based hand sanitizer. These alcohol-based products can help reduce the number of germs on your hands, but they are not a substitute for washing with soap and water.

- Take care in the kitchen. Carefully rinse fruits and vegetables, and cook oysters and other shellfish thoroughly before eating.

- Do not prepare food while infected. People with norovirus illness should not prepare food for others while they have symptoms and for at least 2 days after they recover from their illness.

- Clean and disinfect contaminated surfaces. After throwing up or having diarrhea, immediately clean and disinfect contaminated surfaces using a bleach-based household cleaner as directed on the product label. If no such cleaning product is available, you can use a solution made with 5 tablespoons to 1.5 cups of household bleach per 1 gallon of water.

• Wash laundry thoroughly. Immediately remove and wash clothing or linens that may be contaminated with vomit or stool. Handle soiled items carefully—try not to shake them—to avoid spreading virus. If available, wear rubber or disposable gloves while handling soiled clothing or linens and wash your hands after handling. Wash soiled items with detergent at the maximum available cycle length and then machine dry.

Common Norovirus Outbreak Settings

Norovirus spreads quickly from person to person in enclosed places like nursing homes, daycare centers, schools, and cruise ships. It is also a major cause of outbreaks in restaurants and catered-meal settings if contaminated food is served.

Many Names, Same Symptoms

You may hear norovirus illness called "food poisoning" or "stomach flu." Norovirus can cause foodborne illness, as can other germs and chemicals.

Norovirus illness is not related to the flu (influenza). Though they may share some of the same symptoms, the flu is a respiratory illness caused by influenza virus.

For most people norovirus illness is not serious and they get better in 1 to 3 days. But it can be serious in young children, the elderly, and people with other health conditions. It can lead to severe dehydration, hospitalization and even death.

Chapter 40

Pinworms

What Is a Pinworm?

A pinworm ("threadworm") is a small, thin, white roundworm (nematode) called *Enterobius vermicularis* that sometimes lives in the colon and rectum of humans. Pinworms are about the length of a staple. While an infected person sleeps, female pinworms leave the intestine through the anus and deposit their eggs on the surrounding skin.

What Are the Symptoms of a Pinworm Infection?

Pinworm infection (called enterobiasis or oxyuriasis) causes itching around the anus which can lead to difficulty sleeping and restlessness. Symptoms are caused by the female pinworm laying her eggs. Symptoms of pinworm infection usually are mild and some infected people have no symptoms.

Who Is at Risk for Pinworm Infection?

Pinworm infection occurs worldwide and affects persons of all ages and socioeconomic levels. It is the most common worm infection in the United States. Pinworm infection occurs most commonly among:

- school-aged and preschool-aged children

This chapter includes text excerpted from "Parasites-Enterobiasis (Also Known as Pinworm Infection)," Centers for Disease Control and Prevention (CDC), January 10, 2013.

- institutionalized persons

- household members and caretakers of persons with pinworm infection

Pinworm infection often occurs in more than one person in household and institutional settings. Child care centers often are the site of cases of pinworm infection.

How Is Pinworm Infection Spread?

Pinworm infection is spread by the fecal-oral route, that is by the transfer of infective pinworm eggs from the anus to someone's mouth, either directly by hand or indirectly through contaminated clothing, bedding, food or other articles.

Pinworm eggs become infective within a few hours after being deposited on the skin around the anus and can survive for 2 to 3 weeks on clothing, bedding or other objects. People become infected, usually unknowingly, by swallowing (ingesting) infective pinworm eggs that are on fingers, under fingernails or on clothing, bedding, and other contaminated objects and surfaces. Because of their small size, pinworm eggs sometimes can become airborne and ingested while breathing.

Can My Family Become Infected with Pinworms from Swimming Pools?

Pinworm infections are rarely spread through the use of swimming pools. Pinworm infections occur when a person swallows pinworm eggs picked up from contaminated surfaces or fingers. Although chlorine levels found in pools are not high enough to kill pinworm eggs, the presence of a small number of pinworm eggs in thousands of gallons of water (the amount typically found in pools) makes the chance of infection unlikely.

My Little Kids Like to Co-Bathe—Could This Be How They Are Becoming Infected?

During this treatment time and two weeks after final treatment, it is a good idea to avoid co-bathing and the reuse or sharing of washcloths. Showering may be preferred to avoid possible contamination of bath water. Careful handling and frequent changing of underclothing, night clothes, towels, and bedding can help reduce infection, reinfection, and environmental contamination with pinworm eggs. These items should be laundered in hot water, especially after each treatment of the infected person and after each usage of washcloths until infection is cleared.

Did My Pets Give Me Pinworms / Can I Give Pinworms to My Pets?

No. Humans are considered to be the only hosts of *E. vermicularis* which is also known as the human pinworm.

How Is Pinworm Infection Diagnosed?

Itching during the night in a child's perianal area strongly suggests pinworm infection. Diagnosis is made by identifying the worm or its eggs. Worms can sometimes be seen on the skin near the anus or on underclothing, pajamas or sheets about 2 to 3 hours after falling asleep.

Pinworm eggs can be collected and examined using the "tape test" as soon as the person wakes up. This "test" is done by firmly pressing the adhesive side of clear, transparent cellophane tape to the skin around the anus. The eggs stick to the tape and the tape can be placed on a slide and looked at under a microscope. Because washing/bathing or having a bowel movement can remove eggs from the skin, this test should be done as soon as the person wakes up in the morning before they wash, bathe, go to the toilet, or get dressed. The "tape test" should be done on three consecutive mornings to increase the chance of finding pinworm eggs.

Because itching and scratching of the anal area is common in pinworm infection, samples taken from under the fingernails may also contain eggs. Pinworm eggs rarely are found in routine stool or urine samples.

How Is Pinworm Infection Treated?

Pinworm can be treated with either prescription or over-the-counter medications. A healthcare provider should be consulted before treating a suspected case of pinworm infection.

Treatment involves two doses of medication with the second dose being given 2 weeks after the first dose. All household contacts and caretakers of the infected person should be treated at the same time. Reinfection can occur easily so strict observance of good hand hygiene is essential (e.g., proper handwashing, maintaining clean short fingernails, avoiding nail biting, avoiding scratching the perianal area).

Daily morning bathing and daily changing of underwear helps removes a large proportion of eggs. Showering may be preferred to avoid possible contamination of bath water. Careful handling and frequent changing of underclothing, night clothes, towels, and bedding can help reduce infection, reinfection, and environmental contamination with pinworm eggs. These items should be laundered in hot water, especially after each treatment of the infected person and after each usage of washcloths until infection is cleared.

Should Family and Other Close Contacts of Someone with Pinworm Also Be Treated for Pinworm?

Yes. The infected person and all household contacts and caretakers of the infected person should be treated at the same time.

What Should Be Done If the Pinworm Infection Occurs Again?

Reinfection occurs easily. Prevention always should be discussed at the time of treatment. Good hand hygiene is the most effective means of prevention. If pinworm infection occurs again, the infected person should be retreated with the same two-dose treatment. The infected person's household contacts and caretakers also should be treated. If pinworm infection continues to occur, the source of the infection should be sought and treated. Playmates, schoolmates, close contacts outside the home, and household members should be considered possible sources of infection. Each infected person should receive the recommended two-dose treatment.

How Can Pinworm Infection and Reinfection Be Prevented?

Strict observance of good hand hygiene is the most effective means of preventing pinworm infection. This includes washing hands with soap and warm water after using the toilet, changing diapers, and before handling food. Keep fingernails clean and short, avoid fingernail-biting, and avoid scratching the skin in the perianal area. Teach children the importance of washing hands to prevent infection.

Daily morning bathing and changing of underclothes helps remove a large proportion of pinworm eggs and can help prevent infection and reinfection. Showering may be preferred to avoid possible contamination of bath water. Careful handling (avoid shaking) and frequent laundering of underclothes, night clothes, towels, and bed sheets using hot water also helps reduce the chance of infection and reinfection by reducing environmental contamination with eggs.

Control can be difficult in child care centers and schools because the rate of reinfection is high. In institutions, mass and simultaneous treatment, repeated in 2 weeks, can be effective. Hand hygiene is the most effective method of prevention. Trimming and scrubbing the fingernails and bathing after treatment is important to help prevent reinfection and spread of pinworms.

Chapter 41

Pneumonia

Pneumonia is a general term for lung infections that can be caused by a variety of germs (viruses, bacteria, fungi, and parasites). Most cases, though, are caused by viruses, including adenoviruses, rhinovirus, influenza virus (flu), respiratory syncytial virus (RSV), human metapneumovirus, and parainfluenza virus (which causes croup).

Often, pneumonia begins after an upper respiratory tract infection (an infection of the nose and throat), with symptoms starting after 2 or 3 days of a cold or sore throat. It then moves to the lungs. Fluid, white blood cells, and debris start to gather in the air spaces of the lungs and block the smooth passage of air, making it harder for the lungs to work well.

Signs and Symptoms

Symptoms vary depending on a child's age and what caused the pneumonia, but can include:

- fever

- shaking chills

- cough

- stuffy nose

- very fast breathing (in some cases, this is the only symptom)

- breathing with grunting or wheezing sounds

- working hard to breathe; this can include flaring of the nostrils, belly breathing, or movement of the muscles between the ribs

- vomiting

- chest pain

- abdominal pain, which often happens because a child is coughing and working hard to breathe

- less activity

- loss of appetite (in older kids) or poor feeding (in infants), which may lead to dehydration

- in extreme cases, bluish or gray color of the lips and fingernails

If the pneumonia is in the lower part of the lungs near the abdomen, a child might have a fever and abdominal pain or vomiting but no breathing problems.

Kids with **pneumonia caused by bacteria** usually become sick fairly quickly, starting with a sudden high fever and unusually fast breathing. Kids with **pneumonia caused by viruses** probably will have symptoms that appear more gradually and are less severe, though wheezing can be more common.

Some symptoms give important clues about which germ is causing the pneumonia. For example, in older kids and teens, pneumonia due to *Mycoplasma* (also called walking pneumonia) is notorious for causing a sore throat, headache, and rash in addition to the usual symptoms of pneumonia.

In babies, pneumonia due to chlamydia may cause conjunctivitis (pinkeye) with only mild illness and no fever. When pneumonia is due to whooping cough (pertussis), a child may have long coughing spells, turn blue from lack of air or make the classic "whoop" sound when trying to take a breath.

Start of Symptoms

The length of time between exposure to the germ and when someone starts feeling sick varies, depending on which virus or bacteria is causing the pneumonia (for instance, 4 to 6 days for RSV, but just 18 to 72 hours for the flu).

Duration

With treatment, most types of bacterial pneumonia can be cured within 1 to 2 weeks, although walking pneumonia may take 4 to 6 weeks to go away completely. Viral pneumonia may last longer.

Contagiousness

The viruses and bacteria that cause pneumonia are contagious. They're usually found in fluid from the mouth or nose of someone who's infected, so that person can spread the illness by coughing or sneezing. Sharing drinking glasses and eating utensils, and touching the used tissues or handkerchiefs of an infected person also can spread pneumonia.

Prevention

Some types of pneumonia can be prevented by vaccines. Kids usually get routine immunizations against *Haemophilus influenzae* and whooping cough (pertussis) beginning at 2 months of age. Vaccines are now also given against the pneumococcus, a common cause of bacterial pneumonia. Children with chronic illnesses can be at special risk for certain types of pneumonia, so they might need additional vaccines or protective immune medication. ("Chronic" means an ongoing illness or one that goes away and keeps coming back.) The flu vaccine is recommended for all healthy kids ages 6 months through 19 years, but especially for kids with chronic illnesses such as heart or lung disorders or asthma.

Because they're at higher risk for serious complications, babies born prematurely may get treatments that temporarily protect against RSV because it can lead to pneumonia in younger kids. Doctors may give antibiotics to prevent pneumonia in kids who have been exposed to someone with certain types of pneumonia, such as pertussis.

Those with HIV infection might be given antibiotics to prevent pneumonia caused by *Pneumocystis jirovecii*. Antiviral medicine is now available, too, and can be used to prevent some types of viral pneumonia or to make symptoms less severe.

In general, pneumonia is not contagious, but the upper respiratory viruses and bacteria that lead to it are. So it's best to keep kids away from anyone with symptoms (stuffy or runny nose, sore throat, cough, etc.) of a respiratory infection. If someone in your home has a respiratory infection or throat infection, keep his or her drinking glasses

263

and eating utensils separate from those of other family members, and wash your hands often, especially if you are handling used tissues or dirty handkerchiefs.

When to Call the Doctor

Call your doctor immediately if your child has any of the signs and symptoms of pneumonia, but especially if he or she:

- is having trouble breathing or is breathing too fast
- has a bluish or gray color to the fingernails or lips
- has a fever of 102°F (38.9°C), or above 100.4°F (38°C) in babies younger than 6 months old

Professional Treatment

Doctors usually make a pneumonia diagnosis after a physical examination. They'll check a child's appearance, breathing pattern, and vital signs, and listen to the lungs for abnormal sounds. They might order a chest X-ray, blood tests, and (sometimes) bacterial cultures of mucus produced by coughing.

In most cases, pneumonia is treated with antibiotics taken by mouth at home. The type of antibiotic used depends on the type of pneumonia. In some cases, other members of the household might be treated with medication to prevent illness.

Children might be treated in a hospital if the pneumonia is caused by whooping cough, if another kind of bacterial pneumonia is causing a high fever and breathing problems, or if they:

- need oxygen therapy
- have a lung infection that may have spread to the bloodstream
- have a chronic illness that affects the immune system
- are vomiting so much that they cannot take medicine by mouth
- have frequent episodes of pneumonia

Hospital treatment can include intravenous (IV) antibiotics (given through a needle into a vein) and respiratory therapy (breathing treatments). More severe cases might be treated in the intensive care unit (ICU).

Home Care

- Anyone with pneumonia needs to get plenty of rest and drink lots of fluids while the body works to fight the infection.

- If your child has bacterial pneumonia and the doctor has prescribed antibiotics, give the medicine on schedule for as long as directed. This will help your child recover faster and help prevent the infection from spreading to other household members. For wheezing, the doctor might recommend using a nebulizer or an inhaler.

- Ask the doctor before you use a medicine to treat your child's cough because cough suppressants stop the lungs from clearing mucus, which isn't helpful in some types of pneumonia. Over-the-counter cough and cold medications are not recommended for any kids under 6 years old.

- Take your child's temperature at least once each morning and each evening, and call the doctor if it goes above 102°F (38.9°C) in an older infant or child, or above 100.4°F (38°C) in a baby under 6 months of age.

- Check your child's lips and fingernails to make sure they are rosy and pink. Call your doctor if they are bluish or gray, which is a sign that the lungs are not getting enough oxygen.

Chapter 42

Polio

What Is Polio?

Polio, or poliomyelitis, is a crippling and potentially deadly infectious disease. It is caused by the poliovirus. The virus spreads from person to person and can invade an infected person's brain and spinal cord, causing paralysis (can't move parts of the body).

Symptoms

Most people who get infected with poliovirus (about 72 out of 100) will not have any visible symptoms. About 1 out of 4 people with poliovirus infection will have flu-like symptoms that may include:

- Sore throat
- Fever
- Tiredness
- Nausea
- Headache
- Stomach pain

This chapter contains text excerpted from the following sources: Text beginning with the heading "What Is Polio?" is excerpted from "Global Health-Polio," Centers for Disease Control and Prevention (CDC), October 3, 2014; Text beginning with the heading "Why Get Vaccinated?" is excerpted from "Polio VIS," Centers for Disease Control and Prevention (CDC), June 13, 2014.

These symptoms usually last 2 to 5 days then go away on their own.

A smaller proportion of people with poliovirus infection will develop other more serious symptoms that affect the brain and spinal cord:

- Paresthesia (feeling of pins and needles in the legs)

- Meningitis (infection of the covering of the spinal cord and/or brain) occurs in about 1 out of 25 people with poliovirus infection

- Paralysis (can't move parts of the body) or weakness in the arms, legs, or both, occurs in about 1 out of 200 people with poliovirus infection

Paralysis is the most severe symptom associated with polio because it can lead to permanent disability and death. Between 2 and 10 out of 100 people who have paralysis from poliovirus infection die because the virus affects the muscles that help them breathe.

Even children who seem to fully recover can develop new muscle pain, weakness, or paralysis as adults, 15 to 40 years later. This is called post-polio syndrome. Note that "poliomyelitis" (or "polio" for short) is defined as the paralytic disease. So only people with the paralytic infection are considered to have the disease.

Transmission

Poliovirus only infects humans. It is very contagious and spreads through person-to-person contact. The virus lives in an infected person's throat and intestines. It enters the body through the mouth and spreads through contact with the feces (poop) of an infected person and, though less common, through droplets from a sneeze or cough. You can get infected with poliovirus if you have feces on your hands and you touch your mouth.

Also, you can get infected if you put in your mouth objects like toys that are contaminated with feces (poop). An infected person may spread the virus to others immediately before and about 1 to 2 weeks after symptoms appear. The virus can live in an infected person's feces for many weeks. It can contaminate food and water in unsanitary conditions. People who don't have symptoms can still pass the virus to others and make them sick.

Prevention

Polio vaccine protects children by preparing their bodies to fight the polio virus. Almost all children (99 children out of 100) who get all the recommended doses of vaccine will be protected from polio.

There are two types of vaccine that can prevent polio:

1. inactivated poliovirus vaccine (IPV)

2. oral poliovirus vaccine (OPV)

Only IPV has been used in the United States since 2000; OPV is still used throughout much of the world.

Why Get Vaccinated?

Vaccination can protect people from **polio**. Polio is a disease caused by a virus. It is spread mainly by person-to-person contact. It can also be spread by consuming food or drinks that are contaminated with the feces of an infected person.

Most people infected with polio have no symptoms, and many recover without complications. But sometimes people who get polio develop paralysis (cannot move their arms or legs). Polio can result in permanent disability. Polio can also cause death, usually by paralyzing the muscles used for breathing.

Polio used to be very common in the United States. It paralyzed and killed thousands of people every year before polio vaccine was introduced in 1955. There is no cure for polio infection, but it can be prevented by vaccination.

Polio has been eliminated from the United States. But it still occurs in other parts of the world. It would only take one person infected with polio coming from another country to bring the disease back here if we were not protected by vaccination. If the effort to eliminate the disease from the world is successful, some day we won't need polio vaccine. Until then, we need to keep getting our children vaccinated.

Who Should Get Polio Vaccine and When?

Inactivated Polio Vaccine (**IPV**) can prevent polio.

Children

Most people should get IPV when they are children. Doses of IPV are usually given at 2, 4, 6 to 18 months, and 4 to 6 years of age. The schedule might be different for some children (including those traveling to certain countries and those who receive IPV as part of a combination vaccine). Your healthcare provider can give you more information.

Adults

Most adults do not need IPV because they were already vaccinated against polio as children. But some adults are at higher risk and should consider polio vaccination, including:

- people traveling to certain parts of the world
- laboratory workers who might handle polio virus
- healthcare workers treating patients who could have polio

These higher-risk adults may need 1 to 3 doses of IPV, depending on how many doses they have had in the past. There are no known risks to getting IPV at the same time as other vaccines.

Some People Should Not Get IPV or Should Wait

Tell the person who is giving the vaccine:

- **If the person getting the vaccine has any severe, life-threatening allergies.**

  If you ever had a life-threatening allergic reaction after a dose of IPV, or have a severe allergy to any part of this vaccine, you may be advised not to get vaccinated. Ask your healthcare provider if you want information about vaccine components.

- **If the person getting the vaccine is not feeling well.**

- If you have a mild illness, such as a cold, you can probably get the vaccine today. If you are moderately or severely ill, you should probably wait until you recover. Your doctor can advise you.

Risks of a Vaccine Reaction

With any medicine, including vaccines, there is a chance of side effects. These are usually mild and go away on their own, but serious reactions are also possible. Some people who get IPV get a sore spot where the shot was given. IPV has not been known to cause serious problems, and most people do not have any problems with it.

Other problems that could happen after this vaccine:

- People sometimes faint after a medical procedure, including vaccination. Sitting or lying down for about 15 minutes can help prevent fainting and injuries caused by a fall. Tell your provider if you feel dizzy, or have vision changes or ringing in the ears.

- Some people get shoulder pain that can be more severe and longer-lasting than the more routine soreness that can follow injections. This happens very rarely.

- Any medication can cause a severe allergic reaction. Such reactions from a vaccine are very rare, estimated at about 1 in a million doses, and would happen within a few minutes to a few hours after the vaccination.

As with any medicine, there is a very remote chance of a vaccine causing a serious injury or death.

What If There Is a Serious Reaction?

What Should I Look For?

- Look for anything that concerns you, such as signs of a severe allergic reaction, very high fever or behavior changes.

  Signs of a **severe allergic reaction** can include hives, swelling of the face and throat, difficulty breathing, a fast heartbeat, dizziness, and weakness. These would start a few minutes to a few hours after the vaccination.

What Should I Do?

- If you think it is a **severe allergic reaction** or other emergency that can't wait, call 9-1-1 or get the person to the nearest hospital. Otherwise, call your doctor.

  Afterward, the reaction should be reported to the Vaccine Adverse Event Reporting System (VAERS). Your doctor might file this report, or you can do it yourself through the VAERS website, or by calling **1-800-822-7967.**

The National Vaccine Injury Compensation Program

Persons who believe they may have been injured by a vaccine can learn about the program and about filing a claim by calling **1-800-338-2382** or visiting the VICP website. There is a time limit to file a claim for compensation.

Chapter 43

Respiratory Syncytial Virus (RSV) Infection

Respiratory syncytial virus (RSV) is a respiratory virus that infects the lungs and breathing passages. Healthy people usually experience mild, cold-like symptoms and recover in a week or two. But RSV can be serious, especially for infants and older adults. In fact, RSV is the most common cause of bronchiolitis (inflammation of the small airways in the lung) and pneumonia in children younger than one year of age in the United States. In addition, RSV is being recognized more often as a significant cause of respiratory illness in older adults.

Infection and Incidence

RSV can cause upper respiratory infections (such as colds) and lower respiratory tract infections (such as bronchiolitis and pneumonia). In children younger than 1 year of age, RSV is the most common cause of bronchiolitis, an inflammation of the small airways in the lung, and pneumonia, an infection of the lungs. Almost all children will have had an RSV infection by their second birthday.

When infants and children are exposed to RSV for the first time:

- 25 to 40 out of 100 of them have signs or symptoms of bronchiolitis or pneumonia

---

This chapter includes text excerpted from "Respiratory Syncytial Virus Infection (RSV)," Centers for Disease Control and Prevention (CDC), November 4, 2014.

- 5 to 20 out of 1,000 will require hospitalization. Most children hospitalized for RSV infection are younger than 6 months of age

Infants and children infected with RSV usually show symptoms within 4 to 6 days of infection. Most will recover in 1 to 2 weeks. However, even after recovery, very young infants and children with weakened immune systems can continue to spread the virus for 1 to 3 weeks.

People of any age can get another RSV infection, but infections later in life are generally less severe. Premature infants, children younger than 2 years of age with congenital heart or chronic lung disease, and children with compromised (weakened) immune systems due to a medical condition or medical treatment are at highest risk for severe disease. Adults with compromised immune systems and those 65 and older are also at increased risk of severe disease.

In the United States and other areas with similar climates, RSV infections generally occur during fall, winter, and spring. The timing and severity of RSV circulation in a given community can vary from year to year.

Symptoms and Care

Symptoms of RSV infection are similar to other respiratory infections. Illness usually begins 4 to 6 days after exposure (range: 2 to 8 days) with a runny nose and decrease in appetite. Coughing, sneezing, and fever typically develop 1 to 3 days later. Wheezing may also occur. In very young infants, irritability, decreased activity, and breathing difficulties may be the only symptoms of infection. Most otherwise healthy infants infected with RSV do not need to be hospitalized. In most cases, even among those who need to be hospitalized, hospitalization usually only lasts a few days, and full recovery from illness occurs in about 1 to 2 weeks.

Visits to a healthcare provider for an RSV infection are very common. During such visits, the healthcare provider will assess the severity of disease to determine if the patient should be hospitalized. In the most severe cases of disease, infants may require supplemental oxygen, suctioning of mucus from the airways, or intubation (have breathing tubes inserted) with mechanical ventilation.

There is no specific treatment for RSV infection.

Transmission

People infected with RSV are usually contagious for 3 to 8 days. However, some infants and people with weakened immune systems can be contagious for as long as 4 weeks. Children are often exposed to and infected with RSV outside the home, such as in school or child-care. They can then transmit the virus to other members of the family.

RSV can be spread when an infected person coughs or sneezes into the air, creating virus-containing droplets that can linger briefly in the air. Other people can become infected if the droplet particles contact their nose, mouth, or eye.

Infection can also result from direct and indirect contact with nasal or oral secretions from infected people. Direct contact with the virus can occur, for example, by kissing the face of a child with RSV. Indirect contact can occur if the virus gets on an environmental surface, such as a doorknob, that is then touched by other people. Direct and indirect transmissions of virus usually occur when people touch an infectious secretion and then rub their eyes or nose.

RSV can survive on hard surfaces such as tables and crib rails for many hours. RSV typically lives on soft surfaces such as tissues and hands for shorter amounts of time.

Prevention

Researchers are working to develop RSV vaccines, but none is available yet. However, there are steps that can be taken to help prevent the spread of RSV. Specifically, people who have cold-like symptoms should:

- Cover their coughs and sneeze
- Wash their hands frequently and correctly (with soap and water for 20 seconds)
- Avoid sharing their cups and eating utensils with others
- Refrain from kissing others

In addition, cleaning contaminated surfaces (such as doorknobs) may help stop the spread of RSV. Parents should pay special attention to protecting children at high risk for developing severe disease if infected with RSV. Such children include premature infants, children younger than 2 years of age with chronic lung or heart conditions, and children with weakened immune systems.

Ideally, people with cold-like symptoms should not interact with children at high risk for severe disease. If this is not possible, these people should carefully follow the prevention steps mentioned above and wash their hands before interacting with children at high risk.

They should also refrain from kissing high-risk children while they have cold-like symptoms. When possible, limiting the time that high-risk children spend in child-care centers or other potentially contagious settings may help prevent infection and spread of the virus during the RSV season.

A drug called palivizumab is available to prevent severe RSV illness in certain infants and children who are at high risk. The drug can help prevent development of serious RSV disease, but it cannot help cure or treat children already suffering from serious RSV disease and it cannot prevent infection with RSV. If your child is at high risk for severe RSV disease, talk to your healthcare provider to see if palivizumab can be used as a preventive measure.

Chapter 44

Rubella

Rubella in the United States

Rubella is a contagious disease caused by a virus. It is also called "German measles", but it is caused by a different virus than measles. Rubella was eliminated from the United States in 2004. Rubella elimination is defined as the absence of continuous disease transmission for 12 months or more in a specific geographic area. Rubella is no longer endemic (constantly present) in the United States. However, rubella remains a problem in other parts of the world. It can still be brought into the United States by people who get infected in other countries.

Before the rubella vaccination program started in 1969, rubella was a common and widespread infection in the United States. During the last major rubella epidemic in the United States from 1964 to 1965, an estimated 12.5 million people got rubella, 11,000 pregnant women lost their babies, 2,100 newborns died, and 20,000 babies were born with congenital rubella syndrome (CRS). Once the vaccine became widely used, the number of people infected with rubella in the United States dropped dramatically.

Today, less than ten people in the United States are reported as having rubella each year. Since 2012, all rubella cases had evidence

This chapter contains text excerpted from the following sources: Text beginning with the heading "Rubella in the U.S." is excerpted from "Rubella (German Measles, Three-Day Measles)," Centers for Disease Control and Prevention (CDC), March 31, 2016; Text under the heading "Rubella and the Vaccine (Shot) to Prevent It" is excerpted from "For Parents: Vaccines for Your Children," Centers for Disease Control and Prevention (CDC), November 10, 2014.

that they were infected when they were living or traveling outside the United States. To maintain rubella elimination, it is important that children and women of childbearing age are vaccinated against rubella.

Signs and Symptoms

In children, rubella is usually mild, with few noticeable symptoms. For children who do have symptoms, a red rash is typically the first sign. The rash generally first appears on the face and then spreads to the rest of the body, and lasts about three days. Other symptoms that may occur 1 to 5 days before the rash appears include:

- a low-grade fever
- headache
- mild pinkeye (redness or swelling of the white of the eye)
- general discomfort
- swollen and enlarged lymph nodes
- cough
- runny nose

Most adults who get rubella usually have a mild illness, with low-grade fever, sore throat, and a rash that starts on the face and spreads to the rest of the body. Some adults may also have a headache, pinkeye, and general discomfort before the rash appears. About 25 to 50% of people infected with rubella will not experience any symptoms.

Complications

Up to 70% of women who get rubella may experience arthritis; this is rare in children and men. In rare cases, rubella can cause serious problems, including brain infections and bleeding problems. The most serious complication from rubella infection is the harm it can cause a pregnant woman's developing baby. If an unvaccinated pregnant woman gets infected with rubella virus she can have a miscarriage or her baby can die just after birth.

Also, she can pass the virus to her developing baby who can develop serious birth defects such as:

- heart problems
- loss of hearing and eyesight

- intellectual disability

- liver or spleen damage

Serious birth defects are more common if a woman is infected early in her pregnancy, especially in the first trimester. These severe birth defects are known as congenital rubella syndrome (CRS).

Transmission

Rubella spreads when an infected person coughs or sneezes. Also, if a woman is infected with rubella while she is pregnant, she can pass it to her developing baby and cause serious harm. A person with rubella may spread the disease to others up to one week before the rash appears, and remain contagious up to 7 days after. However, 25% to 50% of people infected with rubella do not develop a rash or have any symptoms. People infected with rubella should tell friends, family, and people they work with, especially pregnant women, if they have rubella. If your child has rubella, it's important to tell your child's school or daycare provider.

Treatment

There is no specific medicine to treat rubella or make the disease go away faster. In many cases, symptoms are mild. For others, mild symptoms can be managed with bed rest and medicines for fever, such as acetaminophen. If you are concerned about your symptoms or your child's symptoms, contact your doctor.

Rubella and the Vaccine (Shot) to Prevent It

The best way to protect against rubella is by getting the measles-mumps-rubella shot (called the MMR shot). Doctors recommend that all children get the MMR shot.

Why Should My Child Get the MMR Vaccine?

The MMR shot:

- Protects your child from rubella, a potentially serious disease (and also protects against measles and mumps).

- Prevents your child from spreading rubella to a pregnant woman, whose unborn baby could develop serious birth defects or die if his mother gets rubella.

- Prevents your child from getting a rash and fever from rubella.

- Keeps your child from missing school or childcare (and keeps you from missing work to care for your sick child).

Is the MMR Shot Safe?

Yes. The MMR shot is very safe, and it is effective at preventing measles, mumps, and rubella. Vaccines, like any medicine, can have side effects. Most children who get the MMR shot have no side effects.

What Are the Side Effects?

Most children don't have any side effects from the shot. When side effects do occur, they are usually very mild, such as a fever or rash. More serious side effects are rare. These may include high fever that could cause a seizure (in about 1 out of every 3,000 people who get the shot) and temporary pain and stiffness in joints (mostly in teens and adults).

Is There a Link between the MMR Shot and Autism?

No. Scientists in the United States and other countries have carefully studied the MMR shot. None has found a link between autism and the MMR shot.

Is It Serious?

Rubella is usually mild in children. Complications are not common, but they occur more often in adults. In rare cases, rubella can cause serious problems, including brain infections and bleeding problems. Rubella is most dangerous for a pregnant woman's unborn baby. Infection during pregnancy can cause miscarriage, or birth defects like deafness, blindness, intellectual disability, and heart defects. As many as 85 out of 100 babies born to mothers who had rubella in the first 3 months of pregnancy will have a birth defect.

How Does Rubella Spread?

Rubella spreads when an infected person coughs or sneezes. The disease is most contagious when the infected person has a rash. But it can spread up to seven days before the rash appears. People without symptoms can still spread rubella.

Chapter 45

Scabies

Scabies is a parasitic infection of the skin. It is caused by the mite, *Sarcoptes scabiei var. hominis*. Averaging 0.3 x 0.35 mm, female scabies mites cannot be seen with the naked eye. This round, eight-legged mite burrows into the host's superficial skin, laying 1–3 eggs per day during its 30–60 day lifetime. On average, a typical patient harbors 12 minutes at a time. Host sensitization to the scabies mite, eggs, and excreta develops over 2–6 weeks. Crusted scabies, also known as Norwegian scabies, is an aggressive infestation of *Sarcoptes scabiei var. hominis*. Due to host immunodeficiency, malnourishment, and/or debilitation, thousands of mites are present in the patient's skin. In a healthy patient, the mite can survive up to 3 days off the host. In contrast, mites in crusted scabies can survive up to 7 days off the host.

Clinical Presentation

Typical Infestation: After acquiring the scabies mite, a patient (without prior infestation) typically develops pruritus after 2–6 weeks.

This chapter contains text excerpted from the following sources: Text in this chapter begins with excerpts from "Scabies Protocol," Federal Bureau of Prisons (BOP), October 2014; Text beginning with the heading "Life Cycle" is excerpted from "Scabies," Centers for Disease Control and Prevention (CDC), November 29, 2013.

Previously exposed patients develop pruritus within 24–48 hours of re-infestation.

Typical lesions are symmetrically distributed on the hands (especially the interdigital spaces), wrists, elbows, waist, legs, and feet. In men, lesions are frequently around the beltline, thigh, and external genitalia. In women, they are often located on the areola, nipples, buttocks, and vulvar areas.

Burrows can be observed at these sites; however, many patients will not have observable burrows. Burrows appear as 1–10 mm, flesh-colored to erythematous, wavy, raised, and threadlike lines on the skin surface. Excoriations are commonly found at these sites and may be the only clinical findings. The mites may be found under the distal fingernails secondary to scratching. Pruritus is worse at night and after a hot shower or bath. Lesions can become secondarily infected and present as pustules or cellulitis.

Crusted Scabies: The usual crusted scabies patient is bedridden or with severe disability or immunosuppression. Pruritus is not present or is a minor concern. The lesions are commonly found on the hands and extremities, but can be located anywhere on the body. Unlike a typical scabies infestation, crusted scabies can involve the face and scalp. The lesions are thickened, scaly crusts that may encompass a large body surface area. Due to the patient's decreased immunity, impaired sensation, and/or physical inability to scratch, the scabies mites number in the thousands.

Diagnosis

The rendering of a presumptive scabies diagnosis is often based on the following: clinical suspicion, severe pruritus, typical distribution of lesions, and response to treatment.

If available, microscopic examination of mineral oil preparations can identify the mite. This is accomplished by applying mineral oil and gently scraping the suspected lesions with a surgical blade. The collected skin debris is placed on a microscope slide with a coverslip and examined under low power. Identification of the mites confirms the diagnosis, while the eggs or scybala (fecal pellets) provide indirect confirmation. A skin biopsy is rarely helpful in diagnosing scabies, but may be considered in unusual cases. Given the consequences of scabies in the correctional setting and the minimal risks associated with treatment, presumptive treatment should be strongly considered if scabies is in the differential diagnosis.

Mode of Transmission

- **Typical Scabies Infestation:** Direct skin-to-skin contact is needed for transmission, and 15–20 minutes of skin-to-skin contact is generally required. Overcrowding and sexual contact increases transmission. Sharing of clothing or bedding and towels can transmit the mite—especially if used immediately after the infested person. Asymptomatic patients, or patients with minimal symptoms, can unknowingly transmit mites.

- **Crusted Scabies:** In contrast to typical scabies infestations, persons with crusted scabies are highly contagious because of the large number of mites, skin sloughing, and increased mite survival. With crusted scabies, there is a much higher risk of transmission of scabies from contaminated clothing, bedding, and towels. Close contacts and staff taking care of patients with crusted scabies are at higher risk of acquiring scabies than in the case of a typical scabies infestation.

Infectious Period

Scabies remains communicable until all mites and eggs are eradicated from the host. In the absence of treatment, individuals can remain infectious for prolonged periods. Fomites can be a source of infection because the mites can live up to 3 days off the host (up to 7 days, in the case of crusted scabies).

Treatment

Typical Scabies Infestation

Inmates with a typical infestation of scabies should be isolated in a single cell until 24 hours after treatment. Topical permethrin 5% cream is a highly efficacious, U.S. Food and Drug Administration (FDA)-approved scabicide that should be applied contiguously from the neck to the toes. Clothing, linens, and towels should be washed at the same time that treatment is applied, in order to prevent reinfection. After leaving the medication on the body for 8–14 hours, the inmate should be allowed to shower off the cream and put on clean clothes. Two separate applications, 7 days apart, are recommended—with clothing, linens, and towels cleaned in the same time-frame as treatment.

- The most common cause of treatment failure is the failure to adequately apply the scabicide. Therefore, it is emphasized that the patient's application of the scabicide should be directly observed.

Most patients have significant improvement within 3 days of treatment. Inmates treated for scabies should be advised that the rash and itching may persist for 2–4 weeks, and that antipruritic medications may help minimize this discomfort.

Symptoms or signs of scabies that persist beyond 2 weeks can be attributed to several factors:

- Misapplication of scabicide

- Reinfection from other inmates, which may be evidenced by new burrows

- Exposure to infected fomites (clothing or bed linens)

- Host allergic dermatitis

The healthcare provider may consider an alternative diagnosis if an inmate is still symptomatic after two completed treatments.

Crusted (Norwegian) Scabies

Any case of crusted scabies requires aggressive treatment, infection control measures, and long term surveillance. Because crusted scabies is highly communicable, strict isolation and contact precautions are critical. A treatment regimen of permethrin should be initiated, including application of the cream to the face and scalp.

In addition, oral ivermectin is strongly recommended for treatment of crusted scabies. It is administered as a single dose, with a repeat dose of both permethrin and ivermectin in 7 days. Isolation is continued for at least 7 days—until after the second treatment and until after resolution of scabies-related skin lesions (i.e., burrows, new bumpy rashes, scales, crusts, and excoriations). Inmates with crusted scabies shall be provided with clean linens and clothing each day while isolated (in order to remove contaminated skin crusts and scales that contain many mites).

Life Cycle

Sarcoptes scabiei undergoes four stages in its life cycle: egg, larva, nymph and adult. Females deposit 2–3 eggs per day as they burrow under the skin. Eggs are oval and 0.10 to 0.15 mm in length and hatch in 3 to 4 days.

After the eggs hatch, the larvae migrate to the skin surface and burrow into the intact stratum corneum to construct almost invisible, short burrows called molting pouches. The larval stage, which emerges from the eggs, has only 3 pairs of legs and lasts about 3 to 4 days. After the larvae molt, the resulting nymphs have 4 pairs of legs. This form molts into slightly larger nymphs before molting into adults. Larvae and nymphs may often be found in molting pouches or in hair follicles and look similar to adults, only smaller. Adults are round, sac-like eyeless mites. Females are 0.30 to 0.45 mm long and 0.25 to 0.35 mm wide, and males are slightly more than half that size.

Mating occurs after the active male penetrates the molting pouch of the adult female. Mating takes place only once and leaves the female fertile for the rest of her life. Impregnated females leave their molting pouches and wander on the surface of the skin until they find a suitable site for a permanent burrow. While on the skin's surface, mites hold onto the skin using sucker-like pulvilli attached to the two most anterior pairs of legs. When the impregnated female mite finds a suitable location, it begins to make its characteristic serpentine burrow, laying eggs in the process.

After the impregnated female burrows into the skin, she remains there and continues to lengthen her burrow and lay eggs for the rest of her life (1–2 months). Under the most favorable of conditions, about 10% of her eggs eventually give rise to adult mites. Males are rarely seen; they make temporary shallow pits in the skin to feed until they locate a female's burrow and mate.

Transmission occurs primarily by the transfer of the impregnated females during person-to-person, skin-to-skin contact. Occasionally transmission may occur via fomites (e.g., bedding or clothing). Human scabies mites often are found between the fingers and on the wrists.

Geographic Distribution

Scabies mites are distributed worldwide, affecting all races and socioeconomic classes in all climates.

Chapter 46

Shigellosis

What Is Shigella?

Shigellosis is a diarrheal disease caused by a group of bacteria called *Shigella*. *Shigella* causes about 500,000 cases of diarrhea in the United States annually. There are four different species of Shigella:

- *Shigella sonnei* (the most common species in the United States)
- *Shigella flexneri*
- *Shigella boydii*
- *Shigella dysenteriae*

S. dysenteriae and *S. boydii* are rare in the United States, though they continue to be important causes of disease in the developing world. *Shigella dysenteriae* type 1 can cause deadly epidemics.

What Are the Symptoms of Shigella?

Symptoms of shigellosis typically start 1–2 days after exposure and include:

- Diarrhea (sometimes bloody)
- Fever

This chapter includes text excerpted from "Shigella–Shigellosis," Centers for Disease Control and Prevention (CDC), April 2, 2015.

- Abdominal pain

- Tenesmus (a painful sensation of needing to pass stools even when bowels are empty)

How Long after Infection Do Symptoms Appear?

Symptoms of shigellosis generally begin 1 to 2 days after becoming infected with the bacteria.

How Long Will Symptoms Last?

In persons with healthy immune systems, symptoms usually last about 5 to 7 days. Persons with diarrhea usually recover completely, although it may be several months before their bowel habits are entirely normal. Once someone has had shigellosis, they are not likely to get infected with that specific type again for at least several years. However, they can still get infected with other types of *Shigella*.

Can There Be Any Complications from Shigella Infections?

Possible complications from *Shigella* infections include:

- **Post-infectious arthritis**. About 2% of persons who are infected with *Shigella flexneri* later develop pains in their joints, irritation of the eyes, and painful urination. This is called post-infectious arthritis. It can last for months or years, and can lead to chronic arthritis. Post-infectious arthritis is caused by a reaction to *Shigella* infection that happens only in people who are genetically predisposed to it.

- **Blood stream infections**. Although rare, blood stream infections are caused either by *Shigella* organisms or by other germs in the gut that get into the bloodstream when the lining of the intestines is damaged during shigellosis. Blood stream infections are most common among patients with weakened immune systems, such as those with HIV, cancer, or severe malnutrition.

- **Seizures**. Generalized seizures have been reported occasionally among young children with shigellosis, and usually resolve without treatment. Children who experience seizures while infected with *Shigella* typically have a high fever or abnormal blood electrolytes (salts), but it is not well understood why the seizures occur.

• **Hemolytic-uremic syndrome or HUS**. HUS occurs when bacteria enter the digestive system and produce a toxin that destroys red blood cells. Patients with HUS often have bloody diarrhea. HUS is only associated with Shiga-toxin producing *Shigella*, which is found most commonly in *Shigella dysenteriae*.

How Can Shigella Infections Be Diagnosed?

Many different kinds of germs can cause diarrhea, so establishing the cause will help guide treatment. Healthcare providers can order laboratory tests to identify *Shigella* in the stools of an infected person. The laboratory can also do special tests to determine which antibiotics, if any, would be best to treat the infection.

How Can Shigella Infections Be Treated?

Diarrhea caused by *Shigella* usually resolves without antibiotic treatment in 5 to 7 days. People with mild shigellosis may need only fluids and rest. Bismuth subsalicylate (e.g., Pepto-Bismol®) may be helpful but medications that cause the gut to slow down, such as loperamide (e.g., Imodium®) or diphenoxylate with atropine (e.g., Lomotil®), should be avoided. Antibiotics are useful for severe cases of shigellosis because they can reduce the duration of symptoms.

However, *Shigella* is often resistant to antibiotics. If you require antibiotic treatment for shigellosis, your healthcare provider can culture your stool and determine which antibiotics are likely to work. Tell your healthcare provider if you do not get better within a couple of days after starting antibiotics. He or she can do additional tests to learn whether your strain of *Shigella* is resistant to the antibiotic you are taking.

Is Antibiotic Resistance a Problem with Shigella?

In 2013, Centers for Disease Control and Prevention (CDC) declared antibiotic-resistant *Shigella* an urgent threat in the United States. Resistance to traditional first-line antibiotics like ampicillin and trimethoprim-sulfamethoxazole is common among *Shigella* globally, and resistance to some other important antibiotics is increasing.

While travelers to the developing world are at particular risk of acquiring antibiotic-resistant shigellosis, outbreaks of shigellosis resistant to ciprofloxacin or azithromycin—the two antibiotics most commonly used to treat shigellosis—have been reported recently within the United States and other industrialized countries. About 27,000 *Shigella* infections in the United States every year are resistant to one or both of these antibiotics. When pathogens are resistant to common antibiotic medications, patients may need to be treated with medications that may be less effective, but more toxic and expensive.

How Will I Know If I Have an Antibiotic-Resistant Shigella Infection?

Shigella infections are diagnosed through laboratory testing of stool specimens (feces). Healthcare providers can order tests to check which antibiotics are likely to help treat a particular patient's infection. If you were treated with antibiotics for shigellosis but do not feel better within a couple of days, tell your healthcare provider. You may need additional tests to check whether your *Shigella* strain is resistant to the antibiotics.

What Should I Do If I Have an Antibiotic-Resistant Shigella Infection?

Please follow the advice of your healthcare provider. If you do not feel better within a couple of days after beginning treatments, tell your healthcare provider. Protect others by washing your hands carefully with soap after using the toilet, and wait until your diarrhea has stopped before preparing food for others, swimming or having sex.

How Can We Reduce the Spread of Antibiotic-Resistant Shigella?

Reducing the spread of antibiotic-resistant *Shigella* requires a multi-pronged approach:

- preventing infections
- tracking resistance
- improving antibiotic use
- developing new treatments

How Is Shigella Spread?

Shigella germs are present in the stools of infected persons while they have diarrhea and for up to a week or two after the diarrhea has gone away. *Shigella* is very contagious; exposure to even a tiny amount of contaminated fecal matter—too small to see—can cause infection. Transmission of *Shigella* occurs when people put something in their mouths or swallow something that has come into contact with stool of a person infected with *Shigella*. This can happen when:

- Contaminated hands touch your food or mouth. Hands can become contaminated through a variety of activities, such as touching surfaces (e.g., toys, bathroom fixtures, changing tables, diaper pails) that have been contaminated by stool from an infected person. Hands can also become contaminated with *Shigella* while changing the diaper of an infected child or caring for an infected person.

- Eating food contaminated with *Shigella*. Food may become contaminated if food handlers have shigellosis. Produce can become contaminated if growing fields contain human sewage. Flies can breed in infected feces and then contaminate food when they land on it.

- Swallowing recreational (for example, lake or river water while swimming) or drinking water that was contaminated by infected fecal matter.

- Exposure to feces through sexual contact.

How Can I Reduce My Risk of Getting Shigellosis?

Currently, there is no vaccine to prevent shigellosis. However, you can reduce your risk of getting shigellosis by:

- Carefully washing your hands with soap during key times:
  - Before eating.
  - After changing a diaper or helping to clean another person who has defecated (pooped).

- If you care for a child in diapers who has shigellosis, promptly discard the soiled diapers in a lidded, lined garbage can, and wash your hands and the child's hands carefully with soap and water immediately after changing the diapers. Any leaks or spills of diaper contents should be cleaned up immediately.

- Avoid swallowing water from ponds, lakes, or untreated swimming pools.

- When traveling internationally, follow food and water precautions strictly and wash hands with soap frequently.

- Avoid sexual activity with those who have diarrhea or who recently recovered from diarrhea.

I Was Diagnosed with Shigellosis. What Can I Do to Avoid Giving It to Other People?

- Wash your hands with soap carefully and frequently, especially after using the toilet.

- Do not prepare food for others while you are sick. After you get better, wash your hands carefully with soap before preparing food for others.

- For those who work in healthcare, food service, or childcare facilities should not prepare or handle food for others until their local health department has authorized them to return to work. Improvements in worker sick leave policies and providing adequate hygiene facilities and education for food service workers may prevent shigellosis caused by contaminated foods.

- Avoid swimming until you have fully recovered.

- Don't have sex until several days after you no longer have diarrhea.

My Child Was Diagnosed with Shigellosis. How Can I Keep Others from Catching It?

- Supervise handwashing of toddlers and small children after they use the toilet. Wash infants' hands with soap and water after diaper changes.

- Dispose of soiled diapers properly, and clean diaper changing areas after using them.

- Keep the child out of childcare and group play settings while ill with diarrhea, and follow the guidance of your local health department about returning your child to his or her childcare facility.

- Avoid taking your child swimming or to group water play venues until after he or she has fully recovered.

Should an Infected Person Be Excluded from School or Work?

School and work exclusion policies differ by local jurisdiction. Check with your local or state health department to learn more about the laws where you live. It is critical to practice good hand-washing after changing diapers, after using the toilet, and before preparing or eating food to prevent the spread of these and many other infections.

What Else Can Be Done to Prevent Shigellosis?

- Providing municipal water service, this may be lacking in many lower income countries. Making municipal water supplies available and safe and treating sewage are highly effective prevention measures that have been in place for many years.

- Following these guidelines to make your food safer to eat. People with shigellosis should not prepare food or drinks for others until they are well. Food service workers should not prepare or handle food for others until their local health department has authorized them to return to work. Improvements in worker sick leave policies and providing adequate hygiene facilities and education for food service workers may prevent shigellosis caused by contaminated foods.

- At swimming beaches, providing enough bathrooms and hand-washing stations with soap near the swimming area helps keep the water from becoming contaminated.

What Can Be Done If an Outbreak of Shigella Occurs in the Childcare Setting?

- Exclude any child with diarrhea from the childcare setting until the diarrhea has stopped.
  - Children who have recently recovered from shigellosis can be grouped together in one classroom (cohorted) to minimize exposing uninfected children and staff to Shigella.
- Assign separate staff to change diapers and prepare or serve food.
- Reassign adults with diarrhea to jobs that minimize opportunities for spreading infection (for example, administrative work instead of food preparation).

- Establish, implement, and enforce policies on water-play and swimming that:

  - Exclude children ill with diarrhea from water-play and swimming activities.

  - Exclude children diagnosed with Shigella from water-play and swimming activities for an additional week after their diarrhea has resolved.

  - Have children and staff wash their hands before using water tables.

  - Have children and staff shower with soap before swimming in the water.

  - If a child is too young to shower independently, have staff wash the child, particularly the rear end, with soap and water.

  - Take frequent bathroom breaks or check their diapers often.

  - Change children's diapers in a diaper-changing area or bathroom and not by the water.

  - Discourage children from getting the water in their mouths and swallowing it.

  - Prohibit the use of temporary inflatable or rigid fill-and-drain swimming pools and slides because they can spread germs in childcare facilities.

People at Risk

- **Young children** are the most likely to get shigellosis, but people from all age groups are affected. Many outbreaks are related to childcare settings and schools, and illness commonly spreads from young children to their family members and others in their communities because it is so contagious.

- **Gay, bisexual, and other men who have sex with men (MSM)**† are more likely to acquire shigellosis than the general adult population. Shigella passes from stools [poop] or soiled fingers of one person to the mouth of another person, which can happen during sexual activity. Many shigellosis outbreaks among MSM have been reported in the United States, Canada, Tokyo, and Europe since 1999.

- **HIV-infected persons** can have more severe and prolonged shigellosis, including having the infection spread into the blood, which can be life-threatening.

- Large outbreaks of *Shigella* have occurred in **traditionally observant Jewish communities**. Documented outbreaks in traditionally observant Jewish communities often begin in child-care settings and spread within and between households during social gatherings.

- **Travelers** to developing countries may be more likely to get shigellosis, and to become infected with strains of *Shigella* that are resistant to important antibiotics. Travelers may be exposed through contaminated food, water (both drinking and recreational water), or surfaces. Travelers can protect themselves by strictly following food and water precautions, and washing hands with soap frequently.

† The term men who have sex with men is used in CDC surveillance systems because it indicates the behaviors that transmit *Shigella* infection, rather than how individuals self-identify in terms of their sexuality.

Statistics

Estimates

Every year, there are about 500,000 cases of shigellosis in the United States. Shigellosis does not have a marked seasonality, likely reflecting the importance of person-to-person transmission.

Incidence

In 2013, the average annual incidence of shigellosis in the United States was 4.82 cases per 100,000 individuals.

Trends

Shigella infections have not declined appreciably over the past ten years. The incidence rate of infection with Shigella sonnei decreased from 2008 through 2011, but increased in 2012.

Antibiotic Resistance

Resistance to traditional first-line drugs such as ampicillin and trimethoprim-sulfamethoxazole is common. Healthcare providers now rely on alternative drugs like ciprofloxacin and azithromycin to treat infections. However, strains of *Shigella* resistant to these antibiotics are becoming more common in the United States. Infections caused by antibiotic-resistant *Shigella* strains can last longer than infections caused by antibiotic-susceptible bacteria (bacteria that can be treated effectively with antibiotics). Because initial treatment can fail, costs are expected to be higher for resistant infections.

Chapter 47

Shingles

Almost 1 out of every 3 people in the United States will develop shingles, also known as zoster or herpes zoster, in their lifetime. There are an estimated 1 million cases of shingles each year in this country. Anyone who has recovered from chickenpox may develop shingles; even children can get shingles. However the risk of shingles increases as you get older. About half of all cases occur in men and women 60 years old or older.

Some people have a greater risk of getting shingles. This includes people who:

- have medical conditions that keep their immune systems from working properly, such as certain cancers like leukemia and lymphoma, and human immunodeficiency virus (HIV)

- receive immunosuppressive drugs, such as steroids and drugs that are given after organ transplantation

People who develop shingles typically have only one episode in their lifetime. However, a person can have a second or even a third episode.

Cause

Shingles is caused by the *Varicella zoster* virus (VZV), the same virus that causes chickenpox. After a person recovers from chickenpox,

This chapter includes text excerpted from "Shingles (Herpes Zoster)," Centers for Disease Control and Prevention (CDC), May 1, 2014.

the virus stays dormant (inactive) in the body. For reasons that are not fully known, the virus can reactivate years later, causing shingles. Shingles is not caused by the same virus that causes genital herpes, a sexually transmitted disease.

Signs and Symptoms

Shingles is a painful rash that develops on one side of the face or body. The rash forms blisters that typically scab over in 7 to 10 days and clears up within 2 to 4 weeks. Before the rash develops, people often have pain, itching or tingling in the area where the rash will develop. This may happen anywhere from 1 to 5 days before the rash appears.

Most commonly, the rash occurs in a single stripe around either the left or the right side of the body. In other cases, the rash occurs on one side of the face. In rare cases (usually among people with weakened immune systems), the rash may be more widespread and look similar to a chickenpox rash. Shingles can affect the eye and cause loss of vision.

Other symptoms of shingles can include:

• Fever

• Headache

• Chills

• Upset stomach

Transmission

Shingles cannot be passed from one person to another. However, the virus that causes shingles, the *Varicella zoster* virus, can be spread from a person with active shingles to another person who has never had chickenpox. In such cases, the person exposed to the virus might develop chickenpox, but they would not develop shingles.

The virus is spread through direct contact with fluid from the rash blisters caused by shingles. A person with active shingles can spread the virus when the rash is in the blister-phase. A person is not infectious before the blisters appear. Once the rash has developed crusts, the person is no longer contagious. Shingles is less contagious than chickenpox and the risk of a person with shingles spreading the virus is low if the rash is covered.

If you have shingles:

• Keep the rash covered.

- Avoid touching or scratching the rash.
- Wash your hands often to prevent the spread of *Varicella zoster* virus.
- Until your rash has developed crusts, avoid contact with:
- pregnant women who have never had chickenpox or the chickenpox vaccine
- premature or low birth weight infants
- people with weakened immune systems, such as people receiving immunosuppressive medications or undergoing chemotherapy, organ transplant recipients, and people with human immunodeficiency virus (HIV) infection

Prevention

The only way to reduce the risk of developing shingles and the long-term pain from postherpetic neuralgia (PHN) is to get vaccinated. Centers for Disease Control and Prevention (CDC) recommends that people aged 60 years and older get one dose of shingles vaccine. Shingles vaccine is available in pharmacies and doctor's offices. Talk with your healthcare professional if you have questions about shingles vaccine.

Treatment

Several antiviral medicines—acyclovir, valacyclovir, and famciclovir—are available to treat shingles. These medicines will help shorten the length and severity of the illness. But to be effective, they must be started as soon as possible after the rash appears. Thus, people who have or think they might have shingles should call their healthcare provider as soon as possible to discuss treatment options. Analgesics (pain medicine) may help relieve the pain caused by shingles. Wet compresses, calamine lotion, and colloidal oatmeal baths may help relieve some of the itching.

Chapter 48

Staph Infections: Group A

Chapter Contents

Section 48.1

Staphylococcal Infections

Amy was used to the occasional outbreak of zits, but the bump on her neck was different. It started out fairly small and itchy, but now was big and red and sore. Amy's mom took her to the doctor and they were surprised to hear that the bump was a boil, an infection usually caused by **staph** bacteria.

What Is a Staph Infection?

Staph is the shortened name for **Staphylococcus**, a type of bacteria. These bacteria can live harmlessly on many skin surfaces, especially around the nose, mouth, genitals, and anus. But when the skin is punctured or broken for any reason, staph bacteria can enter the wound and cause an infection. The staph family of bacteria has more than 30 species, which can cause different kinds of illnesses. For example, one kind of staph can cause urinary tract infections. But most staph infections are caused by the species *Staphylococcus aureus (S. aureus)*.

S. aureus most commonly causes skin infections like folliculitis, boils, impetigo, and cellulitis that are limited to a small area of a person's skin. *S. aureus* can also release toxins (poisons) that may lead to illnesses like food poisoning or toxic shock syndrome.

How Do People Get Staph Infections?

In teens, most staph infections are minor skin infections. People with skin problems like burns or eczema may be more likely to get staph skin infections. People can get staph infections from contaminated objects, but staph bacteria often spread through skin-to-skin contact—the bacteria can be spread from one area of the body to another if someone touches the infected area. Staph infections can spread from person to person in group living situations (like college dorms). Usually this happens when people with skin infections share personal things like bed linens, towels, or clothing. Warm, humid environments can contribute to staph infections, so excessive sweating can increase someone's chances of developing an infection.

Serious Staph Infections

Infections caused by *S. aureus* can occasionally become serious. This happens when the bacteria move from a break in the skin into the bloodstream. This can lead to infections in other parts of the body, such as the lungs, bones, joints, heart, blood, and central nervous system. Staph infections in other parts of the body are less common than staph skin infections. They are more likely in people whose immune systems have been weakened by another disease—or by certain medications, like chemotherapy for cancer.

Sometimes, patients having surgery may get more serious types of staph infections. The good news is that hospital staff take many steps to avoid infection in someone having surgery. That's why they carefully clean the area being operated on, use sterile equipment, and sometimes give a person antibiotics. You may also have heard about **methicillin-resistant** *Staphylococcus aureus* or MRSA for short. MRSA is a type of staph that has built up a resistance to the antibiotics usually used to treat staph infections. Although MRSA can be harder to treat, in most cases the infection heals with the right treatment.

What Are the Signs of a Staph Skin Infection?

Staph skin infections show up in lots of different ways. Some of the more common conditions often caused by *S. aureus* skin infections are:

- **Folliculitis** is an infection of the hair follicles, the tiny pockets under the skin where hair shafts (strands) grow. In folliculitis, tiny white-headed pimples appear at the base of hair shafts, sometimes with a small red area around each pimple. This happens often where people shave or have irritated skin from rubbing against clothing.

- A **furuncle**, commonly known as a boil, is a swollen, red, painful lump in the skin, usually due to an infected hair follicle. The lump usually fills with pus, growing larger and more painful until it ruptures and drains. Furuncles often begin as folliculitis and then worsen. They most often appear on the face, neck, buttocks, armpits, and inner thighs, where small hairs can be irritated. A cluster of several furuncles is called a **carbuncle**. A person with a carbuncle may feel ill and feverish.

• **Impetigo** is a superficial skin infection that mostly happens in young children, but it can sometimes affect teens and adults. Most impetigo infections affect the face, hands, or feet. An impetigo skin infection begins as a small blister or pimple, and then develops a honey-colored crust. Impetigo doesn't usually cause pain or fever, although the blisters may itch and can be spread to other parts of the body by scratching.

• **Cellulitis** is an infection involving the skin and areas of tissue below the skin surface. It begins as a small area of redness, pain, swelling, and warmth on the skin. As this area begins to spread, a person may feel feverish and ill. Cellulitis can affect any area of the body, but it's most common on the legs.

• A **hordeolum**, commonly known as a stye (or sty), is a red, painful bump on the eyelid. It develops when glands connected to the base of the eyelash become swollen and irritated. A person with a stye will usually notice a red, warm, uncomfortable swelling near the edge of the eyelid.

• Many of these staph infections are minor and can be treated at home. If a minor infection gets worse—for example, you start feeling feverish or ill or the area spreads and gets very red or and hot—it's a good idea to see a doctor.

• **Wound infections** generally show up 2 or more days after the injury or surgery. The signs of a wound infection (redness, pain, swelling, and warmth) are similar to those found in cellulitis. A person might have fever and feel sick in general. Pus or a cloudy fluid can drain from the wound and a yellow crust (like that in impetigo) can develop. If you think you have a wound infection after surgery, or you have a serious wound that seems to be infected, call your doctor.

Can I Prevent a Staph Skin Infection?

Staphylococcus aureus bacteria are everywhere. Many healthy people carry staph bacteria without getting sick. Cleanliness and good hygiene are the best way to protect yourself against getting staph (and other) infections—including MRSA.

You can help prevent staph skin infections by washing your hands often and by bathing or showering daily. Make sure to clean and cover areas of injured skin (such as cuts, scrapes, eczema, and rashes caused by allergic reactions or poison ivy). Use any antibiotic ointments or other treatments that your doctor suggests. If someone in your family has a staph infection, don't share towels, sheets, or clothing until the infection has been fully treated.

If you develop a staph infection, you can prevent spreading it to other parts of your body by being careful not to touch the infected skin, keeping it covered whenever possible, and using a towel only once when you clean the area. Make sure to wash the towel in hot water afterwards or use disposable towels.

What Can I Do to Feel Better?

How long it takes for a staph skin infection to heal depends on the type of infection and whether a person gets treatment for it. A boil, for example, may take 10 to 20 days to heal without treatment, but treatment may speed up this process. Most styes, on the other hand, go away on their own within several days. To help relieve pain from a skin infection, and to help pus drain out, try soaking the affected area in warm water or applying warm, moist washcloths. Use a clean washcloth each time—wash used cloths in soap and hot water and dry them fully in a clothes dryer. You can also apply a heating pad or a hot water bottle to the skin for about 20 minutes, three or four times a day.

Pain relievers like acetaminophen or ibuprofen can help reduce pain until the infection subsides. For some skin infections, it can also help to wash the area with an antibacterial cleanser and apply an antibiotic ointment. Cover the skin with a clean dressing. A stye can be treated using warm compresses over the eye (with the eye closed) three or four times a day. Be sure you always use a clean washcloth each time. Occasionally, a stye will require a topical antibiotic. See your doctor if a stye doesn't go away in a few days.

If you get a staph infection on skin areas that you normally shave, avoid shaving, if possible, until the infection clears up. If you do have to shave the area, use a clean disposable razor or clean your electric razor after each use.

Section 48.2

Staphylococcus aureus *and Pregnancy*

"*Staphylococcus aureus* and Pregnancy,"
© 2017 Omnigraphics. Reviewed August 2016.

Staphylococcus aureus

Staphylococcus aureus is a type of bacteria that causes a condition known as staph infection. These bacteria are usually found on the surface of the skin or in the nasal passages and ears of even a healthy person and do not generally cause any harm. But an infection can occur if the skin is cut or wounded and the bacteria enter the wound, making it inflamed, red, and painful. These bacteria are quite hardy in nature and can survive for some time on hard surfaces, withstanding dryness, high levels of salt, and extremes of temperature until a person comes in contact with them. Approximately 500,000 patients in American hospitals are affected annually by *Staphylococcus*, making it one of the primary causes of infection after injury or surgery.

Symptoms of Staph Infection

Staph infection often affects the skin, in which case some of its symptoms include:

- large blisters that ooze fluids (impetigo)

- redness and swelling in layers of skin (cellulitis)

- abscesses on the skin

Staph infection can also be transmitted through food. The symptoms in such cases include:

- nausea and vomiting

- dehydration

- low blood pressure

- diarrhea

Severe symptoms may occur when the bacteria enter the bloodstream. Toxins produced by strains of staph bacteria may develop such symptoms as:

- high fever
- low blood pressure
- rashes on the palms and soles
- muscle aches
- abdominal pain
- diarrhea
- confusion

Staph infection may also cause coughing because of infection in the lungs (pneumonia).

Treatment for Staph Infection

Staph infection is treated mainly with antibiotics, such as methicillin, penicillin, oxacillin, and amoxicillin. For staph skin infection, treatment would likely also include draining the abscesses.

Methicillin-Resistant Staphylococcus aureus (MRSA)

Methicillin-resistant *Staphylococcus aureus* (MRSA) is a variant that resists the antibiotic methicillin. Improper or overuse of antibiotics can increase the chances of MRSA bacteria developing. It is more difficult to treat than normal staph bacteria since commonly used antibiotics for staph infection may not work for MRSA infection.

Transmission of MRSA

MRSA, which in recent years has become a major health concern, is transmitted through physical contact or by touching objects that carry the bacteria. It is generally classified into two types:

- **Hospital-Acquired Methicillin-resistant *Staphylococcus aureus* (HA-MRSA)**

  HA-MRSA primarily affects people who are in hospitals, nursing homes, or other medical-care facilities. People who are most prone to getting HA-MRSA are the elderly, people with

307

compromised immune systems, those who have undergone recent surgery, or people undergoing kidney dialysis or using venous catheters or prosthetics. Studies suggest that at least one percent of in-patients contract HA-MRSA.

• **Community-Associated Methicillin-resistant** *Staphylococcus aureus* **(CA-MRSA)**

CA-MRSA has posed great threats to public health. The CA-MRSA often cannot be traced back to a specific place of origin, unlike the case with HA-MRSA, which is specific to healthcare settings. It tends to spread in overpopulated and unhygienic places, by physical touch or by sharing equipment or personal items. CA-MRSA can be more severe in children, as their immune systems are not fully developed. If a child's skin is infected because of insect-bite, cuts, or scrapes, a doctor needs to be consulted.

Treatment for MRSA Infection

MRSA is not resistant to all antibiotics. Similar to any staph infection, MRSA may be treated with medication and by the draining of any boils by a healthcare provider. Antibiotics that may be prescribed include clindamycin, tetracycline, doxycycline, trimethoprim-sulfamethoxazole, linezolid, vancomycin, and ciprofloxacin.

Staph or MRSA Infection and Pregnancy

Reports suggest that staph or MRSA infections have very low probability of affecting an unborn child. However, these bacteria can make a pregnant woman more susceptible to other infections, so treatment is important to ensure a safer pregnancy.

If infected with staph or MRSA during pregnancy, a healthcare provider should be consulted. For staph infection, certain antibiotics may be prescribed, and for MRSA infection, in which antibiotics do not work, or for people allergic to these medications, other treatments may be recommended by the doctor. If the prescribed antibiotics result in symptoms like rashes, hives or diarrhea, a healthcare provider must be contacted immediately.

Staph or MRSA Infection While Breastfeeding

If either a mother or child is infected with staph or MRSA, it is possible to transmit the infection whenever they come in contact with each other, including during breastfeeding. While a baby is breastfed, the bacteria in its nasal passages can spread to the mother, and that could cause mastitis (breast infection), especially if she has some nipple damage. Bacteria can also be spread to the baby through pumped breast milk if it is stored in contaminated containers or by using unsterilized pumping equipment. Hence, a thorough cleaning of storage containers and pumping materials is crucial to help prevent the infection.

Prevention of Staph or MRSA Infection

Practicing good hygiene is the best way to prevent staph or MRSA infection:

- Wash hands regularly with soap and water. After washing, wipe them dry with a clean towel or napkin. And it is always a good idea to use a hand sanitizer regularly.

- Take regular showers to help decrease the risk of infection.

- Do not share personal items, such as razors, towels, bedsheets, clothes, and sports equipment. Avoid touching other people's wounds and bandages.

- Regularly wash clothes, towels, and sheets, and dry them in the sun or hot dryer to destroy bacteria.

References

1. "Methicillin-Resistant *Staphylococcus aureus* (MRSA)," National Institute of Allergy and Infectious Diseases (NIAID), February 18, 2009.

2. "*Staphylococcus aureus* and Pregnancy," Organization of Teratology and Information Specialists, October 2007.

3. Davis, Charles Patrick. "Methicillin-Resistant *Staphylococcus aureus* (MRSA)," eMedicineHealth.com, January 20, 2016.

4. Mandal, Ananya. "What is *Staphylococcus aureus*?" News Medical, December 9, 2012.

5. Bernstein, Lisa. "Understanding MRSA Infection—The Basics," WebMD, March 18, 2015.

6. "Staph Infections," Mayo Clinic, June 11, 2014.

7. Reichstetter, Sandra. "Staph Infection and Pregnancy" Steady-Health, n.d.

Section 48.3

Vancomycin-Intermediate/Resistance S. Aureus (VISA/VRSA)

Text in this section is excerpted from "General Information about VISA/VRSA," Centers for Disease Control and Prevention (CDC), July 21, 2015.

Vancomycin-intermediate *Staphylococcus aureus* (also called VISA) and Vancomycin-resistant *Staphylococcus aureus* (also called VRSA) are specific types of antimicrobial-resistant bacteria. However, as of October 2010, all VISA and VRSA isolates have been susceptible to other U.S. Food and Drug Administration (FDA)-approved drugs. Persons who develop this type of staph infection may have underlying health conditions (such as diabetes and kidney disease), tubes going into their bodies (such as catheters), previous infections with methicillin-resistant *Staphylococcus aureus* (MRSA), and recent exposure to vancomycin and other antimicrobial agents.

What Is Staphylococcus Aureus*?*

Staphylococcus aureus is a bacterium commonly found on the skin and in the nose of about 30% of individuals. Most of the time, staph does not cause any harm. These infections can look like pimples, boils, or other skin conditions and most are able to be treated. Sometimes staph bacteria can get into the bloodstream and cause serious infections which can be fatal, including:

- Bacteremia or sepsis when bacteria spread to the bloodstream usually as a result of using catheters or having surgery.

- Pneumonia which predominantly affects people with underlying lung disease including those on mechanical ventilators.

- Endocarditis (infection of the heart valves) which can lead to heart failure.

- Osteomyelitis (bone infection) which can be caused by staph bacteria traveling in the bloodstream or put there by direct contact such as following trauma (puncture wound of foot or intravenous (IV) drug abuse).

How Do VISA and VRSA Get Their Names?

Staph bacteria are classified as VISA or VRSA based on laboratory tests. Laboratories perform tests to determine if staph bacteria are resistant to antimicrobial agents that might be used for treatment of infections. For vancomycin and other antimicrobial agents, laboratories determine how much of the agent it requires to inhibit the growth of the organism in a test tube. The result of the test is usually expressed as a minimum inhibitory concentration (MIC) or the minimum amount of antimicrobial agent that inhibits bacterial growth in the test tube. Therefore, staph bacteria are classified as VISA if the MIC for vancomycin is 4–8μg/ml, and classified as VRSA if the vancomycin MIC is ≥16μg/ml.

What Should a Patient Do If They Suspect They Have a Staph, MRSA, VISA or VRSA Infection?

See a healthcare provider.

Are VISA and VRSA Infections Treatable?

Yes. As of October 2010, all VISA and VRSA isolates have been susceptible to several U.S. Food and Drug Administration (FDA)-approved drugs.

How Can the Spread of VISA and VRSA Be Prevented?

Use of appropriate infection control practices (such as wearing gloves before and after contact with infectious body substances and adherence to hand hygiene) by healthcare personnel can reduce the spread of VISA and VRSA.

What Should a Person Do If a Family Member or Close Friend Has VISA or VRSA?

VISA and VRSA are types of antibiotic-resistant staph bacteria. Therefore, as with all staph bacteria, spread occurs among people having close physical contact with infected patients or contaminated material, such as bandages. Persons having close physical contact with infected patients while they are outside of the healthcare setting should:

1. keep their hands clean by washing thoroughly with soap and water

2. avoid contact with other people's wounds or material contaminated from wounds

If they go to the hospital to visit a friend or family member who is infected with VISA or VRSA, they must follow the hospital's recommended precautions.

What Is CDC Doing to Address VISA and VRSA?

In addition to providing guidance for clinicians and infection control personnel, Centers for Disease Control and Prevention (CDC) is also working with state and local health agencies, healthcare facilities, and clinical microbiology laboratories to ensure that laboratories are using proper methods to detect VISA and VRSA.

Chapter 49

Streptococcal Infections: Group A

Chapter Contents

Section 49.1

Strep Throat

This section includes text excerpted from "Is It Strep Throat?"
Centers for Disease Control and Prevention (CDC), October 19, 2015.

Many things can cause that unpleasant, scratchy, and sometimes painful condition known as a sore throat. Viruses, bacteria, allergens, environmental irritants (such as cigarette smoke), chronic postnasal drip, and fungi can all cause a sore throat. While many sore throats will get better without treatment, some throat infections—including strep throat—may need antibiotic treatment.

How You Get Strep Throat

Strep throat is an infection in the throat and tonsils caused by group A *Streptococcus* bacteria (called "group A strep"). Group A strep bacteria can also live in a person's nose and throat without causing illness. The bacteria are spread through contact with droplets after an infected person coughs or sneezes. If you touch your mouth, nose or eyes after touching something that has these droplets on it, you may become ill. If you drink from the same glass or eat from the same plate as the infected person, you could also become ill. It is also possible to get strep throat from contact with sores from group A strep skin infections.

Common Symptoms of Strep Throat

The most common symptoms of strep throat include:

- sore throat, usually starts quickly and can cause severe pain when swallowing
- fever (101°F or above)
- red and swollen tonsils, sometimes with white patches or streaks of pus
- tiny, red spots (petechiae) on the roof of the mouth (the soft or hard palate)

314

- headache, nausea, or vomiting

- swollen lymph nodes in the front of the neck

- sandpaper-like rash

A Simple Test Gives Fast Results

Healthcare professionals can test for strep by swabbing the throat to quickly see if group A strep bacteria are causing a sore throat. **A strep test is needed to tell if you have strep throat; just looking at your throat is not enough to make a diagnosis.** If the test is positive, your healthcare professional can prescribe antibiotics. If the strep test is negative, but your clinician still strongly suspects you have this infection, then they can take a throat culture swab to test for the bacteria, but those results will take a little longer to come back.

Antibiotics Get You Well Fast

The strep test results will help your healthcare professional decide if you need antibiotics, which can:

- decrease the length of time you're sick

- reduce your symptoms

- help prevent the spread of infection to friends and family members

- prevent more serious complications, such as tonsil and sinus infections, and acute rheumatic fever (a rare inflammatory disease that can affect the heart, joints, skin, and brain)

You should start feeling better in just a day or two after starting antibiotics. Call your healthcare professional if you don't feel better after taking antibiotics for 48 hours. People with strep throat should stay home from work, school or daycare until they have taken antibiotics for at least 24 hours so they don't spread the infection to others.

Be sure to finish the entire prescription, even when you start feeling better, unless your healthcare professional tells you to stop taking the medicine. When you stop taking antibiotics early, you risk getting an infection later that is resistant to antibiotic treatment.

315

More Prevention Tips: Wash Those Hands

The best way to keep from getting strep throat is to wash your hands often and avoid sharing eating utensils, like forks or cups. It is especially important for anyone with a sore throat to wash their hands often and cover their mouth when coughing and sneezing. There is no vaccine to prevent strep throat.

Section 49.2

Scarlet Fever

This section includes text excerpted from "Scarlet Fever: A Group A Streptococcal Infection," Centers for Disease Control and Prevention (CDC), January 19, 2016.

Scarlet fever results from group A strep infection. If your child has a sore throat and rash, their doctor can test for strep. Quick treatment with antibiotics can protect your child from possible long-term health problems.

Scarlet fever—or scarlatina—is a bacterial infection caused by group A *Streptococcus* or "group A strep." This illness affects a small percentage of people who have strep throat or, less commonly, streptococcal skin infections. Scarlet fever is treatable with antibiotics and usually is a mild illness, but it needs to be treated to prevent rare but serious long-term health problems. Treatment with antibiotics also helps clear up symptoms faster and reduces spread to other people.

Although anyone can get scarlet fever, it usually affects children between 5 and 15 years old. The classic symptom of the disease is a certain type of red rash that feels rough, like sandpaper.

How Do You Get Scarlet Fever?

Group A strep bacteria can live in a person's nose and throat. The bacteria are spread through contact with droplets from an infected person's cough or sneeze. If you touch your mouth, nose, or eyes after touching something that has these droplets on it, you may become ill. If you drink from the same glass or eat from the same plate as the sick person, you could also become ill. It is possible to get scarlet fever from contact with sores from group A strep skin infections.

What to Expect

Illness usually begins with a fever and sore throat. There also may be chills, vomiting, and abdominal pain. The tongue may have a whitish coating and appear swollen. It may also have a "strawberry"-like (red and bumpy) appearance. The throat and tonsils may be very red and sore, and swallowing may be painful.

One or two days after the illness begins, **the characteristic red rash** appears (although the rash can appear before illness or up to 7 days later). Certain strep bacteria produce a toxin (poison) which causes some people to break out in the rash—the "scarlet" of scarlet fever. The rash may first appear on the neck, underarm, and groin (the area where your stomach meets your thighs), then spread over the body. Typically, the rash begins as small, flat red blotches which gradually become fine bumps and feel like sandpaper.

Although the cheeks might have a flushed appearance, there may be a pale area around the mouth. Underarm, elbow, and groin skin creases may become brighter red than the rest of the rash. These are called Pastia's lines. The scarlet fever rash generally fades in about 7 days. As the rash fades, the skin may peel around the fingertips, toes, and groin area. This peeling can last up to several weeks.

Scarlet fever is treatable with antibiotics. Since either viruses or other bacteria can also cause sore throats, it's important to ask the doctor about getting a strep test (a simple swab of the throat) if your child complains of having a sore throat. If the test is positive, meaning your child is infected with group A strep bacteria, your child's doctor will prescribe antibiotics to avoid possible, although rare, long-term health problems, reduce symptoms, and prevent further spread of the disease.

Long-Term Health Problems from Scarlet Fever

Long-term health problems from scarlet fever may include:

- rheumatic fever (an inflammatory disease that can affect the heart, joints, skin, and brain)

- kidney disease (inflammation of the kidneys, called poststreptococcal glomerulonephritis)

- otitis media (ear infections)

- skin infections

- abscesses of the throat

- pneumonia (lung infection)

- arthritis (joint inflammation)

Most of these health problems can be prevented by treatment with antibiotics.

Preventing Infection: Wash Those Hands

The best way to keep from getting infected is to wash your hands often and avoid sharing eating utensils, linens, towels or other personal items. It is especially important for anyone with a sore throat to wash his or her hands often. There is no vaccine to prevent strep throat or scarlet fever. Children with scarlet fever or strep throat should stay home from school or daycare for at least 24 hours after starting antibiotics.

Section 49.3

Severe/Invasive Group A Streptococcal (GAS) Disease

This section includes text excerpted from "Group a Streptococcal (GAS) Disease," Centers for Disease Control and Prevention (CDC), January 19, 2016.

What Is Group-A Streptococcus?

Group A *Streptococcus* (group A strep) are bacteria that can cause a wide range of infections. People may also carry group A strep in the throat or on the skin and have no symptoms of illness. Most group A strep infections are relatively mild illnesses, such as "strep throat" or impetigo (a skin infection). Occasionally these bacteria can cause serious and even life-threatening diseases. These diseases can sometimes lead to sepsis, the body's overwhelming and life-threatening response to infection that can cause tissue damage, organ failure, and death.

How Are Group-A Strep Spread?

These bacteria are spread through direct contact with mucus from the nose or throat of people who are sick with a group A strep infection or through contact with infected wounds or sores on the skin. The bacteria may also be spread through contact with people without symptoms but who carry the bacteria in their throat or on their skin. Ill people, such as those who have strep throat or skin infections, are most likely to spread the infection. People who carry the bacteria but have no symptoms are much less contagious. Treating an infected person with an antibiotic for 24 hours or longer generally prevents the spread of the bacteria to others.

However, it is important to complete the entire course of antibiotics as prescribed. It is not likely that household items, like toys, spread these bacteria. However, it is possible to spread these bacteria by drinking from the same glass or eating from the same plate as someone who is ill with a group A strep infection like strep throat.

What Kind of Illnesses Are Caused by Group-A Strep?

Infection with group A strep can result in a range of illnesses:

- mild illness such as strep throat or impetigo

- serious illness such as pneumonia (lung infection), necrotizing fasciitis or streptococcal toxic shock syndrome (STSS)

Serious, sometimes life-threatening group A strep disease may occur when these bacteria get into parts of the body where bacteria usually are not found, such as the blood, muscle, or the lungs. These infections are called "invasive group A strep disease." Two of the most serious, but least common, forms of invasive group A strep disease are necrotizing fasciitis and STSS. Necrotizing fasciitis (occasionally described by the media as "the flesh-eating bacteria") rapidly destroys muscles, fat, and skin tissue. STSS causes blood pressure to drop rapidly and organs (e.g., kidney, liver, lungs) to fail. STSS is not the same as the staphylococcal toxic shock syndrome that has been associated with tampon usage. Less serious invasive illnesses caused by group A strep include cellulitis and pneumonia. In the United States, about

1 out of 4 patients with necrotizing fasciitis due to group A strep and approximately 4 out of 10 with STSS die. About 10 to 15 out of 100 patients with any form of invasive group A strep disease die.

How Common Is Invasive Group-A Strep Disease?

Approximately 9,000 to 11,500 cases of invasive group A strep disease occur each year in the United States, resulting in 1,000 to 1,800 deaths annually. Most of these cases are less serious invasive infections, like cellulitis. STSS and necrotizing fasciitis are each responsible for an average of about 6 to 7 out of 100 of these invasive cases. In contrast, there are several million cases of non-invasive group A strep infections, like strep throat and impetigo, each year.

Who Is Most at Risk of Getting Invasive Group-A Strep Disease?

Few people who come in contact with group A strep will develop invasive group A strep disease. Most people will have a throat or skin infection, and some may have no symptoms at all. Although healthy people can get invasive group A strep disease, people with chronic illnesses like cancer, diabetes, and chronic heart or lung disease, and those who use medicines, such as steroids, have an increased risk. People with skin lesions (such as cuts, chickenpox or surgical wounds), the elderly, and adults with a history of alcohol abuse or injection drug use also have an increased risk for disease.

What Are the Early Signs and Symptoms of Necrotizing Fasciitis and Streptococcal Toxic Shock Syndrome?

Early signs and symptoms of necrotizing fasciitis include:

- Severe pain and swelling, often rapidly increasing
- Fever
- Redness at a wound site

Early signs and symptoms of STSS include:

- Sudden onset of generalized or localized severe pain, often in an arm or leg
- Dizziness

- Flu-like symptoms such as fever, chills, muscle aches, nausea, vomiting

- Confusion

- A flat red rash over large areas of the body (only occurs in 1 out of 10 cases)

How Is Invasive Group-A Strep Disease Treated?

Group A strep infections can be treated with many different antibiotics (medicines that kill bacteria in the body). For STSS and necrotizing fasciitis, high dose penicillin and clindamycin are recommended. For those with very serious illness, supportive care in an intensive care unit may also be needed. For people with necrotizing fasciitis, early and aggressive surgery is often needed to remove damaged tissue and stop disease spread. Early treatment may reduce the risk of death from invasive group A strep disease. However, even the best medical care does not prevent death in every case.

What Can Be Done to Help Prevent Group-A Strep Infections?

The spread of all types of group A strep infection can be reduced by good hand washing, especially after coughing and sneezing and before preparing foods or eating. People with sore throats should be seen by a doctor who can perform tests to find out whether the illness is strep throat. If the test result shows strep throat, the person should stay home from work, school or daycare until 24 hours after taking an antibiotic.

All wounds should be kept clean and watched for possible signs of infection such as redness, swelling, drainage, and pain at the wound site. A person with signs of an infected wound, especially if fever occurs, should immediately seek medical care. It is not necessary for all people exposed to someone with an invasive group A strep infection (i.e., necrotizing fasciitis or STSS) to receive antibiotic therapy to prevent infection. However, in some situations, antibiotic therapy may be recommended. That decision should be made after talking with your doctor.

Chapter 50

Streptococcal Infections: Group B

Chapter Contents

Section 50.1

Streptococcus pneumoniae

This section includes text excerpted from "Pneumococcal Disease," Centers for Disease Control and Prevention (CDC), June 10, 2015.

Streptococcus pneumoniae (S. pneumoniae) are lancet-shaped, gram-positive, facultative anaerobic bacteria with over 90 known serotypes. Most *S. pneumoniae* serotypes have been shown to cause disease, but only a minority of serotypes produce the majority of pneumococcal infections.

Pneumococci are common inhabitants of the respiratory tract and may be isolated from the nasopharynx of 5–90% of healthy persons, depending on the population and setting. Only 5–10% of adults without children are carriers. Among school-aged children, 20–60% may be carriers. On military installations, as many as 50-60% of service personnel may be carriers. The duration of carriage varies and is generally longer in children than adults. In addition, the relationship of carriage to the development of natural immunity is poorly understood.

Transmission

Transmission of *Streptococcus pneumoniae* occurs as a result of direct person-to-person contact via respiratory droplets and by autoinoculation in persons carrying the bacteria in their upper respiratory tract. The pneumococcal serotypes most often responsible for causing infection are those most frequently found in carriers.

The spread of the organism within a family or household is influenced by such factors as crowding, season, and the presence of upper respiratory infections or pneumococcal disease, such as pneumonia or otitis media. The spread of pneumococcal disease is usually associated with increased carriage rates. However, high carriage rates do not appear to increase the risk of disease transmission in households.

Temporal Pattern

Pneumococcal infections are more common during the winter and in early spring when respiratory diseases are more prevalent.

Communicability

The period of communicability for pneumococcal disease is unknown, but presumably transmission can occur as long as the organism appears in respiratory secretions.

Risk Factors

Conditions that increase the risk of invasive pneumococcal disease among adults include:

- decreased immune function from disease or drugs
- functional or anatomic asplenia
- chronic heart, lung (including asthma), liver or renal disease
- cigarette smoking
- cerebrospinal fluid leak

Children with functional or anatomic asplenia, particularly those with sickle cell disease, and children with HIV infection are at very high risk for invasive disease, with some studies reporting rates more than 50 times higher than those among children of the same age without these conditions. Rates are also increased among children of certain racial and ethnic groups, in particular Alaska Natives, African American, and certain American Indian groups. The reason for this increased risk by race and ethnicity is not known with certainty but was also noted for invasive *Haemophilus influenzae* infection (which is also caused by an encapsulated bacterium).

Attendance at a childcare center has been shown to increase the risk of invasive pneumococcal disease and acute otitis media 2–3-fold among children younger than 59 months old. Children with a cochlear implant are also at increased risk for pneumococcal meningitis.

Diagnosis

A definitive diagnosis of infection with *Streptococcus pneumoniae* generally relies on isolation of the organism from blood or other normally sterile body sites. Tests are also available to detect capsular polysaccharide antigen in body fluids.

A urinary antigen test based on immunochromatographic membrane technique to detect the C-polysaccharide antigen of *Streptococcus pneumoniae* as a cause of community-acquired pneumonia among adults is commercially available and has been cleared by the Food and

Drug Administration. The test is rapid and simple to use, has a reasonable specificity in adults, and has the ability to detect pneumococcal pneumonia after antibiotic therapy has been started.

Medical Management

Pneumococcal bacteria are resistant to one or more antibiotics in 30% of cases. Treatment will usually include a broad-spectrum cephalosporin, and often vancomycin, until results of antibiotic sensitivity testing are available. Resistance to penicillin and other antibiotics was previously very common.

However, following introduction of the 7-valent pneumococcal conjugate vaccine (PCV7) in 2000, antibiotic resistance declined and then began to increase again. Then, in 2008, the definition of penicillin resistance was changed such that a much larger proportion of pneumococci are now considered susceptible to penicillin. The revised susceptibility breakpoints for *Streptococcus pneumoniae*, published by the Clinical and Laboratory Standards Institute (CLSI) in January 2008, were the result of a reevaluation that showed clinical response to penicillin was being preserved in clinical studies of pneumococcal infection, despite reduced susceptibility response in vitro.

Prevention

Vaccine

The best way to prevent pneumococcal disease is to vaccinate your patients. The pneumococcal conjugate vaccine (PCV13 or Prevnar 13®) provides protection against the 13 serotypes responsible for most severe illness. The vaccine can also help prevent some ear infections. PCV13 is administered as a four-dose series at 2, 4, 6, and 12 through 15 months of life. It has been shown to be very effective in preventing infection resulting from the serotypes contained in the vaccine. PCV13 should also be administered to all adults 65 years or older and to some adults 19 through 64 years of age with immunocompromising conditions and other high-risk conditions (i.e., cerebrospinal fluid leaks, cochlear implants, sickle cell disease and other hemoglobinopathies, and congenital or acquired asplenia).

The pneumococcal polysaccharide vaccine (PPSV23 or Pneumovax 23®) is a 23-valent polysaccharide vaccine that is currently recommended for use in all adults who are 65 years or older and for persons who are 2 years or older and at high risk for disease. It is also recommended for use in adults 19 through 64 years of age who smoke cigarettes or who have asthma.

It is also important to administer an influenza vaccination every year because having the flu increases your patient's chances of getting pneumococcal disease.

Chemoprophylaxis

For children with functional or anatomic asplenia, especially those with sickle-cell disease, daily antimicrobial prophylaxis with oral penicillin V or G is typically recommended. In general, antimicrobial prophylaxis (in addition to immunization) should be considered for all children with asplenia younger than 5 years of age and for at least 1 year after splenectomy. Because secondary cases of invasive pneumococcal infection are uncommon, chemoprophylaxis is not indicated for contacts of patients with such infection.

Section 50.2

Group B Strep in Pregnancy and Newborns

This section includes text excerpted from "Group B Strep in Newborns," Centers for Disease Control and Prevention (CDC), May 23, 2016.

About Group B Strep

Group B Streptococcus (group B strep) is a type of bacteria that causes illness in people of all ages. Also known as GBS, group B strep disease can be especially severe in newborns, most commonly causing sepsis (infection of the blood), pneumonia (infection in the lungs), and sometimes meningitis (infection of the fluid and lining around the brain and spinal cord). The most common problems caused by group B strep bacteria in adults are bloodstream infections, pneumonia, skin and soft-tissue infections, and bone and joint infections.

Types of Infection

Among babies, there are 2 main types of group B strep disease:

- Early-onset—occurs during the first week of life

- Late-onset—occurs from the first week through three months of life

Early-onset disease used to be the most common type of disease in babies. Today, because of effective early-onset disease prevention, early and late-onset disease occur at similar low rates.

For early-onset disease, group B strep most commonly causes sepsis (infection of the blood), pneumonia (infection in the lungs), and sometimes meningitis (infection of the fluid and lining around the brain). Similar illnesses are associated with late-onset group B strep disease. Meningitis is more common with late-onset group B strep disease than with early-onset group B strep disease.

How It Spreads

In cases of early-onset disease (occurs in babies younger than 1 week old), group B strep bacteria are most often passed from mother to baby during labor and birth. Antibiotics given to the mother during labor can be very effective at preventing the spread of group B strep bacteria to the baby.

Late-onset disease (occurs in babies 1 week through 3 months old) is sometimes due to passing of the bacteria from mother to newborn, but the bacteria may come from another source. For a baby whose mother does not test positive for group B strep bacteria, the source of infection for late-onset disease can be hard to figure out and is often unknown.

Risk Factors

Some pregnant women are at an increased risk of having a baby who develops early-onset group B strep disease. Some risk factors include:

- Testing positive for group B strep bacteria late in the current pregnancy (35–37 weeks pregnant)

- Detecting group B strep bacteria in urine (pee) during the current pregnancy

- Delivering early (before 37 weeks of pregnancy)

- Developing a fever during labor
- Having a long time between water breaking and delivering (18 hours or more)
- Having a previous baby who developed early-onset disease

The risk factors for late-onset group B strep disease are not as well understood as those for early-onset disease. Late-onset disease is more common among babies who are born prematurely (before 37 weeks of pregnancy). Babies whose mothers tested positive for group B strep bacteria also are at increased risk of late-onset disease.

Symptoms

The symptoms of group B strep (GBS) disease can seem like other health problems in newborns and babies. Most newborns with early-onset disease (occurs in babies younger than 1 week old) have symptoms on the day of birth. Babies who develop late-onset disease may appear healthy at birth and develop symptoms of group B strep disease after the first week through the first three months of life.

Some symptoms include:

- fever
- difficulty feeding
- irritability or lethargy (limpness or hard to wake up the baby)
- difficulty breathing
- blue-ish color to skin

Complications

For both early-and late-onset group B strep disease, and particularly for babies who had meningitis (infection of the fluid and lining around the brain and spinal cord), there may be long-term problems such as deafness and developmental disabilities. Care for sick babies has improved a lot in the United States. However, 2 to 3 out of every 50 babies (4 to 6%) who develop group B strep disease will die.

On average, about 1,000 babies in the United States get early-onset group B strep disease each year, with rates higher among prematurely born babies (born before 37 weeks) and blacks. Group B strep bacteria may also cause some miscarriages, stillbirths, and preterm deliveries. However, there are many different factors that lead to stillbirth, preterm delivery, or miscarriage and, most of the time, the cause is not known.

Diagnosis

Group B strep disease is diagnosed by taking samples of a baby's sterile body fluids, such as blood or spinal fluid. These samples are cultured (bacteria grown in the laboratory) to see if group B strep bacteria are present, which can take a few days. If a mother who tested positive for group B strep bacteria received antibiotics during labor, doctors will check on the baby once he or she is born. The baby likely won't need extra antibiotics or other medicine after birth, unless the doctor says they are needed.

For both early-onset (occurs in babies younger than 1 week old) and late-onset (occurs in babies 1 week through 3 months old) disease, if a group B strep infection is suspected, doctors will take a sample of the baby's blood and spinal fluids or take a chest X-ray to confirm the diagnosis.

Treatment

Group B strep disease in newborns and older babies is treated with antibiotics (medicine used to kill bacteria in the body), such as penicillin or ampicillin, given through a vein (IV). For babies with severe illness, other procedures, in addition to antibiotics, may be needed.

Prevention in Newborns

Preventing Early-Onset Group B Strep Disease (GBS)

The two most important ways to prevent early-onset (occurs in babies younger than 1 week old) group B strep disease include:

- Testing all pregnant women for group B strep bacteria late in pregnancy (ideally between 35 and 37 weeks pregnant)

- Giving antibiotics during labor to women who test positive for group B strep bacteria

Testing Pregnant Women

Pregnant women should be tested, or screened, for group B strep bacteria in her vagina and rectum when she is 35 to 37 weeks pregnant. The test is simple and does not hurt. A sterile swab ("Q-tip") is used to collect a sample from the vagina and the rectum and is then sent to a laboratory for testing.

About 1 out of every 4 (about 25%) pregnant women carry group B strep bacteria in their rectum or vagina. Those women are considered group B strep positive. A woman may test positive for the bacteria at some times and not others. That's why it's important for all pregnant women to be tested for group B strep bacteria between 35 to 37 weeks of every pregnancy.

A woman who has group B strep bacteria in her body usually does not feel sick or have any symptoms (asymptomatic). However, she is at an increased risk for passing the bacteria to her baby during birth.

Women should talk to their doctor about their group B strep status.

Antibiotics during Labor

To help protect their babies from infection, pregnant women who test positive for group B strep bacteria in the current pregnancy should receive antibiotics (medicine that kills bacteria in the body) through the vein (IV) during labor. Also, pregnant women who have group B strep bacteria in their urine during the current pregnancy or who had a previous baby develop group B strep disease should get antibiotics during labor. These women do not need to be screened at 35 to 37 weeks because they should receive antibiotics no matter the results. Pregnant women who do not know if they are positive for group B strep bacteria when labor starts should be given antibiotics if they have:

- labor starting at less than 37 weeks (preterm labor)

- prolonged membrane rupture (water breaking 18 or more hours before delivery)

- fever during labor

Antibiotics help to kill some of the group B strep bacteria that are dangerous to the baby during birth. The antibiotics help during labor only—they cannot be taken before labor, because the bacteria can grow back quickly. Penicillin is the most common antibiotic that is given, but women who are severely allergic to penicillin can be given other antibiotics. Women should tell their doctor or nurse about any allergies during a checkup and try to make a plan for delivery. When women get to the hospital, they should remind their doctor and any staff if they have any allergies to medicines.

Penicillin is very safe and effective at preventing the spread of group B strep bacteria to newborns during birth. There can be side effects from penicillin for the mother, including a mild reaction to penicillin (in about 1 out of every 10 women). There is a rare chance (about 1 out of every 10,000 women) of the mother having a severe allergic reaction that requires emergency treatment.

Preventing Late-Onset Disease

Unfortunately, the method recommended to prevent early-onset disease (giving women who are group B strep positive antibiotics through the vein (IV) during labor) does not prevent late-onset disease (occurs in babies 1 week through 3 months old). Although rates of early-onset disease have declined, rates of late-onset disease have remained about the same since 1990. A strategy has not yet been identified for preventing late-onset group B strep disease.

Alternative Prevention Strategies

Currently, there is no vaccine to help mothers protect their newborns from group B strep bacteria and disease. Researchers are working on developing a vaccine, which may become available one day in the future.

Antibiotics taken by mouth instead of through the vein and antibiotics taken before labor and delivery are not effective at preventing group B strep disease in babies. Birth canal washes with the disinfectant chlorhexidine also do not reduce the risk of a mother spreading group B strep bacteria to her baby or her baby developing early-onset disease. To date, receiving antibiotics through the vein during labor is the only proven strategy to protect a baby from early-onset group B strep disease.

Section 50.3

Adult Group B Strep Disease

This section includes text excerpted from "Group B Strep Infection in Adults," Centers for Disease Control and Prevention (CDC), May 23, 2016.

While the rates of serious group B strep infections are higher among newborns than among any other age group, serious group B strep disease can occur in other age groups in both men and women.

Spread to Others

The sources of disease caused by group B strep bacteria are unknown. Group B strep bacteria are common in the gastrointestinal tract (the part of your body that digests food, including the stomach and intestines) of men and women and may be a source of some infection.

Types of Infection and Symptoms

Symptoms depend on the part of the body that is infected. Below are common diseases caused by group B strep bacteria in adults and their symptoms. Bacteremia and sepsis (blood infections) symptoms include:

- Fever
- Chills
- Low alertness

Pneumonia (lung infection) symptoms include:

- Fever and chills
- Cough
- Rapid breathing or difficulty breathing
- Chest pain

Skin and soft-tissue infections often appear as a bump or infected area on the skin that may be:

- Red

- Swollen or painful

- Warm to the touch

- Full of pus or other drainage

These skin infections may also be accompanied by a fever.

Bone and joint infections often appear as pain in the infected area and might also include:

- Fever

- Chills

- Swilling

- Stiffness or inability to use affected limb or joint

Rarely in adults, group B strep bacteria can cause meningitis (infection of the fluid and lining surrounding the brain and spinal cord).

Diagnosis

If doctors suspect an adult has an invasive group B strep infection (infections where the bacteria have entered a part of the body that is normally not exposed to bacteria), they will take a sample of sterile body fluids, such as blood or spinal fluid. These samples are cultured (bacteria grown in the laboratory) to see if group B strep bacteria are present, which can take a few days. Sometimes group B strep bacteria can cause urinary tract infections (UTIs, also called bladder infections), which also can be diagnosed in the lab with a sample of urine.

Treatment

Group B strep disease is usually treated with penicillin or other common antibiotics (medicine that kills bacteria in the body). Sometimes soft tissue and bone infections may need additional treatment, such as surgery. Treatment will depend on the kind of infection caused by group B strep bacteria. Patients should ask their doctor about specific treatment options.

Risk Factors

Most cases of group B strep disease in adults are among those who have other medical conditions that put them at increased risk, such as:

- Diabetes mellitus
- Cardiovascular disease
- Congestive heart failure
- History of cancer
- Obesity

Complications

Serious group B strep infections, such as sepsis (infection of the blood) and pneumonia (infection of the lungs) in adults can be fatal. On average 1 out of every 20 (5%) non-pregnant adults with invasive group B strep infections die. Risk of death is lower among younger adults and adults who do not have other medical conditions.

Disease Trends

The rate of serious group B strep disease among non-pregnant adults increases with age. The rate of invasive disease is about 10 cases out of every 100,000 non-pregnant adults. However, 25 out of every 100,000 adults 65 years or older will get group B strep disease each year.

Chapter 51

Syphilis

Syphilis is a sexually transmitted bacterial disease that causes genital ulcers (sores) in its early stages. If untreated, syphilis can also lead to more serious symptoms. An ancient disease, syphilis is still of major importance today. The Centers for Disease Control and Prevention (CDC) estimates that each year 55,400 people in the United States get new syphilis infections. During 2012, there were 49,903 reported new cases.

In addition, human immunodeficiency virus (HIV) infection and syphilis are linked. Syphilis increases the risk of transmitting as well as getting infected with HIV.

Cause

Syphilis is caused by a bacterium called *Treponema pallidum*.

Transmission

The most common way to get syphilis is by having sexual contact with an infected person. If you are infected, you can pass the bacteria from infected skin or mucous membranes (linings), usually your genital area, lips, mouth, or anus, to the mucous membranes or skin of your sexual partner. The bacteria are fragile, so you cannot get syphilis from sharing food or utensils, or from using tubs, pools or toilets. Syphilis

---

This chapter includes text excerpted from "Syphilis," National Institute of Allergy and Infectious Diseases (NIAID), October 27, 2014.

can be passed from mother to infant during pregnancy, causing a disease called congenital syphilis.

Symptoms

Syphilis is sometimes called "the great imitator." This is because it has so many possible symptoms, and its symptoms are like those of many other diseases. Having HIV infection at the same time as syphilis can change the symptoms of syphilis and how the disease develops.

Stages

Syphilis (other than congenital syphilis) occurs in four stages that sometimes overlap.

Primary Syphilis

The first symptom of primary syphilis is often a small, round, firm ulcer (sore) called a chancre ("shanker") at the place where the bacteria entered your body. This place is usually the penis, vulva, or vagina, but chancres also can develop on the cervix, tongue, lips, or other parts of the body. Usually there is only one chancre, but sometimes there may be many. Nearby lymph glands are often swollen. (Lymph glands, or nodes, are small bean-shaped organs of your immune system containing cells that help fight off germs. They are found throughout your body.)

The chancre usually appears about three weeks after you're infected with the bacteria, but it can occur any time from 9 to 90 days after you have been infected. Because a chancre is usually painless and can appear inside your body, you might not notice it. The chancre disappears in about three to six weeks whether or not you are treated. Therefore, you can have primary syphilis without symptoms or with only brief symptoms that you may overlook. If primary syphilis is not treated, however, the infection moves to the secondary stage.

Secondary Syphilis

Most people with secondary syphilis have a skin rash that doesn't itch. The rash is usually on the palms of your hands and soles of your feet. However, it may cover your whole body or appear only in a few areas. The rash appears 2 to 10 weeks after the chancre, generally when the chancre is healing or already healed. Other common symptoms include:

- Sore throat

- Tiredness

- Headache

- Swollen lymph glands

Other symptoms that happen less often include fever, aches, weight loss, hair loss, aching joints, or lesions (sores) in the mouth or genital area.

Your symptoms may be mild. The lesions of secondary syphilis contain many bacteria, and anyone who has contact with them can get syphilis. As with primary syphilis, secondary syphilis will seem to disappear even without treatment, but secondary syphilis can return. Without treatment, however, the infection will move to the next stages.

Latent Syphilis

The latent (hidden) stage of syphilis begins when symptoms of secondary syphilis are over. In early latent syphilis, you might notice that signs and symptoms disappear, but the infection remains in your body. When you are in this stage, you can still infect a sexual partner. In late part of latent syphilis, the infection is quiet and the risk of infecting a sexual partner is low or not present. If you don't get treated for latent syphilis, you may move on to tertiary syphilis, the most serious stage of the disease.

Tertiary Syphilis

Even without treatment, only a small number of infected people develop the severe complications known as tertiary, or late, syphilis. In this stage, the bacteria will damage your heart, eyes, brain, nervous system, bones, joints, or almost any other part of your body. This damage can happen years or even decades after the primary stage.

Late syphilis can result in mental illness, blindness, deafness, memory loss or other neurologic problems, heart disease, and death. Late neurosyphilis (brain or spinal cord damage) is one of the most severe complications of this stage.

Diagnosis

It can be very difficult for your healthcare provider to diagnose syphilis based on symptoms. This is because symptoms and signs of the disease might be absent, go away without treatment, or be confused with those of other diseases. Because syphilis can be hard to diagnose, you should:

- Visit your healthcare provider if you have a lesion (sore) in your genital area or a widespread rash.

- Get tested periodically for syphilis if your sexual behaviors put you at risk for sexually transmitted diseases (STDs).

- Get tested for syphilis if you have been treated for another STD such as gonorrhea or HIV infection.

Laboratory Tests

Your healthcare provider can diagnose early syphilis by seeing a chancre or rash and then confirming the diagnosis with laboratory tests. Because latent syphilis has no symptoms, it is diagnosed only by laboratory tests.

There are two methods for diagnosing syphilis through a laboratory.

1. Identifying the bacteria under a microscope in a sample of tissue (a group of cells) taken from a chancre.

2. Performing a blood test for syphilis.

If your healthcare provider thinks you might have neurosyphilis, your spinal fluid will be tested as well.

Treatment

- Syphilis is easy to cure in its early stages. Penicillin, an antibiotic, injected into the muscle, is the best treatment for syphilis. If you are allergic to penicillin, your healthcare provider may give you another antibiotic to take by mouth.

- If you have neurosyphilis, you may need to get daily doses of penicillin intravenously (in the vein) and you may need to be treated in the hospital.

- If you have late syphilis, damage done to your body organs cannot be reversed.

While you are being treated, you should abstain from sex until any sores are completely healed. You should also notify your sex partners so they can be tested for syphilis and treated if necessary.

Prevention

To prevent getting syphilis, you must avoid contact with infected tissue and body fluids of an infected person. However, syphilis is usually transmitted by people who have no sores that can be seen or rashes and don't know they are infected. If you aren't infected with syphilis and are sexually active, having mutually monogamous sex with an uninfected partner is the best way to prevent syphilis. Using condoms properly and consistently during sex reduces your risk of getting syphilis. Washing or douching after sex won't prevent syphilis. Even if you have been treated for syphilis and cured, you can be re-infected by having sex with an infected partner.

To prevent passing congenital syphilis to their unborn babies, all pregnant women should be tested for syphilis. Most cases of congenital syphilis can be avoided with appropriate screening and treatment of pregnant women.

Complications

Pregnancy

Syphilis can cause miscarriages, premature births, or stillbirths. It can also cause death of newborn babies. Some infants with congenital syphilis have symptoms at birth, but most develop symptoms later. Untreated babies with congenital syphilis can have deformities, delays in development, or seizures, along with many other problems such as rash, fever, swollen liver and spleen, anemia, and jaundice. Sores on infected babies are infectious. Rarely, the symptoms of early-stage syphilis may go unseen in infants and they may subsequently develop the symptoms of late-stage syphilis, including damage to their bones, teeth, eyes, ears, and brains.

HIV Infection

People infected with syphilis have a two- to five-fold increase risk of getting infected with HIV. Strong evidence shows the increased odds of getting and transmitting HIV in the presence of other STDs as well. You should discuss this and other STDs with your healthcare provider.

Chapter 52

Tinea Infections (Ringworm, Jock Itch, Athlete's Foot)

For active kids, locker-room showers and heaps of sweaty clothes are part of their everyday lives—and so is the risk of getting fungal skin infections. Jock itch, athlete's foot, and ringworm are all types of fungal skin infections known collectively as tinea. They're caused by fungi called dermatophytes that live on skin, hair, and nails and thrive in warm, moist areas.

Symptoms of these infections can vary depending on where they appear on the body. The source of the fungus might be soil, an animal (usually a cat, dog, or rodent), or in most cases, another person. Minor skin injuries (such as scratches) and too much exposure to heat and humidity make a person more likely to get a skin infection.

It's important to teach kids how to avoid fungal skin infections, which can be itchy and uncomfortable. If they do get one, most can be treated with over-the-counter medication, though some might require treatment by a doctor.

Ringworm

Ringworm isn't a worm, but a fungal infection of the scalp or skin that got its name from the ring or series of rings that it can produce.

This chapter includes text excerpted from "Tinea (Ringworm, Jock Itch, Athlete's Foot)," © 1995–2016. The Nemours Foundation/KidsHealth®. Reprinted with permission.

Symptoms of Ringworm

Ringworm of the scalp may start as a small sore that resembles a pimple before becoming patchy, flaky or scaly. These flakes may look like dandruff. It can cause some hair to fall out or break into stubbles. It can also cause the scalp to become swollen, tender, and red. Sometimes, there may be a swollen, inflamed mass known as a kerion, which oozes fluid. This can be confused with impetigo or cellulitis.

When the scalp has this infection, it can sometimes also cause swollen lymph glands at the back of the head. Ringworm of the skin makes the skin itchy and red and creates a round patchy rash that has raised borders and a clear center. Ringworm of the nails may affect one or more nails on the hands or feet. The nails may become thick, white or yellowish, and brittle. If you suspect that your child has ringworm, call your doctor.

Treating Ringworm

Ringworm is fairly easy to diagnose and treat. Most of the time, the doctor can diagnose it by looking at it or by scraping off a small sample of the flaky infected skin to test for the fungus. The doctor may recommend an antifungal ointment for ringworm of the skin. For ringworm of the scalp or nails, where the infection is usually deeper in the skin, the doctor may prescribe a syrup or pill to take by mouth. Whatever treatment is chosen, your child should take the medicine as long as it is prescribed, even if the rash seems to be getting better. If not, the ringworm can come back.

An antifungal shampoo prescribed by the doctor also can help prevent the spread of the fungal spores. If your child was sent home from school for ringworm, he or she should be able to attend school again after starting treatment.

Preventing Ringworm

Ringworm usually spreads from fallen hair or skin cells, so it's important to encourage kids to avoid sharing combs, brushes, pillows, and hats with others. Sometimes, ringworm can be spread from tools at the barber or from furniture or shared towels.

Jock Itch

Jock itch, an infection of the groin and upper thighs, got its name because cases are commonly seen in active kids who sweat a lot while playing sports. But the fungus that causes the jock itch infection can thrive on the skin of any kids who spend time in hot and humid weather, wear tight clothing like bathing suits that cause friction, share towels and clothing, and don't completely dry off their skin. It can last for weeks or months if it goes untreated.

Symptoms of Jock Itch

Symptoms of jock itch may include:

- itching, chafing or burning in the groin, thigh or anal area
- skin redness in the groin, thigh or anal area
- flaking, peeling or cracking skin

Treating Jock Itch

Jock itch can usually be treated with over-the-counter antifungal creams and sprays. When using one of these, kids should:

- Wash and then dry the area with a clean towel
- Apply the antifungal cream, powder or spray as directed on the label
- Change clothing, especially the underwear, every day
- Continue this treatment for 2 weeks, even if symptoms disappear, to prevent the infection from recurring

If the ointment or spray is not effective, call your doctor, who can prescribe other treatment.

Preventing Jock Itch

Jock itch can be prevented by keeping the groin area clean and dry, particularly after showering, swimming, and sweaty activities.

Athlete's Foot

Athlete's foot typically affects the soles of the feet, the areas between the toes, and sometimes the toenails. It can also spread to the palms of the hands, the groin, or the underarms if your child touches the affected foot and then touches another body part. It got its name because it affects people whose feet tend to be damp and sweaty, which is often the case with athletes.

Symptoms of Athlete's Foot

The symptoms of athlete's foot may include itching, burning, redness, and stinging on the soles of the feet. The skin may flake, peel, blister or crack.

Treating Athlete's Foot

A doctor can often diagnose athlete's foot simply by examining the foot or by taking a small scraping of the affected skin to see if it has the fungus that causes athlete's foot. Over-the-counter (OTC) antifungal creams and sprays may effectively treat mild cases of athlete's foot within a few weeks. Athlete's foot can recur or be more serious. If that's the case, ask your doctor about trying a stronger treatment.

Preventing Athlete's Foot

Because the fungus that causes athlete's foot thrives in warm, moist areas, you can prevent infections by keeping feet and the space between the toes clean and dry. Athlete's foot is contagious and can be spread in damp areas, such as public showers or pool areas, so it's wise to take extra precautions.

Encourage kids to:

- Wear waterproof shoes or flip-flops in public showers, like those in locker rooms

- Alternate shoes or sneakers to prevent moisture buildup and fungus growth

- Avoid socks that trap moisture or make the feet sweat, and instead choose cotton or wool socks or socks made of fabric that wicks away the moisture

- Choose sneakers that are well ventilated with small holes to keep the feet dry

By taking the proper precautions and teaching them to your kids, you can prevent these uncomfortable skin infections from putting a crimp in your family's lifestyle.

Chapter 53

Trichomoniasis

What Is Trichomoniasis?

Trichomoniasis (or "trich") is a very common sexually transmitted disease (STD) that is caused by infection with a protozoan parasite called *Trichomonas vaginalis*. Although symptoms of the disease vary, most women and men who have the parasite cannot tell they are infected.

How Common Is Trichomoniasis?

Trichomoniasis is considered the most common curable STD. In the United States, an estimated 3.7 million people have the infection, but only about 30% develop any symptoms of trichomoniasis. Infection is more common in women than in men, and older women are more likely than younger women to have been infected.

How Do People Get Trichomoniasis?

The parasite is passed from an infected person to an uninfected person during sex. In women, the most commonly infected part of the body is the lower genital tract (vulva, vagina, or urethra), and in men, the most commonly infected body part is the inside of the penis (urethra). During sex, the parasite is usually transmitted from a penis to a vagina,

This chapter includes text excerpted from "Trichomoniasis—CDC Fact Sheet," Centers for Disease Control and Prevention (CDC), May 20, 2016.

or from a vagina to a penis, but it can also be passed from a vagina to another vagina. It is not common for the parasite to infect other body parts, like the hands, mouth, or anus. It is unclear why some people with the infection get symptoms while others do not, but it probably depends on factors like the person's age and overall health. Infected people without symptoms can still pass the infection on to others.

What Are the Signs and Symptoms of Trichomoniasis?

About 70% of infected people do not have any signs or symptoms. When trichomoniasis does cause symptoms, they can range from mild irritation to severe inflammation. Some people with symptoms get them within 5 to 28 days after being infected, but others do not develop symptoms until much later. Symptoms can come and go.

Men with trichomoniasis may feel itching or irritation inside the penis, burning after urination or ejaculation or some discharge from the penis. Women with trichomoniasis may notice itching, burning, redness or soreness of the genitals, discomfort with urination, or a thin discharge with an unusual smell that can be clear, white, yellowish or greenish. Having trichomoniasis can make it feel unpleasant to have sex. Without treatment, the infection can last for months or even years.

What Are the Complications of Trichomoniasis?

Trichomoniasis can increase the risk of getting or spreading other sexually transmitted infections. For example, trichomoniasis can cause genital inflammation that makes it easier to get infected with the human immunodeficiency virus (HIV) or to pass the HIV virus on to a sex partner.

How Does Trichomoniasis Affect a Pregnant Woman and Her Baby?

Pregnant women with trichomoniasis are more likely to have their babies too early (preterm delivery). Also, babies born to infected mothers are more likely to have an officially low birth weight (less than 5.5 pounds).

How Is Trichomoniasis Diagnosed?

It is not possible to diagnose trichomoniasis based on symptoms alone. For both men and women, your primary care doctor or another trusted healthcare provider must do a check and a laboratory test to diagnose trichomoniasis.

What Is the Treatment for Trichomoniasis?

Trichomoniasis can be cured with a single dose of prescription antibiotic medication (either metronidazole or tinidazole), pills which can be taken by mouth. It is okay for pregnant women to take this medication. Some people who drink alcohol within 24 hours after taking this kind of antibiotic can have uncomfortable side effects.

People who have been treated for trichomoniasis can get it again. About 1 in 5 people get infected again within 3 months after treatment. To avoid getting reinfected, make sure that all of your sex partners get treated too, and wait to have sex again until all of your symptoms go away (about a week). Get checked again if your symptoms come back.

How Can Trichomoniasis Be Prevented?

Using latex condoms correctly every time you have sex will help reduce the risk of getting or spreading trichomoniasis. However, condoms don't cover everything, and it is possible to get or spread this infection even when using a condom. The only sure way to prevent sexually transmitted infections is to avoid having sex entirely.

Another approach is to talk about these kinds of infections before you have sex with a new partner, so that you can make informed choices about the level of risk you are comfortable taking with your sex life. If you or someone you know has questions about trichomoniasis or any other STD, especially with symptoms like unusual discharge, burning during urination, or a sore in the genital area, check in with a healthcare provider and get some answers.

Chapter 54

Tuberculosis

What Is Tuberculosis (TB)?

Tuberculosis (TB) is a disease caused by bacteria called *Mycobacterium tuberculosis*. The bacteria usually attack the lungs. But TB bacteria can attack any part of the body such as the kidney, spine, and brain. If not treated properly, TB disease can be fatal. TB disease was once the leading cause of death in the United States.

TB is spread through the air from one person to another. The bacteria are put into the air when a person with TB disease of the lungs or throat coughs, sneezes, speaks or sings. People nearby may breathe in these bacteria and become infected.

However, not everyone infected with TB bacteria becomes sick. People who are infected, but not sick, have what is called latent TB infection. People who have latent TB infection do not feel sick, do not have any symptoms, and cannot spread TB to others. But some people with latent TB infection go on to get TB disease.

There is good news. People with TB disease can be treated if they seek medical help. Even better, most people with latent TB infection can take medicine so that they will not develop TB disease.

Why Is TB Still a Problem in the United States?

In the early 1900s, TB killed one out of every seven people living in the United States and Europe. Starting in the 1940s, scientists

This chapter includes text excerpted from "Tuberculosis (TB)," Centers for Disease Control and Prevention (CDC), December 18, 2014.

discovered the first of several medicines now used to treat TB. As a result, TB slowly began to decrease in the United States. But in the 1970s and early 1980s, the country let its guard down and TB control efforts were neglected. This led to an increase in the number of TB cases between 1985 and 1992. However, with increased funding and attention to the TB problem, there has been a steady decline in the number of persons with TB since 1993.

TB continues to be a problem. Multidrug-resistant TB (MDR TB) remains a concern, and extensively drug-resistant TB (XDR TB) has become an important issue. While the number of TB cases in the United States has been declining, there remains a higher burden of TB among racial and ethnic minorities. This is due to uneven distribution of TB risk factors that can increase the chance of developing the disease.

How Is TB Spread?

TB is spread through the air from one person to another. The bacteria are put into the air when a person with TB disease of the lungs or throat coughs, sneezes, speaks or sings. People nearby may breathe in these bacteria and become infected.

When a person breathes in TB bacteria, the bacteria can settle in the lungs and begin to grow. From there, they can move through the blood to other parts of the body, such as the kidney, spine, and brain.

TB disease in the lungs or throat can be infectious. This means that the bacteria can be spread to other people. TB in other parts of the body, such as the kidney or spine, is usually not infectious.

People with TB disease are most likely to spread it to people they spend time with every day. This includes family members, friends, and coworkers or schoolmates.

What Is Latent Infection?

In most people who breathe in TB bacteria and become infected, the body is able to fight the bacteria to stop them from growing. The bacteria become inactive, but they remain alive in the body and can become active later. This is called latent TB infection. People with latent TB infection:

- Have no symptoms
- Don't feel sick
- Can't spread TB bacteria to others

- Usually have a positive skin test reaction or positive TB blood test

- May develop TB disease if they do not receive treatment for latent TB infection

Many people who have latent TB infection never develop TB disease. In these people, the TB bacteria remain inactive for a lifetime without causing disease. But in other people, especially people who have weak immune systems, the bacteria become active, multiply, and cause TB disease.

What Is TB Disease?

If the immune system can't stop TB bacteria from growing, the bacteria begin to multiply in the body and cause TB disease. The bacteria attack the body and destroy tissue. If this occurs in the lungs, the bacteria can actually create a hole in the lung. Some people develop TB disease soon after becoming infected (within weeks) before their immune system can fight the TB bacteria. Other people may get sick years later, when their immune system becomes weak for another reason.

Babies and young children often have weak immune systems. People infected with HIV, the virus that causes AIDS, have very weak immune systems. Other people can have weak immune systems, especially people with any of these conditions:

- Substance abuse

- Diabetes mellitus

- Silicosis

- Cancer of the head or neck

- Leukemia or Hodgkin's disease

- Severe kidney disease

- Low body weight

- Certain medical treatments (such as corticosteroid treatment or organ transplants)

- Specialized treatment for rheumatoid arthritis or Crohn's disease

Symptoms of TB disease depend on where in the body the TB bacteria are growing. TB disease in the lungs may cause symptoms such as:

- A bad cough that lasts 3 weeks or longer

- Pain in the chest

- Coughing up blood or sputum (phlegm from deep inside the lungs)

Other symptoms of TB disease are:

- Weakness or fatigue

- Weight loss

- No appetite

- Chills

- Fever

- Sweating at night

Table 54.1. The Difference between Latent TB Infection and TB Disease

A Person with Latent TB Infection	A Person with TB Disease
Does not feel sick	Usually feels sick
Has no symptoms	Has symptoms that may include: • a bad cough that lasts 3 weeks or longer • pain in the chest • coughing up blood or sputum • weakness or fatigue • weight loss • no appetite • chills • fever • sweating at night
Cannot spread TB bacteria to others	May spread TB bacteria to others
Usually has a positive TB skin test or positive TB blood test	Usually has a positive TB skin test or positive TB blood test
Has a normal chest X-ray and a negative sputum smear	May have an abnormal chest X-ray, or positive sputum smear or culture
Should consider treatment for latent TB infection to prevent TB disease	Needs treatment for TB disease

Chapter 55

Typhoid Fever

Typhoid fever is a life-threatening illness caused by the bacterium *Salmonella typhi*. An estimated 5,700 cases occur each year in the United States. Most cases (up to 75%) are acquired while traveling internationally. Typhoid fever is still common in the developing world, where it affects about 21.5 million people each year. Typhoid fever can be prevented and can usually be treated with antibiotics. If you are planning to travel outside the United States, you should know about typhoid fever and what steps you can take to protect yourself.

How Is Typhoid Fever Spread?

Salmonella typhi lives only in humans. Persons with typhoid fever carry the bacteria in their bloodstream and intestinal tract. In addition, a small number of persons, called carriers, recover from typhoid fever but continue to carry the bacteria. Both ill persons and carriers shed *Salmonella typhi* in their feces (stool). You can get typhoid fever if you eat food or drink beverages that have been handled by a person who is shedding *Salmonella typhi* or if sewage contaminated with *Salmonella typhi* bacteria gets into the water you use for drinking or washing food.

Therefore, typhoid fever is more common in areas of the world where handwashing is less frequent and water is likely to be contaminated with sewage. Once *Salmonella typhi* bacteria are eaten or drunk,

This chapter includes text excerpted from "Tuberculosis (TB)," Centers for Disease Control and Prevention (CDC), May 14, 2013.

they multiply and spread into the bloodstream. The body reacts with fever and other signs and symptoms.

What Are the Signs and Symptoms of Typhoid Fever?

Persons with typhoid fever usually have a sustained fever as high as 103° to 104° F (39° to 40° C). They may also feel weak, or have stomach pains, headache, or loss of appetite. In some cases, patients have a rash of flat, rose-colored spots. The only way to know for sure if an illness is typhoid fever is to have samples of stool or blood tested for the presence of *Salmonella typhi*.

What Do You Do If You Think You Have Typhoid Fever?

If you have a high fever and feel very ill, see a doctor immediately. If you are traveling in a foreign country, you can usually call the U.S. consulate for a list of recommended doctors. Typhoid fever is treated with antibiotics. Resistance to multiple antibiotics is increasing among *Salmonella* that cause typhoid fever. Reduced susceptibility to fluoroquinolones (e.g., ciprofloxacin) and the emergence of multidrug-resistance has complicated treatment of infections, especially those acquired in South Asia. Antibiotic susceptibility testing may help guide appropriate therapy. Choices for antibiotic therapy include fluoroquinolones (for susceptible infections), ceftriaxone, and azithromycin. Persons who do not get treatment may continue to have fever for weeks or months, and as many as 20% may die from complications of the infection.

Typhoid Fever's Danger Doesn't End When Symptoms Disappear

Even if your symptoms seem to go away, you may still be carrying *Salmonella typhi*. If so, the illness could return, or you could pass the disease to other people. In fact, if you work at a job where you handle food or care for small children, you may be barred legally from going back to work until a doctor has determined that you no longer carry any typhoid bacteria. If you are being treated for typhoid fever, it is important to do the following:

- Keep taking the prescribed antibiotics for as long as the doctor has asked you to take them.

- Wash your hands carefully with soap and water after using the bathroom, and do not prepare or serve food for other people.

This will lower the chance that you will pass the infection on to someone else.

- Have your doctor perform a series of stool cultures to ensure that no *Salmonella typhi* bacteria remain in your body.

Where in the World Do You Get Typhoid Fever?

Typhoid fever is common in most parts of the world except in industrialized regions such as the United States, Canada, western Europe, Australia, and Japan. Therefore, if you are traveling to the developing world, you should consider taking precautions. Other areas of risk include East and Southeast Asia, Africa, the Caribbean, and Central and South America.

How Can You Avoid Typhoid Fever?

Two basic actions can protect you from typhoid fever:

1. Avoid risky foods and drinks
2. Get vaccinated against typhoid fever

It may surprise you, but watching what you eat and drink when you travel is as important as being vaccinated. This is because the vaccines are not completely effective. Avoiding risky foods will also help protect you from other illnesses, including travelers' diarrhea, cholera, dysentery, and hepatitis A.

"Boil It, Cook It, Peel It, or Forget It"

- If you drink water, buy it bottled or bring it to a rolling boil for 1 minute before you drink it. Bottled carbonated water is safer than uncarbonated water.

- Ask for drinks without ice unless the ice is made from bottled or boiled water. Avoid popsicles and flavored ices that may have been made with contaminated water.

- Eat foods that have been thoroughly cooked and that are still hot and steaming.

- Avoid raw vegetables and fruits that cannot be peeled. Vegetables like lettuce are easily contaminated and are very hard to wash well.

357

- When you eat raw fruit or vegetables that can be peeled, peel them yourself. (Wash your hands with soap first.) Do not eat the peelings.

- Avoid foods and beverages from street vendors. It is difficult for food to be kept clean on the street, and many travelers get sick from food bought from street vendors.

Vaccination

If you are traveling to a country where typhoid is common, you should consider being vaccinated against typhoid. Visit a doctor or travel clinic to discuss your vaccination options. Remember that you will need to complete your vaccination at least 1–2 weeks (dependent upon vaccine type) before you travel so that the vaccine has time to take effect. Typhoid vaccines lose effectiveness after several years; if you were vaccinated in the past, check with your doctor to see if it is time for a booster vaccination. Taking antibiotics will not prevent typhoid fever; they only help treat it. The table below provides basic information on typhoid vaccines that are available in the United States.

Table 55.1. Typhoid Vaccines Available in the United States

A Person with Latent TB Infection	A Person with TB Disease
Does not feel sick	Usually feels sick
Has no symptoms	Has symptoms that may include: • a bad cough that lasts 3 weeks or longer • pain in the chest • coughing up blood or sputum • weakness or fatigue • weight loss • no appetite • chills • fever • sweating at night
May spread TB bacteria to others	Usually has a positive TB skin test or positive TB blood test
Usually has a positive TB skin test or positive TB blood test	Has a normal chest X-ray and a negative sputum smear
May have an abnormal chest X-ray, or positive sputum smear or culture	Should consider treatment for latent TB infection to prevent TB disease
Needs treatment for TB disease	

Chapter 56

Vaginal and Reproductive Tract Infections

Bacterial Vaginosis

Bacterial vaginosis (BV) is an infection in the vagina. BV is caused by changes in the amount of certain types of bacteria in your vagina. BV is the most common vaginal infection in women ages 15 to 44. BV is easily treatable with medicine from your doctor or nurse. If left untreated, it can raise your risk for sexually transmitted infections (STIs), including human immunodeficiency virus (HIV), genital herpes, chlamydia, and gonorrhea. Women with HIV who get BV are also more likely to pass HIV to a male sexual partner.

How Do You Get BV?

Researchers are still studying how women get BV. You can get BV without having sex, but BV can also be caused by vaginal, oral, or anal sex. You can get BV from male or female partners.

This chapter contains text excerpted from the following sources: Text under the heading "Bacterial Vaginosis" is excerpted from "Bacterial Vaginosis," Office on Women's Health (OWH), U.S. Department of Health and Human Services (HHS), November 19, 2014; Text under the heading "Pelvic Inflammatory Disease" is excerpted from "Pelvic Inflammatory Disease," Office on Women's Health (OWH), U.S. Department of Health and Human Services (HHS), March 25, 2014; Text under the heading "Vaginal Yeast Infections-Women's Health Guide" is excerpted from "Vaginal Yeast Infections," U.S. Department of Veterans Affairs (VA), January 9, 2013.

You may be more at risk for BV if you:

- Have a new sex partner

- Have multiple sex partners

- Douche

- Do not use condoms

- Are pregnant. The Centers for Disease Control and Prevention (CDC) estimates that 1 million pregnant women get BV each year. The risk for BV is higher for pregnant women because of the hormonal changes that happen during pregnancy.

- Are African-American. BV is twice as common in African-American women as in white women.

- Have an intrauterine device (IUD), especially if you also have irregular bleeding.

What Are the Signs and Symptoms of BV?

Many women have no signs or symptoms. If you do have symptoms, they may include:

- Unusual vaginal discharge. The discharge can be white (milky) or gray. It may also be foamy or watery. Some women report a strong fish-like odor, especially after sex.

- Burning when urinating.

- Itching around the outside of the vagina.

- Vaginal irritation.

These symptoms may be similar to vaginal yeast infections and other health problems. Only your doctor or nurse can tell you for sure whether you have BV.

What Should I Do If I Have BV?

BV is easy to treat. If you think you have BV:

- See a doctor or nurse. Antibiotics will treat BV.

- Take all of your medicine. Even if symptoms go away, you need to finish all of the antibiotic.

- Tell any female sex partners so they can be treated. Male sex partners won't need to be treated.

- Avoid sexual contact until you finish your treatment.

- See your doctor or nurse again if you have symptoms that don't go away within a few days after finishing the antibiotic.

How Can I Lower My Risk of BV?

Steps you can take to lower your risk of BV include:

- Help keep your vaginal bacteria balanced. Use only warm water to clean the outside of your vagina. You do not need to use soap. Even mild soap can cause infection or irritate your vagina. Always wipe front to back from your vagina to your anus.

- Do not douche. Douching removes some of the normal bacteria in your vagina that protect you from infection. Doctors do not recommend douching.

- Practice safe sex. The best way to prevent the spread of BV through sex is by not having sex. If you do have sex, you can lower your risk of getting BV, or any STI, with the following steps:

  - Use condoms. Condoms are the best way to prevent BV or STIs when you have sex. Make sure to put on the condom before the penis touches your vagina, mouth, or anus. Other methods of birth control, like birth control pills, shots, implants, or diaphragms, will not protect you from STIs.

  - Get tested. Be sure you and your partner are tested for STIs. Talk to each other about your test results before you have sex.

  - Be monogamous. Having sex with just one partner can lower your risk. Be faithful to each other. That means that you only have sex with each other and no one else.

  - Limit your number of sex partners. Your risk of getting BV and STIs goes up with the number of partners you have.

  - Don't abuse alcohol or drugs, which are linked to sexual risk taking. Drinking too much alcohol or using drugs also puts you at risk of sexual assault and possible exposure to STIs.

Pelvic Inflammatory Disease

Pelvic inflammatory disease (PID) is an infection of a woman's reproductive organs. Usually PID is caused by bacteria from sexually transmitted infections (STIs). Sometimes PID is caused by normal bacteria found in the vagina. If left untreated, PID can cause problems getting pregnant, problems during pregnancy, and long-term pelvic pain.

Who Gets PID?

PID affects about 5 percent of women in the United States. Your risk for PID is higher if you:

- Have had an STI.
- Have had PID before.
- Are younger than 25 and have sex. PID is most common in women 15 to 24 years old.
- Have more than one sex partner or have a partner who has multiple sexual partners.
- Douche. Douching can push bacteria into the reproductive organs and cause PID. Douching can also hide the signs of PID.
- Recently had an intrauterine device (IUD) inserted. The risk of PID is higher for the first few weeks only after insertion of an IUD. PID is rare after that time period. Getting tested for STIs before the IUD is inserted lowers your risk for PID.

What Are the Signs and Symptoms of PID?

Many women do not know they have PID, because they do not have any signs or symptoms. When symptoms do happen, they can be mild or more serious. Signs and symptoms include:

- Pain in the lower abdomen (this is the most common symptom)
- Fever (100.4° F or higher)
- Vaginal discharge that may smell foul
- Painful sex
- Pain when urinating
- Irregular menstrual periods
- Pain in the upper right abdomen (this is rare)

If you think that you may have PID, see a doctor or nurse as soon as possible.

How Is PID Treated?

Your doctor or nurse will give you antibiotics to treat PID. Most of the time, at least two antibiotics are used that work against many different types of bacteria. You must take all of your antibiotics, even if your symptoms go away. This helps to make sure the infection is fully cured. See your doctor or nurse again two to three days after starting the antibiotics to make sure they are working.

How Can I Prevent PID?

You may not be able to prevent PID. It is not always caused by an STI. Sometimes, normal bacteria in your vagina can travel up to your reproductive organs and cause PID. But you can lower your risk of PID by not douching. You can also prevent STIs by not having vaginal, oral, or anal sex. If you do have sex, lower your risk of getting an STI with the following steps:

- Use condoms. Condoms are the best way to prevent STIs when you have sex. Because a man does not need to ejaculate (come) to give or get STIs, make sure to put the condom on before the penis touches the vagina, mouth, or anus. Other methods of birth control, such as birth control pills, shots, implants, or diaphragms, will not protect you from STIs.

- Get tested. Be sure you and your partner are tested for STIs. Talk to each other about the test results before you have sex.

- Be monogamous. Having sex with just one partner can lower your risk for STIs. After being tested for STIs, be faithful to each other. That means that you have sex only with each other and no one else.

- Limit your number of sex partners. Your risk of getting STIs goes up with the number of partners you have.

- Do not douche. Douching removes some of the normal bacteria in the vagina that protect you from infection. Douching may also raise your risk for PID by helping bacteria travel to other areas, like your uterus, ovaries, and fallopian tubes.

- Do not abuse alcohol or drugs. Drinking too much alcohol or using drugs increases risky behavior and may put you at risk of sexual assault and possible exposure to STIs.

The steps work best when used together. No single step can protect you from every single type of STI.

Vaginal Yeast Infections

A vaginal yeast infection is an infection of the vagina and vaginal area. It is caused by a type of fungus called yeast. When this yeast increases it can cause an infection.

Three out of four women will get a vaginal yeast infection during their life. Some women will have it more than once. A vaginal yeast infection is NOT a sexually transmitted disease (STD).

How Is It Spread?

Yeast is not spread from person to person. Small amounts of yeast can be found in the normal vagina. Infection occurs when too much yeast begins to grow. Vaginal yeast infections can increase with:

- Pregnancy
- Illness such as HIV disease or diabetes
- Some medicines such as:
- Antibiotics
- Birth control pills
- Cortisone-type drugs
- Some chemotherapy drugs
- Stress
- Lack of sleep
- Having your period

Having many vaginal yeast infections may be a sign of other health problems.

What Are Signs of Vaginal Yeast Infections?

- Itching in the vaginal area.
- Vaginal discharge. This is mostly white. It can be watery to thick, and even chunky. It does not have a bad smell.
- Redness, swelling, and burning in the vaginal area.
- Pain with urination or during sex.

How Do You Know If You Have an Infection?

Yeast infections can be diagnosed during a medical exam. To check for a vaginal yeast infection, your healthcare provider looks for signs of infection and collects a sample of vaginal fluid for lab tests.

How Is It Treated?

Vaginal yeast infections can be treated with medicines such as pills or creams, ovules, or ointments. Treatment may take from 1 to 7 days.

Women with weak immune systems or other medical problems may need longer treatment. Always finish treatment, even if the signs of a yeast infection go away. Yeast infections can come back if not treated correctly. Infection is more likely to return if some health problems, such as diabetes, are not under control.

What Can Happen If You Don't Get Treated for a Yeast Infection?

Signs of infection may get worse without treatment. Scratching the vaginal area can leave open or raw areas. These can become infected with other germs.

How Can You Avoid Vaginal Yeast Infections?

- Do not douche.
- Avoid scented products such as bubble baths, feminine hygiene sprays, pads or tampons.
- Change pads and tampons often during your period.
- Do not wear tight clothing. This can cause irritation and sweating in the vaginal area.
- Wear cotton underwear.
- Wear pantyhose with a cotton crotch.
- Change out of wet clothing and swimsuits right away.
- Keep blood sugar under control if you have diabetes.

What about Pregnancy?

Pregnancy can increase the risk of vaginal yeast infections. Ask your healthcare provider about safe and effective treatments. Babies born to a mother with a vaginal yeast infection can get a mouth infection (thrush).

Chapter 57

Vancomycin-Resistant Enterococci (VRE)

What Is Vancomycin-Resistant Enterococci?

Enteroccocci are bacteria that are normally present in the human intestines and in the female genital tract and are often found in the environment. These bacteria can sometimes cause infections. Vancomycin is an antibiotic that is used to treat some drug-resistant infections caused by enterococci. In some instances, enterococci have become resistant to this drug and thus are called vancomycin-resistant enterococci (VRE). Most VRE infections occur in hospitals.

What Types of Infections Does VRE Cause?

VRE can live in the human intestines and female genital tract without causing disease (often called colonization). However, sometimes it can cause infections of the urinary tract, the bloodstream or of wounds associated with catheters or surgical procedures.

This chapter includes text excerpted from "Healthcare-Associated Infections," Centers for Disease Control and Prevention (CDC), May 10, 2011. Reviewed August 2016.

Are Certain People at Risk of Getting VRE?

The following persons are at increased risk becoming infected with VRE:

- People who have been previously treated with the antibiotic vancomycin or other antibiotics for long periods of time.
- People who are hospitalized, particularly when they receive antibiotic treatment for long periods of time.
- People with weakened immune systems such as patients in intensive care units, or in cancer or transplant wards.
- People who have undergone surgical procedures such as abdominal or chest surgery.
- People with medical devices that stay in for some time such as urinary catheters or central intravenous (IV) catheters.
- People who are colonized with VRE.

What Is the Treatment for VRE?

People with colonized VRE (bacteria are present, but have no symptoms of an infection) do not need treatment. Most VRE infections can be treated with antibiotics other than vancomycin. Laboratory testing of the VRE can determine which antibiotics will work. For people who get VRE infections in their bladder and have urinary catheters, removal of the catheter when it is no longer needed can also help get rid of the infection.

How Is VRE Spread?

VRE is often passed from person to person by the contaminated hands of caregivers. VRE can get onto a caregiver's hands after they have contact with other people with VRE or after contact with contaminated surfaces. VRE can also be spread directly to people after they touch surfaces that are contaminated with VRE. VRE is not spread through the air by coughing or sneezing.

How Can Patients Prevent the Spread of VRE?

If a patient or someone in their household has VRE, the following are some things they can do to prevent the spread of VRE:

- Keep their hands clean. Always wash their hands thoroughly after using the bathroom and before preparing food. Clean their hands after contact with persons who have VRE. Wash with soap and water (particularly when visibly soiled) or use alcohol-based hand rubs.

- Frequently clean areas of the home, such as bathrooms, that may become contaminated with VRE.

- Wear gloves if hands may come in contact with body fluids that may contain VRE, such as stool or bandages from infected wounds. Always wash their hands after removing gloves.

- If someone has VRE, be sure to tell healthcare providers so that they are aware of the infection. Healthcare facilities use special precautions to help prevent the spread of VRE to others.

What Should Patients Do If They Think They Have Vancomycin-Resistant Enterococci (VRE)?

Anyone who thinks they have VRE must talk with their healthcare provider.

Chapter 58

Whooping Cough (Pertussis)

Causes

Pertussis, a respiratory illness commonly known as whooping cough, is a very contagious disease caused by a type of bacteria called *Bordetella pertussis*. These bacteria attach to the cilia (tiny, hair-like extensions) that line part of the upper respiratory system. The bacteria release toxins (poisons), which damage the cilia and cause airways to swell.

Transmission

Pertussis is a very contagious disease only found in humans. It is spread from person to person. People with pertussis usually spread the disease to another person by coughing or sneezing or when spending a lot of time near one another where you share breathing space. Many babies who get pertussis are infected by older siblings, parents, or caregivers who might not even know they have the disease. Infected people are most contagious up to about 2 weeks after the cough begins. Antibiotics may shorten the amount of time someone is contagious.

While pertussis vaccines are the most effective tool we have to prevent this disease, no vaccine is 100% effective. If pertussis is circulating

This chapter includes text excerpted from "Pertussis (Whooping Cough)," Centers for Disease Control and Prevention (CDC), August 31, 2015.

in the community, there is a chance that a fully vaccinated person, of any age, can catch this very contagious disease. If you have been vaccinated but still get sick, the infection is usually not as bad.

Signs and Symptoms

Pertussis (whooping cough) can cause serious illness in babies, children, teens, and adults. Symptoms of pertussis usually develop within 5 to 10 days after being exposed, but sometimes not for as long as 3 weeks.

Early Symptoms

The disease usually starts with cold-like symptoms and maybe a mild cough or fever. In babies, the cough can be minimal or not even there. Babies may have a symptom known as "apnea." Apnea is a pause in the child's breathing pattern. Pertussis is most dangerous for babies. About half of babies younger than 1 year who get the disease need care in the hospital.

Early symptoms can last for 1 to 2 weeks and usually include:

- Runny nose
- Low-grade fever (generally minimal throughout the course of the disease)
- Mild, occasional cough
- Apnea–a pause in breathing (in babies)

Because pertussis in its early stages appears to be nothing more than the common cold, it is often not suspected or diagnosed until the more severe symptoms appear.

Later-Stage Symptoms

After 1 to 2 weeks and as the disease progresses, the traditional symptoms of pertussis may appear and include:

- Paroxysms (fits) of many, rapid coughs followed by a high-pitched "whoop"
- Vomiting (throwing up) during or after coughing fits
- Exhaustion (very tired) after coughing fits

Pertussis can cause violent and rapid coughing, over and over, until the air is gone from the lungs and you are forced to inhale with a loud "whooping" sound. This extreme coughing can cause you to throw up and be very tired. Although you are often exhausted after a coughing fit, you usually appear fairly well in-between. Coughing fits generally become more common and bad as the illness continues, and can occur more often at night. The coughing fits can go on for up to 10 weeks or more. In China, pertussis is known as the "100 day cough." However, the "whoop" is often not there for people who have milder (less serious) disease. The infection is generally milder in teens and adults, especially those who have been vaccinated.

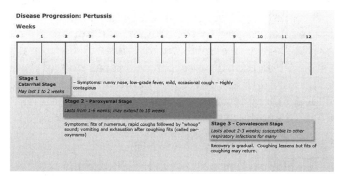

Figure 58.1. *Disease Progression*

Recovery

Recovery from pertussis can happen slowly. The cough becomes milder and less common. However, coughing fits can return with other respiratory infections for many months after the pertussis infection started.

Complications

Babies and Children

Pertussis (whooping cough) can cause serious and sometimes deadly complications in babies and young children, especially those who are not fully vaccinated. In babies younger than 1 year old who get pertussis, about half need care in the hospital. The younger the baby, the more likely treatment in the hospital will be needed. Of those babies who are treated in the hospital with pertussis about:

- 1 out of 4 (23%) get pneumonia (lung infection)

- 1 out of 100 (1.1%) will have convulsions (violent, uncontrolled shaking)

373

- 3 out of 5 (61%) will have apnea (slowed or stopped breathing)

- 1 out of 300 (0.3%) will have encephalopathy (disease of the brain)

- 1 out of 100 (1%) will die

Teens and Adults

Teens and adults can also get complications from pertussis. They are usually less serious in this older age group, especially in those who have been vaccinated with a pertussis vaccine. Complications in teens and adults are often caused by the cough itself. For example, you may pass out or break (fracture) a rib during violent coughing fits.

In one study, less than 1 out of 20 (5%) teens and adults with pertussis needed care in the hospital. Pneumonia (lung infection) was diagnosed in 1 out of 50 (2%) of those patients. The most common complications in another study were:

- Weight loss in 1 out of 3 (33%) adults

- Loss of bladder control in 1 out of 3 (28%) adults

- Passing out in 3 out of 50 (6%) adults

- Rib fractures from severe coughing in 1 out of 25 (4%) adults

Diagnosis

Pertussis (whooping cough) can be diagnosed by taking into consideration if you have been exposed to pertussis and by doing a:

- History of typical signs and symptoms

- Physical examination

- Laboratory test which involves taking a sample of mucus (with a swab or syringe filled with saline) from the back of the throat through the nose.

- Blood test

Treatment

Pertussis is generally treated with antibiotics and early treatment is very important. Treatment may make your infection less serious if it is started early, before coughing fits begin. Treatment can also help prevent spreading the disease to close contacts (people who have spent a lot of time around the infected person). Treatment after three weeks of illness is unlikely to help because the bacteria are gone from your body, even though you usually will still have symptoms. This is because the bacteria have already done damage to your body.

There are several antibiotics (medications that can help treat diseases caused by bacteria) available to treat pertussis. If you or your child is diagnosed with pertussis, your doctor will explain how to treat the infection. Pertussis can sometimes be very serious, requiring treatment in the hospital. Babies are at greatest risk for serious complications from pertussis.

If Your Child Is Treated for Pertussis at Home

Do not give cough medications unless instructed by your doctor. Giving cough medicine probably will not help and is often not recommended for kids younger than 4 years old.

Manage pertussis and reduce the risk of spreading it to others by:

- Following the schedule for giving antibiotics exactly as your child's doctor prescribed.

- Keeping your home free from irritants-as much as possible-that can trigger coughing, such as smoke, dust, and chemical fumes.

- Using a clean, cool mist vaporizer to help loosen mucus and soothe the cough.

- Practicing good hand washing.

- Encouraging your child to drink plenty of fluids, including water, juices, and soups, and eating fruits to prevent dehydration (lack of fluids). Report any signs of dehydration to your doctor immediately. These include dry, sticky mouth, sleepiness or tiredness, thirst, decreased urination or fewer wet diapers, few or no tears when crying, muscle weakness, headache, dizziness or lightheadedness.

- Encouraging your child to eat small meals every few hours to help prevent vomiting (throwing up) from occurring.

If Your Child Is Treated for Pertussis in the Hospital

Your child may need help keeping breathing passages clear, which may require suctioning (drawing out) of mucus. Breathing is monitored and oxygen will be given, if needed. Intravenous (IV, through the vein) fluids might be required if your child shows signs of dehydration or has difficulty eating. Precautions, like practicing good hand hygiene and keeping surfaces clean, should be taken.

Prevention

Vaccines

The best way to prevent pertussis (whooping cough) among babies, children, teens, and adults is to get vaccinated. Also, keep babies and other people at high risk for pertussis complications away from infected people.

In the United States, the recommended pertussis vaccine for babies and children is called DTaP. This is a combination vaccine that helps protect against three diseases: diphtheria, tetanus, and pertussis. Vaccine protection for these three diseases fades with time. Before 2005, the only booster (called Td) available contained protection against tetanus and diphtheria, and was recommended for teens and adults every 10 years. Today there is a booster (called Tdap) for preteens, teens, and adults that contains protection against tetanus, diphtheria and pertussis.

Being up-to-date with pertussis vaccines is especially important for families with and caregivers of new babies.

Infection

If your doctor confirms that you have pertussis, your body will have a natural defense (immunity) to future infections. Some observational studies suggest that pertussis infection can provide immunity for 4 to 20 years. Since this immunity fades and does not offer lifelong protection, vaccination is still recommended.

Antibiotics

If you or a member of your household has been diagnosed with pertussis, your doctor or local health department may recommend preventive antibiotics (medications that can help prevent diseases caused by bacteria) to other members of the household to help prevent the spread of disease. Additionally, some other people outside the household who have been exposed to a person with pertussis may be given preventive antibiotics, including:

- People at risk for serious disease

- People who have routine contact with someone that is considered at high risk of serious disease

Babies younger than one year old are most at risk for serious complications from pertussis. Although pregnant women are not at increased risk for serious disease, those in their third trimester would be considered at increased risk since they could in turn expose their newborn to pertussis. You should discuss whether or not you need preventative antibiotics with your doctor, especially if there is a baby or pregnant woman in your household or you plan to have contact with a baby or pregnant woman.

Hygiene

Like many respiratory illnesses, pertussis is spread by coughing and sneezing while in close contact with others, who then breathe in the pertussis bacteria. Practicing good hygiene is always recommended to prevent the spread of respiratory illnesses. To practice good hygiene you should:

- Cover your mouth and nose with a tissue when you cough or sneeze.

- Put your used tissue in the waste basket.

- Cough or sneeze into your upper sleeve or elbow, not your hands, if you don't have a tissue.

- Wash your hands often with soap and water for at least 20 seconds.

- Use an alcohol-based hand rub if soap and water are not available.

Chapter 59

Zika Virus

How Zika Spreads

Zika can be transmitted through:

- Mosquito bites
- From a pregnant woman to her fetus
- Sex
- Blood transfusion (very likely but not confirmed)

Zika Symptoms

Many people infected with Zika virus won't have symptoms or will only have mild symptoms. The most common symptoms of Zika are:

- Fever
- Rash
- Joint pain
- Conjunctivitis (red eyes)

Other symptoms include:

- Muscle pain
- Headache

This chapter includes text excerpted from "Zika Virus," Centers for Disease Control and Prevention (CDC), July 13, 2016.

Symptoms can last for several days to a week. People usually don't get sick enough to go to the hospital, and they very rarely die of Zika. Once a person has been infected with Zika, they are likely to be protected from future infections.

Why Zika Is Risky for Some People

Zika infection during pregnancy can cause a birth defect of the brain called microcephaly and other severe fetal brain defects. Other problems have been detected among fetuses and infants infected with Zika virus before birth, such as defects of the eye, hearing deficits, and impaired growth. There have also been increased reports of Guillain-Barré syndrome, an uncommon sickness of the nervous system, in areas affected by Zika.

How to Prevent Zika

There is no vaccine to prevent Zika. The best way to prevent diseases spread by mosquitoes is to protect yourself and your family from mosquito bites. Here's how:

Clothing

- Wear long-sleeved shirts and long pants.
- Treat your clothing and gear with permethrin or buy pre-treated items.

Insect repellent

- Use Environmental Protection Agency (EPA)-registered insect repellents with one of the following active ingredients: DEET, picaridin, IR3535, or oil of lemon eucalyptus or para-menthane-diol. Always follow the product label instructions.
- When used as directed, these insect repellents are proven safe and effective even for pregnant and breastfeeding women.
- Do not use insect repellents on babies younger than 2 months old.
- Do not use products containing oil of lemon eucalyptus or para-menthane-diol on children younger than 3 years old.

At Home

- Stay in places with air conditioning and window and door screens to keep mosquitoes outside.

- Take steps to control mosquitoes inside and outside your home.

- Mosquito netting can be used to cover babies younger than 2 months old in carriers, strollers, or cribs.

- Sleep under a mosquito bed net if air conditioned or screened rooms are not available or if sleeping outdoors.

Sexual transmission

- Prevent sexual transmission of Zika by using condoms or not having sex.

How Zika Is Diagnosed

- Diagnosis of Zika is based on a person's recent travel history, symptoms, and test results.

- A blood or urine test can confirm a Zika infection.

- Symptoms of Zika are similar to other illnesses spread through mosquito bites, like dengue and chikungunya.

- Your doctor or other healthcare provider may order tests to look for several types of infections.

What to Do If You Have Zika

There is no specific medicine or vaccine for Zika virus. Treat the symptoms:

- Get plenty of rest.

- Drink fluids to prevent dehydration.

- Take medicine such as acetaminophen to reduce fever and pain.

- Do not take aspirin or other non-steroidal anti-inflammatory drugs (NSAIDs).

- If you are taking medicine for another medical condition, talk to your healthcare provider before taking additional medication.

Part Three

Self-Treatment for Contagious Diseases

Chapter 60

Self-Care for Colds or Flu

Chapter Contents

Section 60.1

What to Do for Colds and Flu

This section includes text excerpted from "Get Set
for a Healthy Winter Season," U.S. Food and Drug
Administration (FDA), January 21, 2016.

Although contagious viruses are active year-round, we're most vulnerable to them in fall and winter. That's because, in large part, we spend more time indoors with other people when the weather gets cold. Fortunately, you can fight back with several U.S. Food and Drug Administration (FDA)-approved medicines and vaccines.

Colds and Flu

Most respiratory bugs come and go within a few days, with no lasting effects. But some cause serious health problems. People who use tobacco or who are exposed to secondhand smoke are more prone to respiratory illnesses and more severe complications than nonsmokers.

Colds usually cause a stuffy or runny nose and sneezing. Other symptoms include coughing, a scratchy throat, and watery eyes. There is no vaccine against colds, which come on gradually and often spread through contact with infected mucus.

Flu comes on suddenly and lasts longer than colds. Flu symptoms include fever, headache, chills, dry cough, body aches, fatigue, and general misery. Like colds, flu can cause a stuffy or runny nose, sneezing, and watery eyes. Young children may also experience nausea and vomiting with flu. Flu viruses spread mainly by droplets made when people with flu cough, sneeze or talk. You also can get flu by touching a surface or object that has flu virus on it. Flu season in the United States may begin as early as October and can last as late as May, and generally peaks between December and February.

According to the Centers for Disease Control and Prevention (CDC):

- More than 200,000 people in the United States are hospitalized from flu-related complications each year, including 20,000 children younger than age 5.

- Between 1976 and 2006, the estimated number of flu-related deaths every year ranged from about 3,000 to about 49,000.

- In the 2014–15 season, there were about 40 million flu-associated illnesses, 19 million flu-associated medical visits, and 970,000 flu-associated hospitalizations—the highest estimate for a single flu season.

Prevention Tips

Get Vaccinated against Flu

With rare exceptions, everyone ages six months and older should be vaccinated against flu. Flu vaccination, available as a shot or a nasal spray, can reduce flu illnesses, doctors' visits, missed work and school, and prevent flu-related hospitalizations and deaths. It's ideal to be vaccinated by October, although vaccination into January and beyond can still offer protection. Annual vaccination is needed because flu viruses are constantly changing, flu vaccines may need to be updated, and because a person's immune protection from the vaccine declines over time. Annual vaccination is especially important for people at high risk for developing serious complications from flu. These people include:

- Children younger than 5 years, but especially those younger than 2

- Pregnant women

- People with certain chronic health conditions (such as asthma, diabetes or heart and lung disease)

- People 65 or older

Vaccination is especially important for healthcare workers, as well as those who live with or care for people at high risk for serious flu-related complications, such as people older than 65 or with compromised immune systems. Because babies younger than 6 months are too young to get a flu vaccine, their mother should get a flu shot during her pregnancy to protect them throughout pregnancy and up to 6 months after birth. Additionally, all of the baby's caregivers and close contacts should be vaccinated.

Although there was a less than ideal match between circulating flu strains and those included in the vaccine during last season, CDC estimates that the vaccines still provided about half the protection they did during the previous season. CDC also reports that this season's vaccines better match circulating viruses.

387

Practice Healthy Habits

Wash your hands often. Teach children to do the same. Both colds and flu can be passed through contaminated surfaces, including the hands. Wash hands with warm water and soap for 20 seconds. **Try to limit exposure to infected people**. Keep infants away from crowds for the first few months of life.

- Eat a balanced diet

- Get enough sleep

- Exercise

- Do your best to keep stress in check

What to Do If You're Already Sick

Usually, colds have to run their course. Gargling with salt water may relieve a sore throat. And a cool-mist humidifier may help relieve stuffy noses. Here are other steps to consider:

- **Call your healthcare professional.** Start the treatment early.

- **Limit your exposure to other people.** Cover your mouth with a tissue when you cough or sneeze.

- **Stay hydrated and rested.** Avoid alcohol and caffeinated products, which may dehydrate you.

- **Talk to your healthcare professional to find out what will work best for you.**

In addition to over-the-counter (OTC) medicines, there are FDA-approved prescription medications for treating flu. Cold and flu complications may include bacterial infections (e.g., bronchitis, sinusitis, ear infections, and pneumonia) that could require antibiotics.

Tips for Taking OTC Products

Read medicine labels carefully and follow the directions. People with certain health conditions, such as high blood pressure and diabetes, should check with a healthcare professional or pharmacist before taking a new cough and cold medicine.

Choose OTC Medicines Appropriate for Your Symptoms

- Nasal decongestants unclog a stuffy nose

- Cough suppressants quiet coughs

- Expectorants loosen mucus

- Antihistamines help stop a runny nose and sneezing

- Pain relievers can ease fever, headaches, and minor aches

Check the medicine's side effects. Medications can cause drowsiness and interact with food, alcohol, dietary supplements, and each other. It's best to tell your healthcare professional and pharmacist about every medical product and supplement you are taking.

Check with a Healthcare Professional before Giving Medicine to Children

See a healthcare professional if you aren't getting any better. With children, be alert for high fevers and for abnormal behavior such as unusual drowsiness, refusal to eat, crying a lot, holding the ears or stomach, and wheezing. **Signs of trouble** for all people can include:

- A cough that disrupts sleep

- A fever that won't respond to treatment

- Increased shortness of breath

- Face pain caused by a sinus infection

- High fever, chest pain or a difference in the mucus you're producing, after feeling better for a short time

Section 60.2

Actions to Fight Flu and FAQs about Preventing Seasonal Flu

This section contains text excerpted from the following sources: Text under the heading "Centers for Disease Control and Prevention (CDC) Says "Take 3" Actions to Fight the Flu" is excerpted from "CDC Says "Take 3" Actions to Fight the Flu," Centers for Disease Control and Prevention (CDC), May 26, 2016; Text under the heading "FAQs for Preventing Seasonal Flu Illness" is excerpted from "Preventing Seasonal Flu Illness," Centers for Disease Control and Prevention (CDC), April 28, 2015.

Centers for Disease Control and Prevention (CDC) Says "Take 3" Actions to Fight the Flu

1. Take Time to Get a Flu Vaccine

- Centers for Disease Control and Prevention (CDC) recommends a yearly flu vaccine as the first and most important step in protecting against flu viruses.

- While there are many different flu viruses, a flu vaccine protects against the viruses that research suggests will be most common.

- Flu vaccination can reduce flu illnesses, doctors' visits, and missed work and school due to flu, as well as prevent flu-related hospitalizations and deaths.

- Everyone six months of age and older should get a flu vaccine as soon as the current season's vaccines are available.

- Vaccination of high risk persons is especially important to decrease their risk of severe flu illness.

- People at high risk of serious flu complications include young children, pregnant women, people with chronic health conditions like asthma, diabetes or heart and lung disease and people 65 years and older.

- Vaccination also is important for healthcare workers, and other people who live with or care for high risk people to keep from spreading flu to them.

- Children younger than 6 months are at high risk of serious flu illness, but are too young to be vaccinated. People who care for infants should be vaccinated instead.

2. Take Everyday Preventive Actions to Stop the Spread of Germs

- Try to avoid close contact with sick people.

- While sick, limit contact with others as much as possible to keep from infecting them.

- If you are sick with flu-like illness, CDC recommends that you stay home for at least 24 hours after your fever is gone except to get medical care or for other necessities. (Your fever should be gone for 24 hours without the use of a fever-reducing medicine.)

- Cover your nose and mouth with a tissue when you cough or sneeze. Throw the tissue in the trash after you use it.

- Wash your hands often with soap and water. If soap and water are not available, use an alcohol-based hand rub.

- Avoid touching your eyes, nose, and mouth. Germs spread this way.

- Clean and disinfect surfaces and objects that may be contaminated with germs like the flu.

3. Take Flu Antiviral Drugs If Your Doctor Prescribes Them

- If you get the flu, antiviral drugs can be used to treat your illness.

- Antiviral drugs are different from antibiotics. They are prescription medicines (pills, liquid or an inhaled powder) and are not available over-the-counter (OTC).

- Antiviral drugs can make illness milder and shorten the time you are sick. They may also prevent serious flu complications. For people with high risk factors, treatment with an antiviral drug can mean the difference between having a milder illness versus a very serious illness that could result in a hospital stay.

- Studies show that flu antiviral drugs work best for treatment when they are started within 2 days of getting sick, but starting them later can still be helpful, especially if the sick person has a high-risk health condition or is very sick from the flu. Follow your doctor's instructions for taking this drug.

- Flu-like symptoms include fever, cough, sore throat, runny or stuffy nose, body aches, headache, chills, and fatigue. Some people also may have vomiting and diarrhea. People may be infected with the flu, and have respiratory symptoms without a fever.

FAQs for Preventing Seasonal Flu Illness

What Can I Do to Protect Myself against the Flu?

The single best way to protect against the flu is to get a flu vaccine each year. CDC recommends that everyone 6 months and older, especially people at high risk for developing serious complications from flu, get vaccinated each season.

What Are Other Steps That Can Be Taken to Prevent Flu Illness?

Take everyday preventive actions to stop the spread of germs.

- Try to avoid close contact with sick people.

- If you are sick with flu–like illness, CDC recommends that you stay home for at least 24 hours after your fever is gone except to get medical care or for other necessities. Your fever should be gone without the use of a fever-reducing medicine.

- While sick, limit contact with others as much as possible to keep from infecting them.

- Cover your nose and mouth with a tissue when you cough or sneeze. Throw the tissue in the trash after you use it.

- Wash your hands often with soap and water. If soap and water are not available, use an alcohol-based hand rub.

- Avoid touching your eyes, nose, and mouth. Germs spread this way.

Also, antiviral medications, which can treat flu illness, may be used in certain circumstances to prevent the flu.

Can Herbal, Homeopathic or Other Folk Remedies Protect against the Flu?

There is no scientific evidence that any herbal, homeopathic or other folk remedies have any benefit against influenza.

How Long Can Influenza Viruses Live on Hard Surfaces (Such as Books or Doorknobs)?

Studies have shown that human influenza viruses generally can survive on surfaces between 2 and 8 hours.

What Kills Influenza Viruses?

Influenza viruses can be destroyed by heat (167–212°F [75–100°C]). In addition, several chemical germicides, including chlorine, hydrogen peroxide, detergents (soap), iodophors (iodine-based antiseptics), and alcohols are effective against influenza viruses if used in proper concentrations for a sufficient length of time. For example, alcohol-based hand rubs can be used in the absence of soap and water for hand washing. Influenza viruses on the surface of objects also can be killed by ultraviolent C (UV-C) radiation (at a wavelength of 200–270 nm; e.g., 254 nm). UV-C may be provided by exposure to direct sunlight or light from a mobile UV-C device. To date, there are no published studies that demonstrate reduced transmission of influenza viruses by using UV-C devices in household settings.

What If Soap and Water Are Not Available and Alcohol-Based Products Are Not Allowed in My Facility?

If soap and water are not available and alcohol-based products are not allowed, other hand sanitizers that do not contain alcohol may be useful.

Section 60.3

Taking Care of Yourself When You Have Seasonal Flu

This section includes text excerpted from "The Flu: What to Do If You Get Sick," Centers for Disease Control and Prevention (CDC), May 26, 2016.

How Do I Know If I Have the Flu?

You may have the flu if you have some or all of these symptoms:

- fever*
- cough
- sore throat
- runny or stuffy nose
- body aches
- headache
- chills
- fatigue
- sometimes diarrhea and vomiting

It's important to note that not everyone with flu will have a fever.

What Should I Do If I Get Sick?

Most people with the flu have mild illness and do not need medical care or antiviral drugs. If you get sick with flu symptoms, in most cases, you should stay home and avoid contact with other people except to get medical care. If, however, you have symptoms of flu and are in a high risk group, or are very sick or worried about your illness, contact your healthcare provider (doctor, physician's assistant, etc.).

Certain people are at high risk of serious flu-related complications (including young children, people 65 and older, pregnant women and people with certain medical conditions) and this is true both for seasonal flu and novel flu virus infections. If you are in a high risk group and develop flu symptoms, it's best for you to contact your doctor. Remind them about your high risk status for flu. Healthcare providers will determine whether influenza testing and treatment are needed. Your doctor may prescribe antiviral drugs that can treat the flu. These drugs work better for treatment the sooner they are started.

Do I Need to Go the Emergency Room If I Am Only a Little Sick?

No. The emergency room should be used for people who are very sick. You should not go to the emergency room if you are only mildly ill. If you have the emergency warning signs of flu sickness, you should go to the emergency room. If you get sick with flu symptoms and are at high risk of flu complications or you are concerned about your illness, call your healthcare provider for advice. If you go to the emergency room and you are not sick with the flu, you may catch it from people who do have it.

What Are the Emergency Warning Signs of Flu Sickness?

In children:

- Fast breathing or trouble breathing
- Bluish skin color
- Not drinking enough fluids
- Not waking up or not interacting
- Being so irritable that the child does not want to be held
- Flu-like symptoms improve but then return with fever and worse cough
- Fever with a rash

In addition to the signs above, get medical help right away for any infant who has any of these signs:

- Being unable to eat
- Has trouble breathing
- Has no tears when crying
- Significantly fewer wet diapers than normal

In adults:

- Difficulty breathing or shortness of breath
- Pain or pressure in the chest or abdomen
- Sudden dizziness

395

- Confusion

- Severe or persistent vomiting

- Flu-like symptoms that improve but then return with fever and worse cough

Are There Medicines to Treat the Flu?

Yes. There are drugs your doctor may prescribe for treating the flu called "antivirals." These drugs can make you better faster and may also prevent serious complications.

How Long Should I Stay Home If I'm Sick?

Centers for Disease Control and Prevention (CDC) recommends that you stay home for at least 24 hours after your fever is gone except to get medical care or other necessities. Your fever should be gone without the use of a fever-reducing medicine, such as Tylenol®. You should stay home from work, school, travel, shopping, social events, and public gatherings.

What Should I Do While I'm Sick?

Stay away from others as much as possible to keep from infecting them. If you must leave home, for example, to get medical care, wear a facemask if you have one, or cover coughs and sneezes with a tissue. Wash your hands often to keep from spreading flu to others.

Section 60.4

Complementary and Alternative Medicine (CAM) for Flu and Colds

This section includes text excerpted from "Flu and Colds: In Depth," National Center for Complementary and Integrative Health (NCCIH), January 2016.

What Do We Know about the Effectiveness of Complementary Approaches for Flu and Colds?

- No complementary health approach has been shown to be helpful for the **flu**.

- For **colds**:

- Complementary approaches that have shown some promise include **oral zinc products, rinsing the nose and sinuses** (with a neti pot or other device), **honey** (as a nighttime cough remedy for children), **vitamin C** (for people under severe physical stress), **probiotics**, and **meditation**.

- Approaches for which the evidence is conflicting, inadequate, or mostly negative include **vitamin C** (for most people), **echinacea**, **garlic**, and **American ginseng**.

What Do We Know about the Safety of Complementary Approaches for Colds and Flu?

- People can get severe infections if they use neti pots or other nasal rinsing devices improperly. Tap water isn't safe **for use as a nasal rinse unless it has been filtered, treated, or processed in specific ways.**

- Zinc products used in the nose (such as nasal gels and swabs) have been linked to a long-lasting or even permanent **loss of the sense of smell.**

- Using a dietary supplement to prevent colds often involves taking it for long periods of time. However, little is known about the long-term safety of some dietary supplements studied for prevention of colds, such as **American ginseng** and **probiotics.**

- Complementary approaches that are safe for some people may not be safe for others. Your age, health, special circumstances (such as pregnancy), and medicines or supplements that you take may affect the safety of complementary approaches.

What the Science Says about Complementary Health Approaches for the Flu

No complementary approach has been shown to prevent the flu or relieve flu symptoms. Complementary approaches that have been studied for the flu include the following:

- American ginseng

- Chinese herbal medicines

- Echinacea

- Elderberry

- Green tea

- Oscillococcinum

- Vitamin C

- Vitamin D

- In all instances, there's not enough evidence to show whether the approach is helpful.

What the Science Says about Complementary Health Approaches for Colds

American Ginseng

- Several studies have evaluated the use of American ginseng (Panax quinquefolius) to prevent colds. A 2011 evaluation of these studies concluded that the herb has not been shown to reduce the number of colds that people catch, although it may shorten the length of colds. The researchers who conducted the evaluation concluded that there was insufficient evidence to support the use of American ginseng for preventing colds.

- Taking American ginseng in an effort to prevent colds means taking it for prolonged periods of time. However, little is known about the herb's long-term safety. American ginseng may interact with the anticoagulant (blood thinning) drug warfarin.

Echinacea

- At least 24 studies have tested echinacea to see whether it can prevent colds or relieve cold symptoms. A comprehensive 2014 assessment of this research concluded that echinacea hasn't been convincingly shown to be beneficial. However, at least some echinacea products might have a weak effect.

- One reason why it's hard to reach definite conclusions about this herb is that echinacea products vary greatly. They may contain different species (types) of the plant and be made from different plant parts (the above-ground parts, the root or both). They also may be manufactured in different ways, and some products contain other ingredients in addition to echinacea. Research findings on one echinacea product may not apply to other products.

- Few side effects have been reported in studies of echinacea. However, some people are allergic to this herb, and in one study in children, taking echinacea was linked to an increase in rashes.

Garlic

- A 2014 evaluation of the research on garlic concluded that there isn't enough evidence to show whether this herb can help prevent colds or relieve their symptoms.

- Garlic can cause bad breath, body odor, and other side effects. Because garlic may interact with anticoagulant drugs (blood thinners), people who take these drugs should consult their healthcare providers before taking garlic.

Honey

- Honey's traditional reputation as a cough remedy has some science to back it up. A small amount of research suggests that honey may help to decrease nighttime coughing in children.

- Honey should never be given to infants under the age of 1 year because it may contain spores of the bacterium that causes infant botulism. Honey is considered safe for older children.

Meditation

- Reducing stress and improving general health may protect against colds and other respiratory infections. In a 2012 study funded by the National Center for Complementary and Integrative Health (NCCIH), adults aged 50 and older were randomly assigned to training in mindfulness meditation, which can reduce stress; an exercise training program, which may improve physical health; or a control group that didn't receive any intervention. The study participants kept track of their illnesses during the cold and flu season. People in the meditation group had shorter and less severe acute respiratory infections (most of which were colds) and lost fewer days of work because of these illnesses than those in the control group. Exercise also had some benefit, but not as much as meditation.

- This study is the first to suggest that meditation may reduce the impact of colds. Because it's the only study of its kind, its results shouldn't be regarded as conclusive.

- Meditation is generally considered to be safe for healthy people. However, there have been reports that it might worsen symptoms in people with certain chronic physical or mental health problems. If you have an ongoing health issue, talk with your healthcare provider before starting meditation.

Probiotics

- A 2015 evaluation of 13 studies found some evidence suggesting that probiotics might reduce the number of colds or other upper respiratory tract infections that people catch and the length of the illnesses, but the quality of the evidence was low or very low.

- In people who are generally healthy, probiotics have a good safety record. Side effects, if they occur at all, usually consist only of mild digestive symptoms such as gas. However, information on the long-term safety of probiotics is limited, and safety may differ from one type of probiotic to another. Probiotics have been linked to severe side effects, such as dangerous infections, in people with serious underlying medical problems.

Saline Nasal Irrigation

- Saline nasal irrigation means rinsing your nose and sinuses with salt water. People may do this with a neti pot (a device that comes from the Ayurvedic tradition) or with other devices, such as bottles, sprays, pumps or nebulizers. Saline nasal irrigation may be used for sinus congestion, allergies, or colds.

- There's limited evidence that saline nasal irrigation can help relieve cold symptoms. Studies of this technique have been too small to allow researchers to reach definite conclusions.

- Saline nasal irrigation used to be considered safe, with only minor side effects such as nasal discomfort or irritation. However, in 2011, a severe disease caused by an amoeba (a type of microorganism) was linked to nasal irrigation with tap water. The U.S. Food and Drug Administration (FDA) has warned that tap water that is not filtered, treated, or processed in specific ways is not safe for use in nasal rinsing devices and has explained how to use and clean these devices safely.

Vitamin C

- An evaluation of the large amount of research done on vitamin C and colds (29 studies involving more than 11,000 people) concluded that taking vitamin C doesn't prevent colds in the general population and shortens colds only slightly. Taking vitamin C only after you start to feel cold symptoms doesn't affect the length or severity of the cold.

- Unlike the situation in the general population, vitamin C does seem to reduce the number of colds in people exposed to short periods of extreme physical stress (such as marathon runners and skiers). In studies of these groups, taking vitamin C cut the number of colds in half.

- Taking too much vitamin C can cause diarrhea, nausea, and stomach cramps. People with the iron storage disease hemochromatosis should avoid high doses of vitamin C. People who are being treated for cancer or taking cholesterol-lowering medications should talk with their healthcare providers before taking vitamin C supplements.

Zinc

- Zinc has been used for colds in forms that are taken orally (by mouth), such as lozenges, tablets, or syrup, or used intranasally (in the nose), such as swabs or gels.

401

- **Oral Zinc**

- A 2013 assessment of 16 clinical trials of oral zinc (lozenges or syrup), involving almost 1,400 people, concluded that zinc helps to reduce the length of colds when taken within 24 hours after symptoms start, but it hasn't been shown to affect the severity of colds. Zinc lozenges may shorten the duration of symptoms affecting the throat, which comes into direct contact with the zinc, as well as other symptoms such as runny nose and sneezing.

- Zinc has not been studied in people for whom cold symptoms might be particularly troublesome, such as those with asthma or immune deficiencies, so its effects in these groups are unknown.

- A few studies have tested the use of zinc, in doses lower than those used for treatment, to try to prevent colds in children, but there aren't enough results to allow conclusions to be reached.

- Oral zinc can cause a bad taste, as well as nausea and other gastrointestinal symptoms. Long-term use of high doses of zinc can cause low copper levels, reduced immunity, and low levels of HDL cholesterol (the "good" cholesterol). Zinc may interact with drugs, including antibiotics and penicillamine (a drug used to treat rheumatoid arthritis).

- **Intranasal Zinc**

- The use of zinc products inside the nose, such as gels or swabs, may cause loss of the sense of smell, which may be long-lasting or permanent. In 2009, the FDA warned consumers to stop using several intranasal zinc products marketed as cold remedies because of this risk.

- Prior to the warnings about effects on the sense of smell, a few studies of intranasal zinc had suggested a possible benefit against cold symptoms. However, the risk of a serious and lasting side effect outweighs any possible benefit in the treatment of a minor illness.

Other Complementary Approaches

In addition to the complementary approaches described above, several other approaches mentioned below have been studied for colds.

- Andrographis (Andrographis paniculata)

- Chinese herbal medicines
- Green tea
- Guided imagery
- Hydrotherapy
- Vitamin D
- Vitamin E
- In all instances, there is insufficient evidence to show whether these approaches help to prevent colds or relieve cold symptoms.

Chapter 61

Sore Throat Care

Causes[1]

Most sore throats are caused by viruses, like ones that cause a cold or the flu, and do not need antibiotic treatment. Some sore throats are caused by bacteria, such as group A Streptococcus (group A strep). Sore throats caused by these bacteria are known as strep throat. In children, 20 to 30 out of every 100 sore throats are strep throat. In adults, only 5 to 15 out of every 100 sore throats is strep throat. Other common causes of sore throats include:

- Allergies
- Dry air
- Pollution (airborne chemicals or irritants)
- Smoking or exposure to second-hand smoke

Risk Factors[1]

There are many things that can increase your risk for a sore throat, including:

- Age (children and teens between 5 and 15 years old are most likely to get a sore throat)

This chapter includes text excerpted from documents published by two public domain sources. Text under headings marked 1 are excerpted from "Get Smart: Know When Antibiotics Work," Centers for Disease Control and Prevention (CDC), July 23, 2015; text under headings marked 2 are excerpted from "Soothing a Sore Throat," *NIH News in Health*, National Institutes of Health (NIA), March 2013.

- Exposure to someone with a sore throat or strep throat

- Time of year (winter and early spring are common times for strep throat)

- Weather (cold air can irritate your throat)

- Irregularly shaped or large tonsils

- Pollution or smoke exposure

- A weak immune system or taking drugs that weaken the immune system

- Post-nasal drip or allergies

- Acid reflux disease

Signs and Symptoms[1]

A sore throat can make it painful to swallow. A sore throat can also feel dry and scratchy, and may be a symptom of the common cold or other upper respiratory tract infection. The following symptoms are often associated with sore throats caused by a viral infection or due to allergies:

- Sneezing

- Coughing

- Watery eyes

- Mild headache or body aches

- Runny nose

- Low fever (less than 101 °F)

Symptoms more commonly associated with strep throat include:

- Red and swollen tonsils, sometimes with white patches or streaks of pus

- Tiny red spots (petechiae) on the soft or hard palate (the roof of the mouth)

- High fever (101 °F or above)

- Nausea

- Vomiting

- Swollen lymph nodes in the neck

- Severe headache or body aches
- Rash

When to Seek Medical Care[1]

See a healthcare professional if you or your child has any of the following:

- Sore throat that lasts longer than 1 week
- Difficulty swallowing or breathing
- Excessive drooling (young children)
- Temperature higher than 100.4 °F
- Pus on the back of the throat
- Rash
- Joint pain
- Hoarseness lasting longer than 2 weeks
- Blood in saliva or phlegm
- Dehydration (symptoms include a dry, sticky mouth; sleepiness or tiredness; thirst; decreased urination or fewer wet diapers; few or no tears when crying; muscle weakness; headache; dizziness or lightheadedness)
- Recurring sore throats

If your child is younger than three months of age and has a fever, it's important to always call your healthcare professional right away.

Diagnosis and Treatment[1]

Antibiotics are not needed to treat most sore throats, which usually improve on their own within 1–2 weeks. Antibiotics will not help if a sore throat is caused by a virus or irritation from the air. Antibiotic treatment in these cases may cause harm in both children and adults. Your healthcare professional may prescribe other medicine or give you tips to help with other symptoms like fever and coughing. Antibiotics are needed if a healthcare professional diagnoses you or your child with strep throat, which is caused by bacteria. This diagnosis can be done using a quick swab of the throat. **Strep throat cannot be diagnosed by looking in the throat—a lab test must be done.** Antibiotics are prescribed for strep throat to prevent rheumatic fever. If diagnosed with strep throat, an infected patient should stay home from work, school, or day care until 24 hours after starting an antibiotic.

Soothing a Sore Throat[2]

We've all had sore throats around this time of year. Your throat feels scratchy and may hurt when you swallow. What can you do to soothe a sore throat? And when is it a sign of a more serious infection?

Most sore throats are caused by viral infections such as the common cold or the flu. These throat problems are generally minor and go away on their own. To soothe your irritated throat, keep it moist. "Ever notice that a sore throat seems worse in the morning? It's because your throat gets so dry overnight," says Dr. Valerie Riddle, an infectious disease expert at National Institutes of Health (NIH). "Having lozenges or hard candies—or anything that stimulates saliva production—will keep your throat moist. It's also important to drink plenty of fluids."

For young children who might choke on hard candies or lozenges, try cold liquids and popsicles. Throat pain might also be soothed by throat sprays and over-the-counter pain relievers such as acetaminophen, ibuprofen or aspirin, but don't give aspirin to young children.

Contact a doctor if your sore throat is severe, doesn't feel better after a few days, or is accompanied by a high fever or swollen glands. These symptoms could be signs of a bacterial infection, such as strep throat. Taking antibiotics won't help at all if your sore throat is caused by viruses, but they're essential for fighting bacterial infections like strep.

Strep is the most common bacterial throat infection. Although it can occur in adults, strep throat is more common in children between ages 5 and 15. Riddle says strep can be harder to detect in younger children, because it can cause a runny nose and other symptoms that make it seem like a cold. "If your child has severe throat pain, a fever above 100.4 degrees, or swollen glands, you should get medical attention right away," advises Riddle. Children with strep also may experience nausea, vomiting, and stomach pain.

To see whether you have strep throat, the doctor will take a throat swab. If test results confirm strep, your doctor will prescribe antibiotics. After 24 hours of taking them, you should no longer be contagious. You'll likely begin feeling better within a couple of days, but to fully recover it's important to finish all of the medicine.

Strep is highly contagious. Treat it quickly to prevent it from spreading to others. Riddle says, "Not only can the infection be transmitted, but there are potential complications from untreated strep throat." These include ear infections, rheumatic fever and kidney problems.

Another fairly common throat infection is tonsillitis, which occurs when you have sore, swollen **tonsils**. It's caused by many of the same viruses and bacteria that cause sore throats. If you have frequent bouts of tonsillitis or strep throat, you may need surgery (called a tonsillectomy) to have your tonsils removed.

The best way to protect yourself from the germs that cause these infections is to wash your hands often. Try to steer clear of people who have colds or other contagious infections. And avoid smoking and inhaling second-hand smoke, which can irritate your throat.

Symptom Relief[1]

Most sore throats will go away on their own without antibiotics. In some cases (like for strep throat), a lab test will need to be done to see if you or your child need antibiotics. Rest, over-the-counter medicines and other self-care methods may help you or your child feel better. For more information about symptomatic relief, talk to your healthcare professional, including your pharmacist. Remember, always use over-the-counter products as directed. Many over-the-counter products are not recommended for children of certain ages.

Prevention[1]

There are steps you can take to help prevent getting a sore throat, including:

- Practice good hand hygiene
- Avoid close contact with people who have sore throats, colds or other upper respiratory infections
- Avoid smoking and exposure to secondhand smoke

Chapter 62

Fever: What You Can Do

What Is a Fever?

A fever—also called high temperature or pyrexia—is a temporary rise in the body's temperature. It is not an illness itself but a natural defense against bacteria or viruses that thrives best at normal body temperature, around 98.6°F.

Hyperthermia is a form of fever in which the body's temperature rises far above normal and can be caused, for example, by side effects of illicit drugs or certain medications, stroke, or by temperature-related conditions like heat stroke. Usually a fever is not considered life-threatening, but hyperthermia can lead to a critical elevation of the body's temperature.

An adult is considered to have a fever if the body temperature is above 99–99.5°F (37.2–37.5°C), depending on the time of the day. (Body temperature is usually highest in late afternoon.) A child is considered to have a fever if the temperature is at or above:

- 100.4°F (38°C) rectally
- 99.5°F (37.5°C) orally
- 99°F (37.2°C) axillary (measured under the arm)

What Causes Fever?

The hypothalamus, a region in the brain that helps the body maintain its normal temperature, may cause temperature to fluctuate in

"Fever: What You Can Do," © 2017 Omnigraphics. Reviewed August 2016.

response to a number of factors, such as eating, heavy clothing, high humidity, medications, physical activity, room temperature, strong emotions, and menstrual cycles in women. The hypothalamus may also cause an increase in the body temperature as a response to an infection or illness.

Although the most frequent causes of fever are common infections, such as colds, other possibilities include:

- appendicitis
- autoimmune or inflammatory conditions
- blood clots or thrombophlebitis
- bone infections (osteomyelitis)
- cancer, particularly leukemia, Hodgkin's disease, and non-Hodgkin's lymphoma
- reaction to medications, such as certain antibiotics, antihistamines, and seizure medicines
- hormone disorders, such as hyperthyroidism
- immunization, in some children
- infections of the bladder or kidney
- meningitis
- respiratory infections, such as flu, sinus infections, mononucleosis, bronchitis, pneumonia, and tuberculosis
- side effects of drugs like amphetamines and cocaine
- skin infections or cellulitis
- teething

Signs and Symptoms of Fever

In addition to an elevated body temperature, other symptoms of fever, depending on its underlying cause, can include headache, sweating, chills, muscle ache, weakness, and dehydration.

In children, symptoms may also include fussiness, lethargy, poor appetite, stiff neck, rashes, earache, sore throat, cough, vomiting, diarrhea, and a weakened immune system.

How Is a Fever Diagnosed?

Once a fever is measured with a thermometer, a physician will attempt to determine its cause by a physical examination (including thorough examination of the skin, eyes, ears, nose, throat, neck, chest, and abdomen) and by asking about recent behavior and interactions, including travel to regions that are known to be sources of infections. For instance, conditions like Lyme disease and Rocky Mountain spotted fever (RMSF) are endemic to certain parts of the United States, while such conditions as malaria are more common in sub-Saharan Africa and southern Asia. In certain cases, a person might be diagnosed with a "fever of unknown origin," one in which the cause is not attributable to an obvious condition.

To diagnose fever, the doctor may order tests that include:

- blood tests (such as a complete blood count or blood differential)

- chest X-ray

- urinalysis

How Is Fever Treated?

A fever is treated based on its duration and cause, along with other symptoms that may accompany the elevated temperature. Typically, medications for fever include over-the-counter (OTC) drugs, such as acetaminophen (Tylenol), and nonsteroidal anti-inflammatory medicines, such as naproxen (Aleve) and ibuprofen (Advil, Motrin). If the fever is the result of a bacterial infection, such as strep throat, antibiotics would be prescribed. Aspirin may be taken by adults but is not recommended for children and teens, as it is associated with Reye's syndrome, which can cause damage to the brain and liver.

Home Care

Fever is not necessarily a symptom of a serious problem. While a simple cold can lead to body temperatures as high as 104°F (40°C), some serious conditions may cause no fever at all.

A mild fever does not generally require treatment; enough rest and proper fluid consumption will usually suffice. The condition is most likely not serious if the patient:

- is alert and active.

- continues to eat and drink well.

- has a normal skin color.

- looks well when the body temperature returns to normal.

413

If a person with high body temperature is uncomfortable and experiences vomiting, dehydration, or inadequate sleep, follow these steps reduce the fever:

- Make the room comfortable. It should neither be too hot nor too cool.

- Remove excess clothing from the person. A single layer of lightweight clothing will be sufficient. If the patient has chills, do not bundle him/her up excessively.

- Cool the person with a lukewarm bath or sponge bath. This may be particularly effective after medication is given.

- Avoid cold baths, ice, or alcohol rubs, as they worsen the situation by making the person shiver, which can increase the core body temperature.

When Taking Medicine to Lower a Fever

- Always consult a doctor before giving medicines to a child 3 months of age or younger.

- In adults and children, acetaminophen and ibuprofen help reduce fever. A doctor may recommend the use of either type of medicine, although ibuprofen is not generally recommended for children under the age of 6 months.

- Aspirin is highly effective for treating fever but is recommended only for adults unless prescribed for a child by a doctor.

- The correct dose of medicine should be given to a child based on the child's weight and per the instructions on the package.

Eating and Drinking

It is important for adults, and even more so for children, to drink plenty of fluids to keep the body hydrated. Water, soup, popsicles, and gelatin are good choices. Consumption of fruit juice should be limited, and sports drinks should be avoided in young children. Eating is fine; however, food should not be forced.

When to Contact a Medical Professional?

Call a doctor immediately if the fever:

- is 100.4°F (38°C) or higher in a child 3 months or younger.

- is 102.2°F (39°C) or higher in children between 3 and 12 months old.

- is 105°F (40.5°C) or higher and does not come down readily when treated, and the person is not comfortable.

- lasts longer than 24 to 48 hours in children 2 years or younger.

- lasts longer than 48 to 72 hours in those older than 2 years.

Medical assistance will also be required if the patient:

- has a fever that stays at 103°F or keeps rising.

- has symptoms (such as a sore throat, cough or earache) that are usually associated with other illnesses.

- has had recurrent mild fevers for a week or more.

- has bruises or a new rash.

- has been vaccinated recently.

- has pain when urinating.

- traveled to another region or country recently.

- is suffering from a serious medical condition, such as diabetes, heart disease, sickle cell anemia, chronic obstructive pulmonary disease (COPD), other chronic lung problems, or cystic fibrosis.

- has problems with the immune system (such as one caused by a bone marrow or organ transplant, cancer treatment, chronic steroid therapy, HIV or spleen removal).

If an infant three months old or younger has a temperature above 100.4°F, or any child has a temperature above 104°F, you should call a doctor or visit an emergency room immediately, since this could be a sign of potentially life-threatening condition. Febrile seizure can occur in some children with such high body temperatures, although this generally does not cause any permanent damage. But brain damage can occur if the fever is above 107.6°F (42°C).

References

1. Kaneshiro, Neil K. "Fever," MedlinePlus, U.S. National Library of Medicine (NLM), August 30, 2014.

2. Blahd, William. "Fever Facts," WebMD, LLC, April 16, 2015.

Chapter 63

Over-the-Counter (OTC) Medications

Chapter Contents

Section 63.1

Over-the-Counter Medicines: What's Right for You?

This section includes text excerpted from "Over-The-Counter Medicines: What's Right for You?" U.S. Food and Drug Administration (FDA), September 3, 2013.

Advice for Americans about Self-Care: Access + Knowledge = Power

American medicine cabinets contain a growing choice of nonprescription, over-the-counter (OTC) medicines to treat an expanding range of ailments. OTC medicines often do more than relieve aches, pains and itches. Some can prevent diseases like tooth decay, cure diseases like athlete's foot and, with a doctor's guidance, help manage recurring conditions like vaginal yeast infection, migraine and minor pain in arthritis.

The U.S. Food and Drug Administration (FDA) determines whether medicines are prescription or nonprescription. The term prescription (Rx) refers to medicines that are safe and effective when used under a doctor's care. Nonprescription or OTC drugs are medicines FDA decides are safe and effective for use without a doctor's prescription.

FDA also has the authority to decide when a prescription drug is safe enough to be sold directly to consumers over the counter. This regulatory process allowing Americans to take a more active role in their healthcare is known as Rx-to-OTC switch. As a result of this process, more than 700 products sold over the counter today use ingredients or dosage strengths available only by prescription 30 years ago.

Increased access to OTC medicines is especially important for our maturing population. Two out of three older Americans rate their health as excellent to good, but four out of five report at least one chronic condition.

Fact is, OTC medicines offer greater opportunity to treat more of the aches and illnesses most likely to appear in our later years. As we live longer, work longer, and take a more active role in our own healthcare, the need grows to become better informed about self-care.

The best way to become better informed—for young and old alike—is to read and understand the information on OTC labels. Next to the medicine itself, label comprehension is the most important part of self-care with OTC medicines.

With new opportunities in self-medication come new responsibilities and an increased need for knowledge. FDA and the Consumer Healthcare Products Association (CHPA) have prepared the following information to help Americans take advantage of self-care opportunities.

OTC Know-How: It's on the Label

You wouldn't ignore your doctor's instructions for using a prescription drug; so don't ignore the label when taking an OTC medicine. Here's what to look for:

- PRODUCT NAME

- "ACTIVE INGREDIENTS": therapeutic substances in medicine

- "PURPOSE": product category (such as antihistamine, antacid, or cough suppressant)

- "USES": symptoms or diseases the product will treat or prevent

- "WARNINGS": when not to use the product, when to stop taking it, when to see a doctor, and possible side effects

- "DIRECTIONS": how much to take, how to take it, and how long to take it

- "OTHER INFORMATION": such as storage information

- "INACTIVE INGREDIENTS": substances such as binders, colors, or flavoring

You can help yourself read the label too. Always use enough light. It usually takes three times more light to read the same line at age 60 than at age 30. If necessary, use your glasses or contact lenses when reading labels. Always remember to look for the statement describing the tamper-evident feature(s) before you buy the product and when you use it.

When it comes to medicines, more does not necessarily mean better. You should never misuse OTC medicines by taking them longer or in higher doses than the label recommends. Symptoms that persist are a clear signal it's time to see a doctor. Be sure to read the label each time you purchase a product. Just because two or more products are

419

from the same brand family doesn't mean they are meant to treat the same conditions or contain the same ingredients.

Remember, if you read the label and still have questions, talk to a doctor, nurse or pharmacist.

Drug Interactions

Although mild and relatively uncommon, interactions involving OTC drugs can produce unwanted results or make medicines less effective. It's especially important to know about drug interactions if you're taking Rx and OTC drugs at the same time. Some drugs can also interact with foods and beverages, as well as with health conditions such as diabetes, kidney disease, and high blood pressure. Here are a few drug interaction cautions for some common OTC ingredients:

- Avoid alcohol if you are taking antihistamines, cough-cold products with the ingredient dextromethorphan, or drugs that treat sleeplessness.

- Do not use drugs that treat sleeplessness if you are taking prescription sedatives or tranquilizers.

- Check with your doctor before taking products containing aspirin if you're taking a prescription blood thinner or if you have diabetes or gout.

- Do not use laxatives when you have stomach pain, nausea, or vomiting.

- Unless directed by a doctor, do not use a nasal decongestant if you are taking a prescription drug for high blood pressure or depression, or if you have heart or thyroid disease, diabetes, or prostate problems.

This is not a complete list. Read the label! Drug labels change as new information becomes available. That's why it's important to read the label each time you take medicine.

Time for a Medicine Cabinet Checkup?

- Be sure to look through your medicine supply at least once a year

- Always store medicines in a cool, dry place or as stated on the label

- Throw away any medicines that are past the expiration date

- To make sure no one takes the wrong medicine, keep all medicines in their original containers

Pregnancy and Breastfeeding

Drugs can pass from a pregnant woman to her unborn baby. A safe amount of medicine for the mother may be too much for the unborn baby. If you're pregnant, always talk with your doctor before taking any drugs, Rx or OTC.

Although most drugs pass into breast milk in concentrations too low to have any unwanted effects on the baby, breast-feeding mothers still need to be careful. Always ask your doctor or pharmacist before taking any medicine while breast-feeding. A doctor or pharmacist can tell you how to adjust the timing and dosing of most medicines so the baby is exposed to the lowest amount possible, or whether the drugs should be avoided altogether.

Child-Resistant Packaging

Child-resistant closures are designed for repeated use to make it difficult for children to open. Remember, if you don't re-lock the closure after each use, the child-resistant device can't do its job—keeping children out!

It's best to store all medicines and dietary supplements where children can neither see nor reach them. Containers of pills should not be left on the kitchen counter as a reminder. Purses and briefcases are among the worst places to hide medicines from curious kids. And since children are natural mimics, it's a good idea not to take medicine in front of them. They may be tempted to "play house" with your medicine later on.

If you find some packages too difficult to open—and don't have young children living with you or visiting—you should know the law allows one package size for each OTC medicine to be sold without child-resistant features. If you don't see it on the store shelf, ask.

Protect Yourself against Tampering

Makers of OTC medicines seal most products in tamper-evident packaging (TEP) to help protect against criminal tampering. TEP works by providing visible evidence if the package has been disturbed. But OTC packaging cannot be 100 percent tamper-proof. Here's how to help protect yourself:

- Be alert to the tamper-evident features on the package before you open it. These features are described on the label.

- Inspect the outer packaging before you buy it. When you get home, inspect the medicine inside.

- Don't buy an OTC product if the packaging is damaged.

- Don't use any medicine that looks discolored or different in any way.

- If anything looks suspicious, be suspicious. Contact the store where you bought the product. Take it back!

- Never take medicines in the dark.

Section 63.2

Kids Are Not Just Small Adults: Tips on Giving OTC Medicine to Children

This section includes text excerpted from "Kids Aren't Just Small Adults—Medicines, Children, and the Care Every Child Deserves," U.S. Food and Drug Administration (FDA), August 28, 2013.

Use care when giving any medicine to an infant or a child. Even over-the-counter (OTC) medicines that you buy are serious medicines. The following is advice for giving OTC medicine to your child, from the U.S. Food and Drug Administration (FDA) and the makers of OTC medicines:

1. Always read and follow the Drug Facts label on your over-the-counter (OTC) medicine. This is important for choosing and safely using all OTC medicines. Read the label every time, before you give the medicine. Be sure you clearly understand how much medicine to give and when the medicine can be taken again.

2. Know the "active ingredient" in your child's medicine. This is what makes the medicine work and is always listed at the top of the Drug Facts label. Sometimes an active ingredient can

treat more than one medical condition. For that reason, the same active ingredient can be found in many different medicines that are used to treat different symptoms. For example, a medicine for a cold and a medicine for a headache could each contain the same active ingredient. So, if you're treating a cold and a headache with two medicines and both have the same active ingredient, you could be giving two times the normal dose. If you're confused about your child's medicines, check with a doctor, nurse, or pharmacist.

3. Give the right medicine, in the right amount, to your child. Not all medicines are right for an infant or a child. Medicines with the same brand name can be sold in many different strengths, such as infant, children, and adult formulas. The amount and directions are also different for children of different ages or weights. Always use the right medicine and follow the directions exactly. Never use more medicine than directed, even if your child seems sicker than the last time.

4. Talk to your doctor, pharmacist, or nurse to find out what mixes well and what doesn't. Medicines, vitamins, supplements, foods, and beverages don't always mix well with each other. Your healthcare professional can help.

5. Use the dosing tool that comes with the medicine, such as a dropper or a dosing cup. A different dosing tool, or a kitchen spoon, could hold the wrong amount of medicine.

6. Know the difference between a tablespoon (TBSP.) and a teaspoon (TSP.) Do not confuse them! A tablespoon holds three times as much medicine as a teaspoon. On measuring tools, a teaspoon (tsp.) is equal to "5 cc" or "5 mL."

7. Know your child's weight. Directions on some OTC medicines are based on weight. Never guess the amount of medicine to give to your child or try to figure it out from the adult dose instructions. If a dose is not listed for your child's age or weight, call your doctor or other members of your healthcare team.

8. Prevent a poison emergency by always using a child-resistant cap. Re-lock the cap after each use. Be especially careful with any products that contain iron; they are the leading cause of poisoning deaths in young children.

9. Store all medicines in a safe place. Today's medicines are tasty, colorful, and many can be chewed. Kids may think that these

products are candy. To prevent an overdose or poisoning emergency, store all medicines and vitamins in a safe place out of your child's (and even your pet's) sight and reach. If your child takes too much, call the Poison Center Hotline at 1-800-222-1222 (open 24 hours every day, 7 days a week) or call 9-1-1.

10. Check the medicine three times. First, check the outside packaging for such things as cuts, slices, or tears. Second, once you are at home, check the label on the inside package to be sure you have the right medicine. Make sure the lid and seal are not broken. Third, check the color, shape, size, and smell of the medicine. If you notice anything different or unusual, talk to a pharmacist or another healthcare professional.

Section 63.3

Nonprescription Cough and Cold Medicine Use in Children

This section includes text excerpted from "OTC Cough and Cold Products: Not for Infants and Children under 2 Years of Age," U.S. Food and Drug Administration (FDA), February 28, 2015.

What Is FDA Recommending about Use of Over-The-Counter Cough and Cold Products for Infants and Children under 2 Years of Age?

U.S. Food and Drug Administration (FDA) strongly recommends that over-the-counter (OTC) cough and cold products should not be used for infants and children under 2 years of age because serious and potentially life-threatening side effects could occur.

What Are These Side Effects?

There are a wide variety of serious adverse events reported with cough and cold products. They include death, convulsions, rapid heart rates, and decreased levels of consciousness.

What Ingredients May Cause These Effects, and What Should I Look for on the Label to Tell If These Ingredients Are Present in an OTC Product?

OTC cough and cold products include these ingredients: deconges-tants (for unclogging a stuffy nose), expectorants (for loosening mucus so that it can be coughed up), antihistamines (for sneezing and runny nose), and antitussives (for quieting coughs). The terms on the label include "nasal decongestants", "cough suppressants", "expectorants", and "antihistamines."

How Did FDA Arrive at Its Decision to Issue These Recommendations?

FDA's recommendation is based on the review of reports the agency has received about serious side effects, as well as a review of informa-tion presented at a joint Nonprescription Drugs and Pediatric Advisory Committee meeting on Oct.18–19, 2007. FDA has determined that OTC cough and cold medicines, which treat symptoms and not the underlying condition, have not been shown to be safe or effective in infants and children under 2.

Not Effective? Does That Mean They Don't Work?

FDA does not have any data to support that these products work in children less than 2 years of age.

My Child Has Allergies. Does This Alert Affect the Medicines for My Child?

This advisory relates only to the use of OTC products for the treat-ment of cough and cold.

What Should Parents Do If Infants and Children under 2 Years of Age Experience Cough and Cold Symptoms?

A cold is a respiratory illness that is usually self-limited and lasts about a week. Cold symptoms typically include sneezing, coughing, runny or stuffy nose, and sore throat. Children may also experience a fever. Most of the time, a cold will go away by itself. If you are concerned about making your child feel more comfortable, talk with your doctor about what approaches to take. Your doctor may recommend drinking plenty of fluids to help loosen mucus and keep children hydrated, and using saline nasal drops and gently suctioning mucus from the nose with a bulb syringe. Your doctor may also recommend fever reducers such as acetaminophen or ibuprofen. If your child's cold symptoms do not improve or get worse, contact your doctor. A persistent cough may signal a more serious condition such as bronchitis or asthma.

Are Particular Products Being Recalled?

No. This public health advisory does not mean that products are being recalled. In October 2007, the Consumer Healthcare Products Association (CHPA), on behalf of leading manufacturers of OTC cough and cold medicines, announced voluntary market withdrawals of OTC products for infants and children under 2 years of age. FDA strongly supports the actions taken by many manufacturers to voluntarily withdraw cough and cold medicines that were being marketed for infants.

Is FDA Making a Recommendation about Whether Cough and Cold Products Should Be Used in Age Groups Other than Infants and Children under 2 Years of Age at This Time?

No. This public health advisory does not include FDA's final recommendation about use of cough and cold medicines in children ages 2 through 11 years. FDA's review of the data for these age groups is continuing. The agency is committed to making a timely and comprehensive review of the safety of OTC cough and cold medicines in children. FDA plans to issue its recommendations on use of the products in children ages 2 to 11 as soon as the review is complete.

While FDA Is Completing Its Review for Children Ages 2 through 11, What Should Parents of Children in This Age Group Know about Using Cough and Cold Products?

Giving too much cough and cold medicine can be dangerous. OTC cough and cold products can be harmful if more than the recommended amount is used, if they are given too often, or if more than one product containing the same active ingredient is being used. Parents need to be aware that many OTC cough and cold products contain multiple ingredients (for nasal congestion, cough, and fever). Giving more than one product could result in an overdose. There are many products that have similar names, so it is critical to identify the active ingredient(s) in the product, select the proper medicine, and use the correct dose. Reading the DRUG FACTS section of the label will help caretakers learn about what active ingredients are in the products. Also, children should not be given medicines that are packaged and made for adults.

Pending completion of its review, FDA recommends these steps for consumers who use OTC cough and cold products in children 2 years of age and older:

- Check the "active ingredients" section of the DRUG FACTS label.

- Be very careful if you are giving more than one OTC cough and cold medicine to a child. If you use two medicines that have the same or similar "active ingredients," a child could get too much of an ingredient which may hurt your child.

- Carefully follow the directions in the DRUG FACTS label.

- Only use the measuring spoons or cups that come with the medicine or those made specially for measuring drugs.

- Choose OTC cough and cold medicines with childproof safety caps, when available, and store the medicines out of reach of children.

- Understand that OTC cough and cold medicines do not cure or shorten the duration of the common cold.

- Do not use these products to sedate your child or make children sleepy.

- Call a physician, pharmacist or other healthcare professional if you have any questions about using cough or cold medicines in children 2 years of age and older.

Chapter 64

Avoid Drug Interactions

Overview

People often combine foods. For example, chocolate and peanut butter might be considered a tasty combination. But eating chocolate and taking certain drugs might carry risks. In fact, eating chocolate and taking monoamine oxidase (MAO) inhibitors, such as Nardil (phenelzine) or Parnate (tranylcypromine), could be dangerous. MAO inhibitors treat depression. Someone who eats an excessive amount of chocolate after taking an MAO inhibitor may experience a sharp rise in blood pressure. Other foods that should be avoided when taking MAO inhibitors:

- aged cheese

- sausage

- bologna

- pepperoni

- salami

These foods can also cause elevated blood pressure when taken with these medications. "Consumers should learn about the warnings for their medications and talk with their healthcare professionals about how to lower the risk of interactions," says Shiew-Mei Huang, Ph.D.,

This chapter includes text excerpted from "Avoiding Drug Interactions," U.S. Food and Drug Administration (FDA), July 25, 2015.

deputy director of the Office of Clinical Pharmacology in U.S. Food and Drug Administration's (FDA) Center for Drug Evaluation and Research (CDER).

There are three main types of drug interactions:

1. Drugs with Food and Beverages

Consequences of drug interactions with food and beverages may include delayed, decreased or enhanced absorption of a medication. Food can affect the bioavailability (the degree and rate at which a drug is absorbed into someone's system), metabolism, and excretion of certain medications. Below are the examples of drug interactions with food and beverages:

Alcohol: If you are taking any sort of medication, it's recommended that you avoid alcohol, which can increase or decrease the effect of many drugs.

Grapefruit juice: Grapefruit juice is often mentioned as a product that can interact negatively with drugs, but the actual number of drugs the juice can interact with is less well-known. Grapefruit juice shouldn't be taken with certain blood pressure-lowering drugs or cyclosporine for the prevention of organ transplant rejection. That's because grapefruit juice can cause higher levels of those medicines in your body, making it more likely that you will have side effects from the medicine. The juice can also interact to cause higher blood levels of the anti-anxiety medicine Buspar (buspirone); the anti-malaria drugs Quinerva or Quinite (quinine); and Halcion (triazolam), a medication used to treat insomnia.

Licorice: This would appear to be a fairly harmless snack food. However, for someone taking Lanoxin (digoxin), some forms of licorice may increase the risk for Lanoxin toxicity. Lanoxin is used to treat congestive heart failure and abnormal heart rhythms. Licorice may also reduce the effects of blood pressure drugs or diuretic (urine-producing) drugs, including Hydrodiuril (hydrochlorothiazide) and Aldactone (spironolactone).

Chocolate: MAO inhibitors are just one category of drugs that shouldn't be consumed with excessive amounts of chocolate. The caffeine in chocolate can also interact with stimulant drugs such as Ritalin (methylphenidate), increasing their effect or by decreasing the effect of sedative-hypnotics such as Ambien (zolpidem).

2. Drugs with Dietary Supplements

Research has shown that 50 percent or more of American adults use dietary supplements on a regular basis, according to congressional testimony by the Office of Dietary Supplements (ODS) in the National Institutes of Health (NIH).

The law defines dietary supplements in part as products taken by mouth that contain a "dietary ingredient." Dietary ingredients include vitamins, minerals, amino acids, and herbs or botanicals, as well as other substances that can be used to supplement the diet. Below are the examples of drug interactions with dietary supplements:

St. John's Wort (Hypericum perforatum): This herb is considered an inducer of liver enzymes, which means it can reduce the concentration of medications in the blood. St. John's Wort can reduce the blood level of medications such as Lanoxin, the cholesterol-lowering drugs Mevacor and Altocor (lovastatin), and the erectile dysfunction drug Viagra (sildenafil).

Vitamin E: Taking vitamin E with a blood-thinning medication such as Coumadin can increase anti-clotting activity and may cause an increased risk of bleeding.

Ginseng: This herb can interfere with the bleeding effects of Coumadin. In addition, ginseng can enhance the bleeding effects of heparin, aspirin, and nonsteroidal anti-inflammatory drugs such as ibuprofen, naproxen, and ketoprofen. Combining ginseng with MAO inhibitors such as Nardil or Parnate may cause headache, trouble sleeping, nervousness, and hyperactivity.

Ginkgo Biloba: High doses of the herb Ginkgo biloba could decrease the effectiveness of anticonvulsant therapy in patients taking the following medications to control seizures: Tegretol, Equetro or Carbatrol (carbamazepine), and Depakote (valproic acid).

3. Drugs with Other Drugs

Two out of every three patients who visit a doctor leave with at least one prescription for medication, according to a 2007 report on medication safety issued by the Institute for Safe Medication Practices. Close to 40 percent of the U.S. population receive prescriptions for four or more medications. And the rate of adverse drug reactions increases dramatically after a patient is on four or more medications.

Drug-drug interactions have led to adverse events and withdrawals of drugs from the market, according to an article on drug interactions co-authored by Shiew-Mei Huang, Ph.D., deputy director of FDA's

Office of Clinical Pharmacology. The paper was published in the June 2008 issue of the Journal of Clinical Pharmacology.

However, market withdrawal of a drug is a fairly drastic measure. More often, FDA will issue an alert warning the public and healthcare providers about risks as the result of drug interactions. Below are the examples of drug interactions with other drugs:

Cordarone (amiodarone): FDA issued an alert in August 2008, warning patients about taking Cordarone to correct abnormal rhythms of the heart and the cholesterol-lowering drug Zocor (Simvastatin). Patients taking Zocor in doses higher than 20 mg while also taking Cordarone run the risk of developing a rare condition of muscle injury called rhabdomyolysis, which can lead to kidney failure or death. "Cordarone also can inhibit or reduce the effect of the blood thinner Coumadin (warfarin)," said Huang. "So if you're using Cordarone, you may need to reduce the amount of Coumadin you're taking."

Lanoxin (digoxin): "Lanoxin has a narrow therapeutic range. So other drugs, such as Norvir (ritonvair), can elevate the level of Lanoxin," says Huang. "And an increased level of Lanoxin can cause irregular heart rhythms." Norvir is a protease inhibitor used to treat HIV, the virus that causes AIDS.

Antihistamines: Over-the-counter (OTC) antihistamines are drugs that temporarily relieve a runny nose, or reduce sneezing, itching of the nose or throat, and itchy watery eyes. If you are taking sedatives, tranquilizers, or a prescription drug for high blood pressure or depression, you should check with a doctor or pharmacist before you start using antihistimines. Some antihistamines can increase the depressant effects (such as sleepiness) of a sedative or tranquilizer. The sedating effect of some antihistamines combined with a sedating antidepressant could strongly affect your concentration level. Operating a car or any other machinery could be particularly dangerous if your ability to focus is impaired. Antihistamines taken in conjunction with blood pressure medication may cause a person's blood pressure to increase and may also speed up the heart rate.

Tips to Avoid Problems

There are lots of things you can do to take prescription or over-the-counter (OTC) medications in a safe and responsible manner.

- Always read drug labels carefully.

- Learn about the warnings for all the drugs you take.

- Keep medications in their original containers so that you can easily identify them.

- Ask your doctor what you need to avoid when you are prescribed a new medication. Ask about food, beverages, dietary supplements, and other drugs.

- Check with your doctor or pharmacist before taking an OTC drug if you are taking any prescription medications.

- Use one pharmacy for all of your drug needs.

- Keep all of your healthcare professionals informed about everything that you take.

- Keep a record of all prescription drugs, OTC drugs, and dietary supplements (including herbs) that you take. Try to keep this list with you at all times, but especially when you go on any medical appointment.

Chapter 65

Complementary and Alternative Medicine (CAM) for Contagious Diseases

Chapter Contents

Section 65.1

Selecting a CAM Practitioner

This section contains text excerpted from the following sources: Text in this section begins with excerpts from "Things to Know When Selecting a Complementary Health Practitioner," National Center for Complementary and Integrative Health (NCCIH), March 24, 2016; Text beginning with the heading "Discuss CAM Use with Your Healthcare Providers" is excerpted from "4 Tips: Start Talking with Your Health Care Providers about Complementary Health Approaches," National Center for Complementary and Integrative Health (NCCIH), September 24, 2015.

If you're looking for a complementary health practitioner to help treat a medical problem, it is important to be as careful and thorough in your search as you are when looking for conventional care.

Here are some tips to help you in your search:

1. **If you need names of practitioners in your area, first check with your doctor or other healthcare provider.** A nearby hospital or medical school, professional organizations, state regulatory agencies or licensing boards, or even your health insurance provider may be helpful.

2. **Find out as much as you can about any potential practitioner, including education, training, licensing, and certifications.** The credentials required for complementary health practitioners vary tremendously from state to state and from discipline to discipline.

Once you have found a possible practitioner, here are some tips about deciding whether he or she is right for you:

1. **Find out whether the practitioner is willing to work together with your conventional healthcare providers.** For safe, coordinated care, it's important for all of the professionals involved in your health to communicate and cooperate.

2. **Explain all of your health conditions to the practitioner, and find out about the practitioner's training**

and experience in working with people who have your conditions. Choose a practitioner who understands how to work with people with your specific needs, even if general well-being is your goal. And, remember that health conditions can affect the safety of complementary approaches; for example, if you have glaucoma, some yoga poses may not be safe for you.

3. **Don't assume that your health insurance will cover the practitioner's services.** Contact your health insurance provider and ask. Insurance plans differ greatly in what complementary health approaches they cover, and even if they cover a particular approach, restrictions may apply.

4. **Tell all your healthcare providers about all complementary approaches you use and about all practitioners who are treating you.** Keeping your healthcare providers fully informed helps you to stay in control and effectively manage your health.

Discuss CAM Use with Your Healthcare Providers

When patients tell their providers about their use of complementary health practices, they can better stay in control and more effectively manage their health. When providers ask their patients, they can ensure that they are fully informed and can help patients make wise healthcare decisions.

Here are four tips to help you and your healthcare providers start talking:

1. **List the complementary health practices you use on your patient history form**. When completing the patient history form, be sure to include everything you use—from acupuncture to zinc. It's important to give healthcare providers a full picture of what you do to manage your health.

2. **At each visit, be sure to tell your providers about what complementary health approaches you are using.** Don't forget to include over-the-counter and prescription medicines, as well as dietary and herbal supplements. Make a list in advance, or download and print this wallet card and take it with you. Some complementary health approaches can have an effect on conventional medicine, so your provider needs to know.

3. **If you are considering a new complementary health practice, ask questions**. Ask your healthcare providers about its safety, effectiveness, and possible interactions with medications (both prescription and nonprescription).

4. **Don't wait for your providers to ask about any complementary health practice you are using. Be proactive.** Start the conversation.

Section 65.2

Getting to Know Probiotics

This section includes text excerpted from "Probiotics: In Depth," National Center for Complementary and Integrative Health (NCCIH), July 2015.

What Are Probiotics?

Probiotics are live microorganisms that are intended to have health benefits. Products sold as probiotics include foods (such as yogurt), dietary supplements, and products that are not used orally, such as skin creams.

Although people often think of bacteria and other microorganisms as harmful "germs," many microorganisms help our bodies function properly. For example, bacteria that are normally present in our intestines help digest food, destroy disease-causing microorganisms, and produce vitamins. Large numbers of microorganisms live on and in our bodies. In fact, microorganisms in the human body outnumber human cells by 10 to 1. Many of the microorganisms in probiotic products are the same as or similar to microorganisms that naturally live in our bodies.

What Do We Know about the Usefulness of Probiotics?

Some probiotics may help to prevent diarrhea that is caused by infections or antibiotics. They may also help with symptoms of irritable bowel syndrome. However, benefits have not been conclusively demonstrated, and not all probiotics have the same effects.

What Do We Know about the Safety of Probiotics?

In healthy people, probiotics usually have only minor side effects, if any. However, in people with underlying health problems (for example, weakened immune systems), serious complications such as infections have occasionally been reported.

What Kinds of Microorganisms Are in Probiotics?

Probiotics may contain a variety of microorganisms. The most common are bacteria that belong to groups called *Lactobacillus* and *Bifidobacterium*. Each of these two broad groups includes many types of bacteria. Other bacteria may also be used as probiotics, and so may yeasts such as *Saccharomyces boulardii*.

Probiotics, Prebiotics, and Synbiotics

Prebiotics are not the same as probiotics. The term "prebiotics" refers to dietary substances that favor the growth of beneficial bacteria over harmful ones. The term "synbiotics" refers to products that combine probiotics and prebiotics.

How Popular Are Probiotics?

Data from the 2012 National Health Interview Survey (NHIS) show that about 4 million (1.6 percent) U.S. adults had used probiotics or prebiotics in the past 30 days. Among adults, probiotics or prebiotics were the third most commonly used dietary supplement other than vitamins and minerals, and the use of probiotics quadrupled between 2007 and 2012. The 2012 NHIS also showed that 300,000 children age 4 to 17 (0.5 percent) had used probiotics or prebiotics in the 30 days before the survey.

What the Science Says about the Effectiveness of Probiotics

Researchers have studied probiotics to find out whether they might help prevent or treat a variety of health problems, including:

- Digestive disorders such as diarrhea caused by infections, antibiotic-associated diarrhea, irritable bowel syndrome, and inflammatory bowel disease

- Allergic disorders such as atopic dermatitis (eczema) and allergic rhinitis (hay fever)

439

- Tooth decay, periodontal disease, and other oral health problems

- Colic in infants

- Liver disease

- The common cold

- Prevention of necrotizing enterocolitis in very low birth weight infants

There's preliminary evidence that some probiotics are helpful in preventing diarrhea caused by infections and antibiotics and in improving symptoms of irritable bowel syndrome, but more needs to be learned. We still don't know which probiotics are helpful and which are not. We also don't know how much of the probiotic people would have to take or who would most likely benefit from taking probiotics. Even for the conditions that have been studied the most, researchers are still working toward finding the answers to these questions.

Probiotics are not all alike. For example, if a specific kind of *Lactobacillus* helps prevent an illness, that doesn't necessarily mean that another kind of *Lactobacillus* would have the same effect or that any of the Bifidobacterium probiotics would do the same thing.

Although some probiotics have shown promise in research studies, strong scientific evidence to support specific uses of probiotics for most health conditions is lacking. The U.S. Food and Drug Administration (FDA) has not approved any probiotics for preventing or treating any health problem. Some experts have cautioned that the rapid growth in marketing and use of probiotics may have outpaced scientific research for many of their proposed uses and benefits.

How Might Probiotics Work?

Many probiotics are sold as dietary supplements, which do not require FDA approval before they are marketed. Dietary supplement labels may make claims about how the product affects the structure or function of the body without FDA approval, but they cannot make health claims (claims that the product reduces the risk of a disease) without the FDA's consent.

If a probiotic is marketed as a drug for specific treatment of a disease or disorder in the future, it will be required to meet more stringent requirements. It must be proven safe and effective for its intended use through clinical trials and be approved by the FDA before it can be sold.

What the Science Says about the Safety and Side Effects of Probiotics

Whether probiotics are likely to be safe for you depends on the state of your health.

- In people who are generally healthy, probiotics have a good safety record. Side effects, if they occur at all, usually consist only of mild digestive symptoms such as gas.

- On the other hand, there have been reports linking probiotics to severe side effects, such as dangerous infections, in people with serious underlying medical problems.

  - The people who are most at risk of severe side effects include critically ill patients, those who have had surgery, very sick infants, and people with weakened immune systems.

Even for healthy people, there are uncertainties about the safety of probiotics. Because many research studies on probiotics haven't looked closely at safety, there isn't enough information right now to answer some safety questions. Most of our knowledge about safety comes from studies of *Lactobacillus* and *Bifidobacterium*; less is known about other probiotics. Information on the long-term safety of probiotics is limited, and safety may differ from one type of probiotic to another. For example, even though a National Center for Complementary and Integrative Health (NCCIH)-funded study showed that a particular kind of *Lactobacillus* appears safe in healthy adults age 65 and older, this does not mean that all probiotics would necessarily be safe for people in this age group.

Section 65.3

Herbal Supplements

This section includes text excerpted from "Herbs at a
Glance," National Center for Complementary and Integrative
Health (NCCIH), April 6, 2016.

This section provides basic information about specific herbs or
botanicals—common names, what the science says, and potential side
effects and cautions.

Echinacea

Common Names: echinacea, purple coneflower, coneflower, American coneflower.

Latin Name: *Echinacea purpurea, Echinacea angustifolia, Echinacea pallida.*

There are nine known species of echinacea, all of which are native
to the United States and southern Canada. The most commonly used
is Echinacea purpurea. Echinacea has traditionally been used for colds,
flu, and other infections, based on the idea that it might stimulate the
immune system to more effectively fight infection. Less common folk
or traditional uses of echinacea include for wounds and skin problems,
such as acne or boils.

The aboveground parts of the plant and roots of echinacea are used
fresh or dried to make teas, squeezed (expressed) juice, extracts, or
preparations for external use.

What the Science Says

- Study results are mixed on whether echinacea can prevent or
  effectively treat upper respiratory tract infections such as the
  common cold. For example, two National Center for Complementary and Integrative Health (NCCIH)-funded studies did
  not find a benefit from echinacea, either as *Echinacea purpurea*
  fresh-pressed juice for treating colds in children, or as an unrefined mixture of *Echinacea angustifolia* root and *Echinacea*

purpurea root and herb in adults. However, other studies have shown that echinacea may be beneficial in treating upper respiratory infections.

- NCCIH is continuing to support the study of echinacea for the treatment of upper respiratory infections. NCCIH is also studying echinacea for its potential effects on the immune system.

Side Effects and Cautions

- When taken by mouth, echinacea usually does not cause side effects. However, some people experience allergic reactions, including rashes, increased asthma, and anaphylaxis (a life-threatening allergic reaction). In clinical trials, gastrointestinal side effects were most common.

- People are more likely to experience allergic reactions to echinacea if they are allergic to related plants in the daisy family, which includes ragweed, chrysanthemums, marigolds, and daisies. Also, people with asthma or atopy (a genetic tendency toward allergic reactions) may be more likely to have an allergic reaction when taking echinacea.

- Tell all your healthcare providers about any complementary health approaches you use. Give them a full picture of what you do to manage your health. This will help ensure coordinated and safe care.

Goldenseal

Common Names: goldenseal, yellow root.
Latin Name: *Hydrastis canadensis.*

Goldenseal is a plant that grows wild in parts of the United States but has become endangered by overharvesting. With natural supplies dwindling, goldenseal is now grown commercially across the United States, especially in the Blue Ridge Mountains. Historically, Native Americans have used goldenseal for various health conditions such as skin diseases, ulcers, and gonorrhea. Currently, folk or traditional uses of goldenseal include colds and other respiratory tract infections, infectious diarrhea, eye infections, vaginitis (inflammation or infection of the vagina), and occasionally, cancer. It is also applied to wounds and canker sores and is used as a mouthwash for sore gums, mouth, and throat.

The underground stems or roots of goldenseal are dried and used to make teas, liquid extracts, and solid extracts that may be made into tablets and capsules. Goldenseal is often combined with echinacea in preparations that are intended to be used for colds.

What the Science Says

- Few studies have been published on goldenseal's safety and effectiveness, and there is little scientific evidence to support using it for any health problem.

- Clinical studies on a compound found in goldenseal, berberine, suggest that the compound may be beneficial for certain infections—such as those that cause some types of diarrhea, as well as some eye infections. However, goldenseal preparations contain only a small amount of berberine, so it is difficult to extend the evidence about the effectiveness of berberine to goldenseal.

- NCCIH is funding research on goldenseal, including studies of antibacterial mechanisms and potential cholesterol-lowering effects. NCCIH is also funding development of research-grade goldenseal, to facilitate clinical studies.

Side Effects and Cautions

- Goldenseal is considered safe for short-term use in adults at recommended dosages. Rare side effects may include nausea and vomiting.

- There is little information about the safety of high dosages or the long-term use of goldenseal.

- Goldenseal may cause changes in the way the body processes drugs, and could potentially alter the effects of many drugs.

- Other herbs containing berberine, including Chinese goldthread (Coptis trifolia) and Oregon grape (Mahonia aquifolium), are sometimes substituted for goldenseal. These herbs may have different effects, side effects, and drug interactions than goldenseal.

- Women who are pregnant or breastfeeding should avoid using goldenseal. Berberine, a chemical in goldenseal, can cause or worsen jaundice in newborns and could lead to a life-threatening problem called kernicterus.

- Goldenseal should not be given to infants and young children.

- Tell all your healthcare providers about any complementary health approaches you use. Give them a full picture of what you

444

do to manage your health. This will help ensure coordinated and safe care.

Licorice Root

Common Names: licorice root, licorice, liquorice, sweet root, gan zao (Chinese licorice)

Latin Name: *Glycyrrhiza glabra, Glycyrrhiza uralensis (Chinese licorice)*

Most licorice is grown in Greece, Turkey, and Asia. Licorice contains a compound called glycyrrhizin (or glycyrrhizic acid). Licorice has a long history of medicinal use in both Eastern and Western systems of medicine. Licorice is used as a folk or traditional remedy for stomach ulcers, bronchitis, and sore throat, as well as infections caused by viruses, such as hepatitis.

Peeled licorice root is available in dried and powdered forms. Licorice root is available as capsules, tablets, and liquid extracts. Licorice can be found with glycyrrhizin removed; the product is called DGL (for "deglycyrrhizinated licorice").

What the Science Says

- An injectable form of licorice extract—not available in the United States—has been shown to have beneficial effects against hepatitis C in clinical trials. There are no reliable data on oral forms of licorice for hepatitis C. More research is needed before reaching any conclusions.

- There are not enough reliable data to determine whether licorice is effective for any condition.

Side Effects and Cautions

- In large amounts, licorice containing glycyrrhizin can cause high blood pressure, salt and water retention, and low potassium levels, which could lead to heart problems. DGL products are thought to cause fewer side effects.

- The safety of using licorice as a dietary supplement for more than 4 to 6 weeks has not been thoroughly studied.

- Taking licorice together with diuretics (water pills), corticosteroids, or other medicines that reduce the body's potassium levels could cause dangerously low potassium levels.

- People with heart disease or high blood pressure should be cautious about using licorice.

- When taken in large amounts, licorice can affect the body's levels of a hormone called cortisol and related steroid drugs, such as prednisone.

- Pregnant women should avoid using licorice as a supplement or consuming large amounts of licorice as food, as some research suggests it could increase the risk of preterm labor.

- Tell all your healthcare providers about any complementary health approaches you use. Give them a full picture of what you do to manage your health. This will help ensure coordinated and safe care.

Milk Thistle

Common Names: milk thistle, Mary thistle, holy thistle. Milk thistle is sometimes called silymarin, which is actually a mixture of the herb's active components, including silybinin (also called silibinin or silybin).

Latin Name: *Silybum marianum*

Milk thistle is a flowering herb native to the Mediterranean region. It has been used for thousands of years as a remedy for a variety of ailments, and historically was thought to have protective effects on the liver and improve its function. Its primary folk uses include liver disorders such as cirrhosis and chronic hepatitis, and gallbladder disorders. Other folk uses include lowering cholesterol levels, reducing insulin resistance in people who have both type 2 diabetes and cirrhosis, and reducing the growth of breast, cervical, and prostate cancer cells.

Silymarin, which can be extracted from the seeds (fruit) of the milk thistle plant, is believed to be the biologically active part of the herb. The seeds are used to prepare capsules, extracts, powders, and tinctures.

What the Science Says

Previous laboratory studies suggested that milk thistle may benefit the liver by protecting and promoting the growth of liver cells, fighting oxidation (a chemical process that can damage cells), and inhibiting inflammation. However, results from small clinical trials of milk thistle for liver diseases have been mixed, and two rigorously designed studies found no benefit.

446

- A 2012 clinical trial, cofunded by NCCIH and the National Institute of Diabetes and Digestive and Kidney Diseases, showed that two higher-than-usual doses of silymarin were no better than placebo for chronic hepatitis C in people who had not responded to standard antiviral treatment.

- The 2008 Hepatitis C Antiviral Long-Term Treatment Against Cirrhosis (HALT-C) study, sponsored by the National Institutes of Health (NIH), found that hepatitis C patients who used silymarin had fewer and milder symptoms of liver disease and somewhat better quality of life but no change in virus activity or liver inflammation.

Side Effects and Cautions

- In clinical trials, milk thistle appears to be well tolerated in recommended doses. Occasionally, people report various gastrointestinal side effects.

- Milk thistle can produce allergic reactions, which tend to be more common among people who are allergic to plants in the same family (for example, ragweed, chrysanthemum, marigold, and daisy).

- Milk thistle may lower blood sugar levels. People with diabetes or hypoglycemia, or people taking drugs or supplements that affect blood sugar levels, should use caution.

- Tell all your healthcare providers about any complementary health approaches you use. Give them a full picture of what you do to manage your health. This will help ensure coordinated and safe care.

Section 65.4

Dietary Supplements

This section includes text excerpted from "Using Dietary
Supplements Wisely," National Center for Complementary and
Integrative Health (NCCIH), June 13, 2016.

Like many Americans, you may take dietary supplements in an
effort to stay healthy. With so many dietary supplements available and
so many claims made about their health benefits, how can you decide
whether a supplement is safe or useful? This section provides a general
overview of dietary supplements, and discusses safety considerations.

What Are Dietary Supplements?

Dietary supplements were defined in a law passed by Congress
in 1994 called the Dietary Supplement Health and Education Act
(DSHEA). According to DSHEA, a dietary supplement is a product
that:

- Is intended to supplement the diet.

- Contains one or more dietary ingredients (including vitamins,
  minerals, herbs or other botanicals, amino acids, and certain
  other substances) or their constituents.

- Is intended to be taken by mouth, in forms such as tablet, cap-
  sule, powder, softgel, gelcap or liquid.

- Is labeled as being a dietary supplement.

Herbal supplements are one type of dietary supplement. An herb
is a plant or plant part (such as leaves, flowers, or seeds) that is used
for its flavor, scent, and/or potential health-related properties. "Botan-
ical" is often used as a synonym for "herb." An herbal supplement may
contain a single herb or mixtures of herbs. The law requires that all
of the herbs be listed on the product label.

Research has shown that some uses of dietary supplements are
beneficial to health. For example, scientists have found that folic acid
(a vitamin) prevents certain birth defects. Other research on dietary

448

supplements has failed to show benefit; for example, several major studies of the herbal supplement echinacea did not find evidence of benefit against the common cold.

Key Facts

- Dietary supplements contain a variety of ingredients, such as vitamins, minerals, amino acids, and herbs or other botanicals. Research has confirmed health benefits of some dietary supplements but not others.

- To use dietary supplements safely, read and follow the label instructions, and recognize that "natural" does not always mean "safe." Be aware that an herbal supplement may contain dozens of compounds and that all of its ingredients may not be known.

- Some dietary supplements may interact with medications or pose risks if you have medical problems or are going to have surgery. Most dietary supplements have not been tested in pregnant women, nursing mothers or children.

- The U.S. Food and Drug Administration (FDA) regulates dietary supplements, but the regulations for dietary supplements are different and less strict than those for prescription or over-the-counter drugs.

- Tell all your healthcare providers about any complementary health approaches you use. Give them a full picture of what you do to manage your health. This will help ensure coordinated and safe care.

Dietary Supplement Use in the United States

According to the 2007 National Health Interview Survey (NHIS), which included questions on Americans' use of natural products (not including vitamins and minerals), 17.7 percent of American adults had used these types of products in the past 12 months. The most popular of these products used by adults in the past 30 days were fish oil/omega 3/DHA (37.4 percent), glucosamine (19.9 percent), echinacea (19.8 percent), flaxseed oil or pills (15.9 percent), and ginseng (14.1 percent). National Health and Nutrition Examination Survey (NHANES) data collected from 2003 to 2006 that covered all types of dietary supplements indicate that 53 percent of American adults took at least one dietary supplement, most commonly multivitamin/

multimineral supplements (taken by 39 percent of all adults). Women were more likely than men to take dietary supplements.

Federal Regulation of Dietary Supplements

The Federal Government regulates dietary supplements through the FDA. The regulations for dietary supplements are not the same as those for prescription or over-the-counter drugs.

- Manufacturers of dietary supplements are responsible for ensuring that their products are safe and that the label information is truthful and not misleading. However, a manufacturer of a dietary supplement does not have to provide the FDA with data that demonstrate the safety of the product before it is marketed. In contrast, manufacturers of drugs have to provide the FDA with evidence that their products are both safe and effective before the drugs can be sold.

- Manufacturers may make three types of claims for their dietary supplements: health claims, structure/function claims, and nutrient content claims. Some of these claims describe the link between a food substance and a disease or health-related condition; the intended benefits of using the product; or the amount of a nutrient or dietary substance in a product. Different requirements apply to each type of claim. If a dietary supplement manufacturer makes a claim about a product's effects, the manufacturer must have data to support the claim. Claims about how a supplement affects the structure or function of the body must be followed by the words "This statement has not been evaluated by the U.S. Food and Drug Administration (FDA). This product is not intended to diagnose, treat, cure, or prevent any disease."

- Manufacturers must follow "current good manufacturing practices" for dietary supplements to ensure that these products are processed, labeled, and packaged consistently and meet quality standards.

- Once a dietary supplement is on the market, the FDA evaluates safety by doing research and keeping track of any side effects reported by consumers, healthcare providers, and supplement companies. If the FDA finds a product to be unsafe, it can take action against the manufacturer and/or distributor, and may issue a warning or require that the product be removed from the marketplace.

450

Also, once a dietary supplement is on the market, the FDA monitors product information, such as label claims and package inserts. The Federal Trade Commission (FTC) is responsible for regulating product advertising; it requires that all information be truthful and not misleading.

The Federal Government has taken legal action against dietary supplement promoters or Websites that promote or sell dietary supplements for making false or deceptive statements about their products or because marketed products have proven to be unsafe. In 2010, an investigation by the U.S. Government Accountability Office found instances in which written sales materials for herbal dietary supplements sold through online retailers included illegal claims that the products could treat, prevent, or cure diseases such as diabetes, cancer, or cardiovascular disease.

Sources of Science-Based Information

It's important to look for reliable sources of information on dietary supplements so you can evaluate the claims that are made about them. The most reliable information on dietary supplements is based on the results of rigorous scientific testing. To get reliable information on a particular dietary supplement:

- Ask your healthcare providers. Even if they don't know about a specific dietary supplement, they may be able to access the latest medical guidance about its uses and risks.

- Look for scientific research findings on the dietary supplement. The National Center for Complementary and Integrative Health (NCCIH) and the National Institutes of Health (NIH) Office of Dietary Supplements (ODS), as well as other Federal agencies, have free publications, clearinghouses, and information on their Websites.

Safety Considerations

If you're thinking about or currently using a dietary supplement, here are some points to keep in mind.

- **Tell all your healthcare providers** about any complementary health approaches you use. Give them a full picture of what you do to manage your health. This will help ensure coordinated and safe care.

- It's especially important to talk to your healthcare providers if you:

451

- Take any medications (whether prescription or over-the-counter). Some dietary supplements have been found to interact with medications. For example, the herbal supplement St. John's wort interacts with many medications, making them less effective.

- Are thinking about replacing your regular medication with one or more dietary supplements.

- Expect to have surgery. Certain dietary supplements may increase the risk of bleeding or affect the response to anesthesia.

- Are pregnant, nursing a baby, attempting to become pregnant, or considering giving a child a dietary supplement. Most dietary supplements have not been tested in pregnant women, nursing mothers, or children.

- Have any medical conditions. Some dietary supplements may harm you if you have particular medical conditions. For example, by taking supplements that contain iron, people with hemochromatosis, a hereditary disease in which too much iron accumulates in the body, could further increase their iron levels and therefore their risk of complications such as liver disease.

- If you're taking a dietary supplement, **follow the label instructions**. Talk to your healthcare provider if you have any questions, particularly about the best dosage for you to take. If you experience any side effects that concern you, stop taking the dietary supplement, and contact your healthcare provider. You can report serious problems suspected with dietary supplements to the U.S. Food and Drug Administration and the National Institutes of Health through the Safety Reporting Portal.

- Keep in mind that although many dietary supplements (and some prescription drugs) come from natural sources, **"natural" does not always mean "safe."** For example, the herbs comfrey and kava can cause serious harm to the liver. Also, a manufacturer's use of the term "standardized" (or "verified" or "certified") does not necessarily guarantee product quality or consistency.

- Be aware that **an herbal supplement may contain dozens of compounds** and that all of its ingredients may not be known. Researchers are studying many of these products in an effort to identify what ingredients may be active and understand their effects in the body. Also consider the possibility that what's

452

on the label may not be what's in the bottle. Analyses of dietary supplements sometimes find differences between labeled and actual ingredients. For example:

- An herbal supplement may not contain the correct plant species.

- The amounts of the ingredients may be lower or higher than the label states. That means you may be taking less—or more—of the dietary supplement than you realize.

- The dietary supplement may be contaminated with other herbs, pesticides, or metals, or even adulterated with unlabeled, illegal ingredients such as prescription drugs.

Section 65.5

CAM and Hepatitis C

This section includes text excerpted from "Hepatitis C: A Focus on Dietary Supplements," National Center for Complementary and Integrative Health (NCCIH), November 2014.

Hepatitis C, a liver disease caused by a virus, is usually chronic (long-lasting), with symptoms ranging from mild (or even none) to severe. Conventional medical treatments are available for hepatitis C; however, some people also try complementary health practices, especially herbal supplements.

What Is Hepatitis C?

Hepatitis C is a contagious liver disease. It's caused by the hepatitis C virus. People can get hepatitis C through contact with blood from a person who's already infected or, less commonly, through having sex with an infected person. The infection usually becomes chronic. Chronic hepatitis C often is treated with drugs that can eliminate the virus. This may slow or stop liver damage, but the drugs may cause side effects, and for some people, treatment is ineffective. An estimated 3.2 million Americans have chronic hepatitis C.

Use of Herbal Supplements and Other Complementary Approaches for Hepatitis C

Several herbal supplements have been studied for hepatitis C, and substantial numbers of people with hepatitis C have tried herbal supplements. For example, a survey of 1,145 participants in the HALT-C (Hepatitis C Antiviral Long-Term Treatment Against Cirrhosis) trial, a study supported by the National Institutes of Health (NIH), found that 23 percent of the participants were using herbal products. Although participants reported using many different herbal products, silymarin (milk thistle) was by far the most common. Another study, which surveyed 120 adults with hepatitis C, found that many used a variety of complementary health approaches, including multivitamins, herbal remedies, massage, deep breathing exercises, meditation, progressive relaxation, and yoga.

What the Science Says

No dietary supplement has been shown to be effective for hepatitis C. This section summarizes what's known about the safety and effectiveness of milk thistle and some of the other dietary supplements studied for hepatitis C.

- **Milk thistle** (scientific name *Silybum marianum*) is a plant from the aster family. Silymarin is an active component of milk thistle believed to be responsible for the herb's health-related properties. Milk thistle has been used in Europe for treating liver disease and jaundice since the 16th century. In the United States, silymarin is the most popular dietary supplement taken by people with liver disease. However, two rigorously designed studies of silymarin in people with hepatitis C didn't show any benefit.

  - A 2012 controlled clinical trial, cofunded by National Center for Complementary and Integrative Health (NCCIH) and National Institute of Diabetes and Digestive and Kidney Diseases (NIDDK), showed that two higher-than-usual doses of silymarin were no better than placebo in reducing the high blood levels of an enzyme that indicates liver damage. In the study, 154 people who hadn't responded to standard antiviral treatment for chronic hepatitis C were randomly assigned to receive 420 mg of silymarin, 700 mg of silymarin, or placebo three times per day for 24 weeks. At the end of the treatment period, blood levels of the enzyme were similar in all three groups.

- Results of the HALT-C study mentioned above suggested that silymarin use by hepatitis C patients was associated with fewer and milder symptoms of liver disease and somewhat better quality of life, but there was no change in virus activity or liver inflammation. The researchers emphasized that this was a retrospective study (one that examined the medical and lifestyle histories of the participants). Its finding of improved quality of life in patients taking silymarin wasn't confirmed in the more rigorous 2012 study described above.

Safety. Available evidence from clinical trials in people with liver disease suggests that milk thistle is generally well-tolerated. Side effects can include a laxative effect, nausea, diarrhea, abdominal bloating and pain, and occasional allergic reactions. In NIH-funded studies of silymarin in people with hepatitis C that were completed in 2010 and 2012, the frequency of side effects was similar in people taking silymarin and those taking placebos. However, these studies were not large enough to show with certainty that silymarin is safe for people with chronic hepatitis C.

Other supplements have been studied for hepatitis C, but overall, no benefits have been clearly demonstrated. These supplements include the following:

- **Probiotics** are live microorganisms that are intended to have a health benefit when consumed. Research hasn't produced any clear evidence that probiotics are helpful in people with hepatitis C. Most people can use probiotics without experiencing any side effects—or with only mild gastrointestinal side effects such as intestinal gas—but there have been some case reports of serious adverse effects in people with underlying serious health conditions.

- Preliminary studies, most of which were conducted outside the United States, have examined the use of **zinc** for hepatitis C. Zinc supplements might help to correct zinc deficiencies associated with hepatitis C or reduce some symptoms, but the evidence for these possible benefits is limited. Zinc is generally considered to be safe when used appropriately, but it can be toxic if taken in excessive amounts.

- A few preliminary studies have looked at the effects of combining supplements such as **lactoferrin, SAMe** or zinc with conventional drug therapy for hepatitis C. The evidence isn't sufficient to draw clear conclusions about benefit or safety.

- **Glycyrrhizin**—a compound found in licorice root—has been tested in a few clinical trials in hepatitis C patients, but there's currently not enough evidence to determine if it's helpful. In large amounts, glycyrrhizin or licorice can be dangerous in people with a history of hypertension (high blood pressure), kidney failure, or cardiovascular diseases.

- Preliminary studies have examined the potential of the following products for treating chronic hepatitis C: **TJ-108** (a mixture of herbs used in Japanese Kampo medicine), **schisandra, oxymatrine** (an extract from the sophora root), and **thymus extract**. The limited research on these products hasn't produced convincing evidence that they're helpful for hepatitis C.

- **Colloidal silver** has been suggested as a treatment for hepatitis C, but there's currently no research to support its use for this purpose. Colloidal silver is known to cause serious side effects, including a permanent bluish discoloration of the skin called argyria.

If You're Considering Taking a Dietary Supplement for Hepatitis C

- Do not use any complementary health approach to replace conventional treatments for hepatitis C or as a reason to postpone seeing your healthcare provider about any medical problem.

- Be aware that dietary supplements may have side effects or interact with conventional medical treatments.

- If you're pregnant or nursing a child, or if you're considering giving a child a dietary supplement, it's especially important to consult your (or your child's) healthcare provider. Supplements can act like drugs, and many have not been tested in pregnant women, nursing mothers or children.

- Tell all your healthcare providers about any complementary health approaches you use. Give them a full picture of what you do to manage your health. This will help ensure coordinated and safe care.

Key Points

- **Are Dietary Supplements for Hepatitis C Safe?**

  - Colloidal silver is not safe; it can cause irreversible side effects.

  - Data on the safety of other supplements is limited. However, some can have side effects or may interact in harmful ways with medications, and some may be unsafe for people with certain health problems.

  - If you have hepatitis C, check with your healthcare provider before using any dietary supplement to make sure that it is safe for you and compatible with any medical treatment that you're receiving for hepatitis C or any other health problem.

- **Are Dietary Supplements for Hepatitis C Effective?**

  - No dietary supplement has been shown to be effective for hepatitis C or its complications.

  - The results of research supported by the National Center for Complementary and Integrative Health (NCCIH) and National Institute of Diabetes and Digestive and Kidney Diseases (NIDDK) have shown that silymarin, the active extract of milk thistle and the most popular complementary health product taken by people with liver disease, was no more effective than placebo in people with hepatitis C.

  - Research on other dietary supplements for hepatitis C, such as zinc, licorice root (or its extract glycyrrhizin), S-adenosyl-L-methionine (SAMe), and lactoferrin, is in its early stages, and no firm conclusions can be reached about the potential effectiveness of these supplements.

Part Four

Medical Diagnosis and Treatment of Contagious Diseases

Chapter 66

Diagnostic Tests for Contagious Diseases

Chapter Contents

Section 66.1

Medical Tests That Diagnose Infection

This section includes text excerpted from "A Directory of Medical Tests," © 1995–2016. The Nemours Foundation/KidsHealth®. Reprinted with permission.

Taking a medical history and performing a physical examination usually provide the information a doctor needs to evaluate or to understand what's causing an illness. But sometimes, doctors need to order tests to find out more. Here are some common tests and what they involve:

Blood Tests

Blood tests usually can be done in a doctor's office or in a lab where technicians are trained to take blood. When only a small amount of blood is needed, the sample can sometimes be taken from a baby by sticking a heel and from an older child by sticking a finger with a small needle.

If a larger blood sample is needed, the technician drawing the blood will clean the skin, insert a needle into a vein (usually in the arm or hand), and withdraw blood. In kids, it sometimes takes more than one try. A bandage and a cotton ball or swab will help stop the flow of blood when the needle is removed.

Blood tests can be scary for kids, so try to be a calming presence during the procedure. Holding your child's hand or offering a stuffed animal or other comforting object can help. Tell your child that it may pinch a little, but that it will be over soon. With younger kids, try singing a song, saying the alphabet or counting together while the blood is being drawn.

Common blood tests include:

- **Complete blood count (CBC).** A CBC measures the levels of different types of blood cells. By determining if there are too many or not enough of each blood cell type, a CBC can help to detect a wide variety of illnesses or signs of infection.

- **Blood chemistry test.** Basic blood chemistry tests measure the levels of certain electrolytes, such as sodium and potassium, in the blood. Doctors typically order them to look for any sign of kidney dysfunction, diabetes, metabolic disorders, and tissue damage.

- **Blood culture.** A blood culture may be ordered when a child has symptoms of an infection—such as a high fever or chills—and the doctor suspects bacteria may have spread into the blood. A blood culture shows what type of germ is causing an infection, which will determine how it should be treated.

- **Lead test.** The American Academy of Pediatrics (AAP) recommends that all toddlers get tested for lead in the blood at 1 and 2 years of age since young kids are at risk for lead poisoning if they eat or inhale particles of lead-based paint. High lead levels can cause stomach problems and headaches and also have been linked to some developmental problems.

- **Liver function test.** Liver function tests check to see how the liver is working and look for any sort of liver damage or inflammation. Doctors typically order one when looking for signs of a viral infection (like mononucleosis or viral hepatitis) or liver damage from other health problems.

Pregnancy and Newborns Tests

State requirements differ regarding tests for newborns and pregnant women, and recommendations by medical experts are often updated. So talk with the doctor if you have questions about what's right for you.

- **Prenatal tests.** From ultrasounds to amniocentesis, a wide array of prenatal tests can help keep pregnant women informed. These tests can help identify—and then treat—health problems that could endanger both mother and baby. Some tests are done routinely for all pregnancies. Others are done if the pregnancy is considered high-risk (e.g., when a woman is 35 or older, is younger than 15, is overweight or underweight, or has a history of pregnancy complications).

- **Multiple marker test.** Most pregnant women are offered a blood-screening test between weeks 15–20. Also known as a "triple marker" or quadruple screen depending on the number of things measured, this blood test can reveal conditions like spina bifida or Down syndrome by measuring certain hormones and protein levels in the mother's blood. Keep in mind that these are screening tests and only show the possibility of a problem existing—they don't provide definitive diagnoses. However, if results show a potential problem, a doctor will recommend other diagnostic tests.

- **Newborn screening tests.** These tests are done soon after a baby is born to detect conditions that can't be easily and safely found before delivery, like sickle cell disease or cystic fibrosis. The conditions included in the test panel are also the type that need to be diagnosed and treated as soon as possible in order to help the child. Blood is drawn (usually from a needle stick on the heel) and spots are placed on special paper, which is then sent to a lab for analysis. In the U.S., states vary somewhat with regard to the number of and specific diseases included in the screening test panel.

- **Bilirubin level.** Bilirubin is a substance in the blood that can build up in babies and cause their skin to appear jaundiced (yellow). Usually jaundice is a harmless condition, but if the bilirubin level gets too high, it can lead to brain damage. A baby who appears jaundiced may have a bilirubin level check, which is done with an instrument placed on the skin or by blood tests.

- **Hearing screen.** The American Academy of Pediatrics (AAP) recommends that all babies have a hearing screen done before discharge from the hospital, and most states have universal screening programs. It's important to find hearing deficits early so that they can be treated as soon as possible. Hearing screens take 5–10 minutes and are painless. Sometimes they involve putting small probes in the ears; other times, they're done with electrodes.

Radiology Tests

- **X-rays.** X-rays can help doctors find a variety of conditions, including broken bones and lung infections. X-rays aren't painful, and typically involve just having the child stand, sit, or lie on a table while the X-ray machine takes a picture of the area the doctor is concerned about. The child is sometimes given a special gown or covering to help protect other areas of the body from radiation.

- **Ultrasound.** Though they're typically associated with pregnancy, doctors order ultrasounds in lots of different cases. For example, ultrasounds can be used to look for collections of fluid in the body, for problems with the kidneys, or to look at a baby's brain. An ultrasound is painless and uses high-frequency sound waves to bounce off organs and create a picture. A special jelly is applied to the skin, and a handheld device is moved over the skin. The sound waves that come back produce an image on a screen. The images seen on most ultrasounds are difficult for the untrained eye to decipher, so a doctor will view the image and interpret it.

- **Computed tomography (CAT scan or CT-Scan).** CAT scans are a kind of X-ray, and typically are ordered to look for things such as appendicitis, internal bleeding or abnormal growths. A scan is not painful, but sometimes can be scary for young kids. A child is asked to lie on a narrow table, which slides into a scanner. A scan may require the use of a contrast material (a dye or other substance) to improve the visibility of certain tissues or blood vessels. The contrast material may be swallowed or given through an IV.

- **Magnetic resonance imaging (MRI).** MRIs use radio waves and magnetic fields to produce an image. MRIs are often used to look at bones, joints, and the brain. The child is asked to lie on a narrow table and it slides in to the middle of an MRI machine. While MRIs are not painful, they can be noisy and take a while, making them scary to some kids. Often, children need to be sedated for MRIs. Contrast material is sometimes given through an IV in order to get a better picture of certain structures.

- **Upper gastrointestinal imaging (upper GI).** An upper GI is a study that involves swallowing contrast material while X-rays are taken of the top part of the digestive system. This allows the doctor to see how a child swallows. Upper GI studies are used to evaluate things like difficulty swallowing and gastroesophageal reflux (GER). An upper GI isn't painful, but some kids don't like to drink the contrast material, which sometimes can be flavored to make it more appealing.

- **Voiding cystourethrogram (VCUG).** A VCUG involves putting dye into the bladder and then watching with continuous X-rays to see where the dye goes. Doctors typically order a VCUG when they are concerned about urinary reflux, which can sometimes

465

lead to kidney damage later. A catheter is inserted through the urethra, into the bladder, which can be uncomfortable and scary for a child, but usually is not painful. The bladder is then filled with contrast material that is put in through the catheter. Images are taken while the bladder is filling and then while the child is urinating, to see where the dye and the urine go.

Other Tests

- **Throat culture (strep screen).** Doctors often order throat cultures to test for the germs that cause strep throat (group A *streptococcus*, or strep, bacteria). The cultures are done in the doctor's office and aren't painful, but can be uncomfortable for a few seconds. The doctor or medical assistant wipes the back of the throat with a long cotton swab. This tickles the back of the throat and can cause a child to gag, but will be over very quickly, especially if your child stays still.

- **Stool test.** Stool (or feces or poop) can provide doctors with valuable information about what's wrong when a child has a problem in the stomach, intestines, or another part of the gastrointestinal system. The doctor may order stool tests if there is suspicion of something like an allergy, an infection, or digestive problems. Sometimes it is collected at home by a parent in a special container that the doctor provides. The doctor also will provide instructions on how to get the most useful sample for analysis.

- **Urine test.** Doctors order urine tests to make sure that the kidneys are functioning properly or when they suspect an infection in the kidneys or bladder. It can be taken in the doctor's office or at home. It's easy for toilet-trained kids to give a urine (pee) sample since they can go in a cup. In other cases, the doctor or nurse will insert a catheter (a narrow, soft tube) through the urinary tract opening into the bladder to get the urine sample. While this can be uncomfortable and scary for kids, it's typically not painful.

- **Lumbar puncture (spinal tap).** During a lumbar puncture a small amount of the fluid that surrounds the brain and spinal cord, the cerebrospinal fluid (CSF), is removed and examined. In kids, a lumbar puncture is often done to look for meningitis, an infection of the meninges (the membrane covering the brain and spinal cord). Other reasons to do lumbar punctures include:

to remove fluid and relieve pressure with certain types of headaches, to look for other diseases in the central nervous system,
or to place chemotherapy medications into the CSF. Spinal taps,
which can be done on an inpatient or outpatient basis, might
be uncomfortable but shouldn't be too painful. Depending on a
child's age, maturity, and size, the test may be done while the
child is sedated.

- **Electroencephalography (EEG).** EEGs often are used to
  detect conditions that affect brain function, such as epilepsy,
  seizure disorders, and brain injury. Brain cells communicate by
  electrical impulses, and an EEG measures and records these
  impulses to detect anything abnormal. The procedure isn't painful but kids often don't like the electrodes being applied to their
  heads. A technician arranges several electrodes at specific sites
  on the head, fixing them in place with sticky paste. The patient
  must remain still and lie down while the EEG is done.

- **Electrocardiography (EKG).** EKGs measure the heart's
  electrical activity to help evaluate its function and identify any
  problems. The EKG can help determine the rate and rhythm of
  heartbeats, the size and position of the heart's chambers, and
  whether there is any damage present. EKGs can detect abnormal heart rhythms, some congenital heart defects, and heart
  tissue that isn't getting enough oxygen. It's not a painful procedure—the child must lie down and a series of small electrodes
  are fixed on the skin with sticky papers on the chest, wrists, and
  ankles. The child must sit still and may be asked to hold his or
  her breath briefly while the heartbeats are recorded.

- **Electromyography (EMG).** An EMG measures the response of
  muscles and nerves to electrical activity. It's used to help determine muscle conditions that might be causing muscle weakness,
  including muscular dystrophy and nerve disorders. A needle
  electrode is inserted into the muscle (the insertion might feel
  similar to a pinch) and the signal from the muscle is transmitted
  from the electrode through a wire to a receiver/amplifier, which
  is connected to a device that displays a readout. EMGs can be
  uncomfortable and scary to kids, but aren't usually painful.
  Occasionally kids are sedated while they're done.

- **Biopsies.** Biopsies are samples of body tissues taken to look
  for things such as cancer, inflammation, celiac disease, or the
  presence or absence of certain cells. Biopsies can be taken from

almost anywhere, including lymph nodes, bone marrow or kidneys. Doctors examine the removed tissue under a microscope to make a diagnosis. Kids are usually sedated for a biopsy.

Section 66.2

Strep Throat Testing and Treatment

This section includes text excerpted from "Is It Strep Throat," Centers for Disease Control and Prevention (CDC), October 19, 2015.

A Simple Test Gives Fast Results

Healthcare professionals can test for strep by swabbing the throat to quickly see if group A strep bacteria are causing a sore throat. A strep test is needed to tell if you have strep throat; just looking at your throat is not enough to make a diagnosis. If the test is positive, your healthcare professional can prescribe antibiotics. If the strep test is negative, but your clinician still strongly suspects you have this infection, then they can take a throat culture swab to test for the bacteria, but those results will take a little longer to come back.

Antibiotics Get You Well Fast

The strep test results will help your healthcare professional decide if you need antibiotics, which can:

- Decrease the length of time you're sick

- Reduce your symptoms

- Help prevent the spread of infection to friends and family members

- Prevent more serious complications, such as tonsil and sinus infections, and acute rheumatic fever (a rare inflammatory disease that can affect the heart, joints, skin, and brain)

You should start feeling better in just a day or two after starting antibiotics. Call your healthcare professional if you don't feel better after taking antibiotics for 48 hours. People with strep throat should stay home from work, school, or daycare until they have taken antibiotics for at least 24 hours so they don't spread the infection to others.

Be sure to finish the entire prescription, even when you start feeling better, unless your healthcare professional tells you to stop taking the medicine. When you stop taking antibiotics early, you risk getting an infection later that is resistant to antibiotic treatment.

Section 66.3

Testing for Influenza, Respiratory Infections, and Drug-Resistant Staph Infections

This section contains text excerpted from the following sources: Text beginning with the heading "Diagnosing Flu" is excerpted from "Influenza (Flu)," Centers for Disease Control and Prevention (CDC), August 13, 2015; Text under the heading "Laboratory Diagnostic Procedures" is excerpted from "Influenza (Flu)," Centers for Disease Control and Prevention (CDC), October 1, 2015; Text under the heading "Laboratory Testing for Methicillin-Resistant *Staphylococcus aureus* (MRSA)" is excerpted from "General Information About MRSA in the Community," Centers for Disease Control and Prevention (CDC), March 25, 2016; Text from "How Should Clinical Laboratories Test for MRSA?" is excerpted from "Methicillin-Resistant *Staphylococcus aureus* (MRSA)," Centers for Disease Control and Prevention (CDC), August 25, 2015.

Diagnosing Flu

How Do I Know If I Have the Flu?

Your respiratory illness might be the flu if you have fever, cough, sore throat, runny or stuffy nose, body aches, headache, chills and fatigue. Some people may have vomiting and diarrhea. People may be infected with the flu and have respiratory symptoms without a fever. Flu viruses usually cause the most illness during the colder months of the year. However, influenza can also occur outside of the typical

469

flu season. In addition, other viruses can also cause respiratory illness similar to the flu. So, it is impossible to tell for sure if you have the flu based on symptoms alone. If your doctor needs to know for sure whether you have the flu, there are laboratory tests that can be done.

What Kinds of Flu Tests Are There?

A number of flu tests are available to detect influenza viruses. The most common are called "rapid influenza diagnostic tests." These tests can provide results in 30 minutes or less. Unfortunately, the ability of these tests to detect the flu can vary greatly. Therefore, you could still have the flu, even though your rapid test result is negative. In addition to rapid tests, there are several more accurate and sensitive flu tests available that must be performed in specialized laboratories, such as those found in hospitals or state public health laboratories. All of these tests require that a healthcare provider swipe the inside of your nose or the back of your throat with a swab and then send the swab for testing. These tests do not require a blood sample.

How Well Can Rapid Tests Detect the Flu?

During an influenza outbreak, a positive rapid flu test is likely to indicate influenza infection. However, rapid tests vary in their ability to detect flu viruses, depending on the type of rapid test used, and on the type of flu viruses circulating. Also, rapid tests appear to be better at detecting flu in children than adults. This variation in ability to detect viruses can result in some people who are infected with the flu having a negative rapid test result. (This situation is called a false negative test result.) Despite a negative rapid test result, your healthcare provider may diagnose you with flu based on your symptoms and their clinical judgment.

Will My Healthcare Provider Test Me for Flu If I Have Flu-Like Symptoms?

Not necessarily. Most people with flu symptoms do not require testing because the test results usually do not change how you are treated.

Your healthcare provider may diagnose you with flu based on your symptoms and their clinical judgment or they may choose to use an influenza diagnostic test. During an outbreak of respiratory illness, testing for flu can help determine if flu viruses are the cause of the outbreak. Flu testing can also be helpful for some people with suspected flu who are pregnant or have a weakened immune system, and for whom a diagnosis of flu can help their doctor make decisions about their care.

Laboratory Diagnostic Procedures

A number of tests can help in the diagnosis of influenza. But, tests do not need to be done on all patients. For individual patients, tests are most useful when they are likely to yield clinically useful results that will help with diagnosis and treatment decisions. During a respiratory illness outbreak in a closed setting (e.g., hospitals, nursing home, cruise ship, boarding school, summer camp) however, testing for influenza can be very helpful in determining if influenza is the cause of the outbreak.

Preferred respiratory samples for influenza testing include naso-pharyngeal or nasal swab, and nasal wash or aspirate, depending on which type of test is used. Samples should be collected within the first 4 days of illness. Rapid influenza diagnostic tests provide results within 20 minutes or less; viral culture provides results in 3–10 days. Most of the rapid influenza diagnostic tests that can be done in a physician's office are approximately 50–70% sensitive for detecting influenza and approximately greater than 90% specific. Therefore, false negative results are more common than false positive results, especially during peak influenza activity.

Diagnostic tests available for influenza include viral culture, serol-ogy, rapid antigen testing, reverse transcription polymerase chain reaction (RT-PCR), immunofluorescence assays, and rapid molecular assays. Sensitivity and specificity of any test for influenza might vary by the laboratory that performs the test, the type of test used, the time from illness onset to specimen collection, and the type of specimen tested. Among respiratory specimens for viral isolation or rapid detec-tion of human influenza viruses, nasopharyngeal specimens typically have higher yield than nasal or throat swab specimens. As with any diagnostic test, results should be evaluated in the context of other clin-ical and epidemiologic information available to healthcare providers.

Viral Culture

Despite the availability of rapid influenza diagnostic tests, col-lecting clinical specimens for viral culture is critical, because only culture isolates can provide specific information regarding circulating strains and subtypes of influenza viruses. This information is needed to compare current circulating influenza virus strains with vaccine strains, to guide decisions regarding influenza antiviral treatment and chemoprophylaxis, and to formulate vaccine for the coming year. Virus isolates also are needed to monitor the emergence of antiviral resistance and the emergence of novel influenza A viruses that might pose a pandemic threat.

During outbreaks of respiratory illness when influenza is suspected, some respiratory samples should be tested by both rapid influenza diagnostic tests and by viral culture. The collection of some respiratory samples for viral culture is essential for determining the influenza A subtypes and influenza A and B virus strains causing illness, and for surveillance of new strains that may need to be included in the next year's influenza vaccine. During outbreaks of influenza-like illness, viral culture also can help identify other causes of illness.

Rapid Influenza Diagnostic Tests (RIDTs)

Commercial rapid influenza diagnostic tests are available that can detect influenza viruses within 20 minutes. Some tests are CLIA-waived and approved for use in any outpatient setting, whereas others must be used in a moderately complex clinical laboratory. These rapid influenza diagnostic tests differ in the types of influenza viruses they can detect and whether they can distinguish between influenza types.

Different tests can detect

1. only influenza A viruses;

2. both influenza A and B viruses, but not distinguish between the two types; or

3. both influenza A and B and distinguish between the two

None of the rapid influenza diagnostic tests provide any information about influenza A virus subtypes. The types of specimens acceptable for use (i.e., throat, nasopharyngeal, or nasal aspirates, swabs, or washes) also vary by test. The specificity and, in particular, the sensitivity of rapid influenza diagnostic tests are lower than for viral culture and RT-PCR and vary by test. Because of the lower sensitivity of the rapid influenza diagnostic tests, physicians should consider confirming negative tests with RT-PCR, viral culture or other means, especially in hospitalized patients or during suspected institutional influenza outbreaks because of the possibility of false-negative rapid test results, especially during periods of peak community influenza activity. In contrast, false-positive rapid test results are less likely, but can occur during periods of low influenza activity. Therefore, when interpreting results of a rapid influenza diagnostic test, physicians should consider the positive and negative predictive values of the test in the context of the level of influenza activity in their community. Package inserts and the laboratory performing the test should be consulted for more details regarding use of rapid influenza diagnostic tests.

Laboratory Testing for Methicillin-Resistant Staphylococcus aureus (MRSA)

MRSA is methicillin-resistant *Staphylococcus aureus*, a type of staph bacteria that is resistant to several antibiotics. In the general community, MRSA most often causes skin infections. In some cases, it causes pneumonia (lung infection) and other issues. If left untreated, MRSA infections can become severe and cause sepsis—a life-threatening reaction to severe infection in the body.

In a healthcare setting, such as a hospital or nursing home, MRSA can cause severe problems such as bloodstream infections, pneumonia and surgical site infections.

Who Is at Risk, and How Is MRSA Spread in The Community?

Anyone can get MRSA on their body from contact with an infected wound or by sharing personal items, such as towels or razors, that have touched infected skin. MRSA infection risk can be increased when a person is in activities or places that involve crowding, skin-to-skin contact, and shared equipment or supplies. People including athletes, daycare and school students, military personnel in barracks, and those who recently received inpatient medical care are at higher risk.

How Common Is MRSA?

Studies show that about one in three people carry staph in their nose, usually without any illness. Two in 100 people carry MRSA. There are not data showing the total number of people who get MRSA skin infections in the community.

Can I Prevent MRSA? How?

There are the steps you can take to reduce your risk of MRSA infection:

- Maintain good hand and body hygiene. Wash hands often, and clean your body regularly, especially after exercise.

- Keep cuts, scrapes and wounds clean and covered until healed.

- Avoid sharing personal items such as towels and razors.

- Get care early if you think you might have an infection.

What are MRSA Symptoms?

Sometimes, people with MRSA skin infections first think they have a spider bite. However, unless a spider is actually seen, the irritation is likely not a spider bite. Most staph skin infections, including MRSA, appear as a bump or infected area on the skin that might be:

- Red

- Swollen

- Painful

- Warm to the touch

- Full of pus or other drainage

- Accompanied by a fever

What Should I Do If I See These Symptoms?

If you or someone in your family experiences these signs and symptoms, cover the area with a bandage, wash your hands, and contact your doctor. It is especially important to contact your doctor if signs and symptoms of an MRSA skin infection are accompanied by a fever.

How Should Clinical Laboratories Test for MRSA?

In addition to broth microdultion testing, the Clinical and Laboratory Standards Institute (CLSI), recommends the cefoxitin disk screen test, the latex agglutination test for PBP2a, or a plate containing 6 μg/ml of oxacillin in Mueller-Hinton agar supplemented with 4% NaCl as alternative methods of testing for MRSA. In addition, there are now several FDA-approved selective chromogenic agars that can be used for MRSA detection.

Is It Difficult to Detect Oxacillin/Methicillin Resistance?

Accurate detection of oxacillin/methicillin resistance can be difficult due to the presence of two subpopulations (one susceptible and the other resistant) that may coexist within a culture of staphylococci.

All cells in a culture may carry the genetic information for resistance, but only a small number may express the resistance *in vitro*. This phenomenon is termed heteroresistance and occurs in staphylococci resistant to penicillinase-stable penicillins, such as oxacillin.

Cells expressing heteroresistance grow more slowly than the oxacillin-susceptible population and may be missed at temperatures above 35°C. This is why CLSI recommends incubating isolates being tested against oxacillin or cefoxitin at 33–35° C (maximum of 35°C) for a full 24 hours before reading.

Can All Susceptibility Tests Detect MRSA?

When used correctly, broth-based and agar-based tests usually can detect MRSA. The cefoxitin disk diffusion method can be used in addition to routine susceptibility test methods or as a back-up method.

Are There Additional Tests to Detect Oxacillin/Methicillin Resistance?

Nucleic acid amplification tests, such as the polymerase chain reaction (PCR), can be used to detect the *mecA* gene, is the most common gene that mediates oxacillin resistance in staphylococci. However, *mecA* PCR tests will not detect novel resistance mechanisms such as *mecC* or uncommon phenotypes such as borderline-resistant oxacillin resistance.

How Is the mecA Gene Involved in the Mechanism of Resistance?

Staphylococcal resistance to oxacillin/methicillin occurs when an isolate produces an altered penicillin-binding protein, PBP2a, which is encoded by the mecA gene. The variant penicillin-binding protein binds beta-lactams with lower avidity, which results in resistance to this class of antimicrobial agents.

Section 66.4

Rapid and Home Tests for Human Immunodeficiency Virus (HIV)

This section contains text excerpted from the following sources:
Text under the heading "Rapid Test for Human Immunodeficiency
Virus (HIV)" is excerpted from "HIV Test Types," AIDS.gov, U.S.
Department of Health and Human Services (HHS), June 5, 2015;
Text beginning with the heading "Home Access HIV-1 Test System"
is excerpted from "HIV Test Types," Centers for Disease Control and
Prevention (CDC), October 16, 2015.

Rapid Test for Human Immunodeficiency Virus (HIV)

The rapid test is an immunoassay used for screening, and it produces quick results, in 30 minutes or less. Rapid tests use blood or
oral fluid to look for antibodies to HIV. If an immunoassay (lab test
or rapid test) is conducted during the window period (i.e., the period
after exposure but before the test can find antibodies), the test may not
find antibodies and may give a false-negative result. All immunoassays
that are positive need a follow-up test to confirm the result.

Follow-up diagnostic testing is performed if the first immunoassay
result is positive. Follow-up tests include: an antibody differentiation
test, which distinguishes HIV-1 from HIV-2; an HIV-1 nucleic acid
test, which looks for virus directly, or the Western blot or indirect
immunofluorescence assay, which detect antibodies.

Immunoassays are generally very accurate, but follow-up testing
allows you and your healthcare provider to be sure the diagnosis is
right. If your first test is a rapid test, and it is positive, you will be
directed to a medical setting to get follow-up testing. If your first test
is a lab test, and it is positive, the lab will conduct follow-up testing,
usually on the same blood specimen as the first test.

Home Tests for HIV

There are only two home HIV tests:

1. Home Access HIV-1 Test System

476

2. OraQuick In-home HIV test

If you buy your home test online make sure the HIV test is U.S. Food and Drug Administration (FDA)-approved.

Home Access HIV-1 Test System

The **Home Access HIV-1 Test System** is a home collection kit, which involves pricking your finger to collect a blood sample, sending the sample to a licensed laboratory, and then calling in for results as early as the next business day. This test is anonymous. If the test is positive, a follow-up test is performed right away, and the results include the follow-up test. The manufacturer provides confidential counseling and referral to treatment. The tests conducted on the blood sample collected at home find infection later after infection than most lab-based tests using blood from a vein, but earlier than tests conducted with oral fluid.

OraQuick In-Home HIV Test

The **OraQuick In-Home HIV Test** provides rapid results in the home. The testing procedure involves swabbing your mouth for an oral fluid sample and using a kit to test it. Results are available in 20 minutes. If you test positive, you will need a follow-up test. The manufacturer provides confidential counseling and referral to follow-up testing sites. Because the level of antibody in oral fluid is lower than it is in blood, oral fluid tests find infection later after exposure than do blood tests. Up to 1 in 12 infected people may test false-negative with this test.

Chapter 67

Prescription Medicines That Treat Contagious Diseases

Chapter Contents

Section 67.1

Antibiotics, Antivirals, and Other Prescription Medicines

"Antibiotics, Antivirals, and Other Prescription Medicines,"
© 2017 Omnigraphics. Reviewed August 2016.

Although evidence suggests that the use of medicines to treat infections, also known as antimicrobial chemotherapy, may date back to ancient times, the modern use of this treatment begins in the early twentieth century when researchers in the lab of Paul Ehrlich, a German physician and scientist, synthesized an arsenical compound called arsphenamine. This drug, manufactured under the trade name Salvarsan, went on to become the first chemotherapeutic agent proven effective against human parasitic disease and was widely used in the treatment of syphilis.

This was followed by the discovery of penicillin in 1928 by Alexander Fleming, a Scottish scientist, who noticed that the accidental growth of *Penicillium* mold in a petri dish inhibited the growth of *Staphylococcus aureus* bacteria. By the forties, this wonder drug was being used to treat a number of infections—some life-threatening—of skin, blood, bone, and vital organs caused by *Staphylococcus*. During the Second World War, penicillin saved millions of lives and prevented the debilitating effects of wounds from dangerous infections. These early discoveries set the stage for the development of numerous anti-infective agents capable of preventing and treating a wide range of microbial infections.

Infections are generally caused when infective agents, such as bacteria, virus, or fungi, invade the tissues of an organism, sometimes called the host. These organisms multiply inside the host and produce toxins, provoking a reaction in the host tissues that could either result in an acute infection (short term) or a chronic infection (long term). There are a number of anti-infective agents that are used to treat infections. These agents work either by killing the infectious agent or pathogen, or by inhibiting its growth. While antimicrobial chemotherapy refers to the treatment of infections caused by infective agents, antimicrobial prophylaxis is used to prevent the spread of infection caused by pathogens. Anti-infective agents are classified on the basis of the infective agents they fight. For example, antibacterials are pharmacologic agents generally used to treat infections caused by bacteria. Antifungals are primarily effective against fungi and include fungistats (which inhibit fungal growth and proliferation) and fungicides (which kill fungal cells and spores). Antivirals and antiprotozoals act against viruses and protozoa, respectively.

Antibiotics

The discovery of antimicrobial agents, particularly the antibiotics, is often regarded as one of the greatest achievements of modern medicine, since it led to a significant decline in mortality rates from infectious diseases. The term "antibiotic" was first suggested by Selman Waksman, a Russian-born American biochemist and microbiologist credited with the discovery of several antibiotics, including streptomycin and neomycin, which have found extensive use in the treatment of many infectious diseases. The term is used to define the activity or application of a chemical compound and it includes any molecule that kills or inhibits the growth of bacteria.

Classes of Antibiotics

Antibiotics may be derived from certain classes of microorganisms or living systems and are used to fight against one or more types of disease-causing microorganisms. They may also be derived from non-organic sources, as in the case of sulphonamides and quinolones. Some antibiotics are effective against a number of bacteria, both gram-positive and gram-negative; these are termed as broad-spectrum antibiotics. Other antibiotics, called narrow-spectrum, are used to treat infections caused by specific families of bacteria

Most antibiotics work by disrupting the bacteria's metabolic processes. Although the exact mechanism of how this is brought about is still under study, it is believed that most antibacterial action either targets enzymes that regulate biosynthesis of the cell wall or cell proteins; others target enzymes that regulate nucleic acid metabolism of the bacterial cell. Some, like ionophores, work by interfering with cell membrane integrity. Antibiotics like penicillin and cephalosporins act on the bacterial cell wall, while quinolones and sulphonamides target the bacterial enzymes. Lincosamides and tetracyclines are examples of antibiotics that interfere with protein synthesis in bacterial cells.

Although the discovery of antibiotics was thought to herald the end of infectious diseases, their rampant misuse and overuse in humans, as well as in food-producing animals, in the last few decades have led to the emergence of antibiotic–resistant strains of bacteria. Antibiotics that were used successfully in the treatment of many infections in the past have now become inefficient against the same infection, and the dire need for new antibiotics—along with a slowdown in antibiotic discovery programs in the pharmaceutical industry—poses a serious challenge to public health worldwide.

Mode of Action

Most antibiotics work by disrupting the bacteria's metabolic processes. Although the exact mechanism of how this is brought about is still under study, it is believed that most antibacterial action either targets enzymes that regulate biosynthesis of the cell wall or cell proteins; others target enzymes that regulate nucleic acid metabolism of the bacterial cell. Some, like ionophores, work by interfering with cell membrane integrity. Antibiotics like penicillin and cephalosporins act on the bacterial cell wall, while quinolones and sulphonamides target the bacterial enzymes. Lincosamides and tetracyclines are examples of antibiotics that interfere with protein synthesis in bacterial cells.

Although the discovery of antibiotics was thought to herald the end of infectious diseases, their rampant misuse and overuse in humans, as well as in food-producing animals, in the last few decades have led to the emergence of antibiotic–resistant strains of bacteria. Antibiotics that were used successfully in the treatment of many infections in the past have now become inefficient against the same infection, and the dire need for new antibiotics—along with a slowdown in antibiotic discovery programs in the pharmaceutical industry—poses a serious challenge to public health worldwide.

Antivirals

Drugs used to treat infections caused by viruses are called antiviral drugs. Unlike bacteria, viruses are difficult to treat because they are obligate parasites, meaning they can grow and multiply only within living host cells. This makes it impossible to use prophylactic measures to contain viral infections. Contrary to popular belief, antibiotics do not treat viral infections, such as influenza, bronchitis, ear infection, or chest cold in otherwise healthy people. Most of the antiviral remedies currently in use include vaccines, which have successfully controlled—and in some cases eradicated—such serious viral infections as smallpox and poliomyelitis. The last few decades have seen growing interest in developing antiviral drugs to prevent the multiplication of the virus and cause the illness to run its course rapidly. Unfortunately, these drugs are only partially effective and work only on a very few specific viruses. The most difficult aspect of developing antiviral agents is the astounding diversity in the structural characteristic of viruses, of which there can be more than 50 different types for any given virus. In addition, the viral antigen, a protein coded by the viral genome that provokes an immune response in the host cell, periodically mutates making it particularly difficult to contain the infection with specific therapy.

Mentioned below are few classes of antiviral drugs.

Anti-Hepatitis

Viral hepatitis can be treated with several antiviral medications, most of which work by preventing viral replication in infected cells. Ribavarin is commonly used to treat hepatitis C, while lamivudine and adefovir are used to treat chronic hepatitis B infections. In addition to treating viral hepatitis, these drugs are also used to treat HIV infections. Interferons are another important class of drugs used in the treatment regimen for hepatitis, and they are commonly used in combination with other antiviral agents, such asribavarin.

Anti-Herpes

Anti-herpes medications like acyclovir, penciclovir, and their respective prodrugs (an inactive form of medication that is metabolized into a pharmacologically active drug inside the body) interfere with viral DNA replication and help control their spread to new cells. While anti-herpes drugs cannot eradicate the virus, they can help control symptoms and reduce the course of infections.

Anti-Influenza

Anti-influenza medications are not substitutes for vaccination but are used in conjunction with vaccines. Some strains of the influenza virus have become resistant to older antiviral drugs, such as amantadine and rimantadine, and are no longer used, although their potential use against new strains of virus that may be susceptible to these drugs cannot be ruled out. Some of the U.S. Food and Drug Administration (FDA)-approved anti-influenza drugs include oseltamivir (Tamiflu), zanamivir (Relenza), and peramivir (Rapivab). These drugs can ease the severity of symptoms and reduce the course of infection. The government maintains a stockpile of anti-influenza medications in preparation for a pandemic emergency.

Antiretroviral (ART)

Antiretroviral drugs work by suppressing a virus and retarding the progression of the disease. Although the antiretroviral drugs do not kill the virus or cure the disease, they slow down viral replication and substantially reduce the amount of virus in the body. This helps the immune system stay healthy and also reduces the risk of transmission to other people. More often than not, a cocktail of drugs from three or more classes of antiretroviral drugs is used for maximum effect. Referred to as Highly Active AntiRetroviral Therapy (HAART), this treatment regimen has substantially reduced HIV-related morbidity and mortality around the world.

Antiprotozoals

These are drugs that are used to treat infections caused by single-celled protozoans, such as *Entamoeba histolytica*, which causes amebiasis, and plasmodium, the pathogen that causes malaria. Like many other infective agents, antiprotozoals work on specific targets and inhibit their growth and reproduction. Antimalarial drugs, which include a diverse class of quinoline derivatives, act by targeting the erythrocytic (red blood cell) stage of the infection, which can be life-threatening, since blood circulates through all tissues and organs. In addition to antimalarials, there are several other classes of antiprotozoals, some of which may also be used to treat certain bacterial infections. Two of the most commonly used drugs in this group are metronidazole and tinidazole, which are used to treat a variety of parasitic and amoebic infections.

Antifungal Drugs

This class of medication controls a diverse range of infections caused by fungi, from simple infections like athlete's foot to extremely dangerous infections, such as cryptococcal meningitis, which affects the brain and spinal cord. Antifungal medications are based on mechanisms that inhibit vital cell processes in the organism. They work by either disrupting the integrity of the fungal cell membrane or cell wall, or by interfering with cell division by preventing DNA replication.

Antifungal agents are broadly classified as topical and systemic drugs. While topical antifungal agents may be directly applied to skin, nails, or hair to treat superficial fungal infections, systemic antifungal agents are used to treat invasive fungal infections that affect body tissues or internal organs. Antifungal drugs come as lotions, sprays, creams, tablets, injections, and pessaries (for vaginal use).

As in the case of antibiotics, drug resistance has become a major concern with a number of antifungal drugs as a result of their indiscriminate use in healthcare settings. For example, low dosage or short-term treatments may be a common cause of antifungal resistance in candidemia—one of the most common bloodstream infections in hospital settings—which incurs substantial healthcare costs. Although, drug resistance in several species of candida is a serious problem, studies show that drug resistance in other fungal species, such as aspergillus, is also becoming a cause for concern. Some studies also show that the overuse of antibiotics could lead to resistance by inhibiting gut bacteria and favoring the growth of fungal species like candida.

References

1. "Antiviral Drug," Encyclopaedia Britannica. n.d.

2. Davies, Julian, and Dorothy Davies. "Origins and Evolution of Antibiotic Resistance," Microbiology and Molecular Biology Reviews, September, 2010.

3. "Mechanisms of Action," Sigma-Aldrich. n.d.

4. Coates, R.M., Gerry Halls and Yanmin Hu. "Novel classes of antibiotics or more of the same?" British Journal of Pharmacology, May, 2011.

Section 67.2

Antibiotic Safety (Using Antibiotics Wisely)

This section contains text excerpted from the following sources: Text
beginning with the heading "Antibiotics Aren't Always the Answer"
is excerpted from "Antibiotics Aren't Always the Answer," Centers
for Disease Control and Prevention (CDC), November 16, 2015; Text
under the heading "The Threat of Antibiotic Resistance" is excerpted
from "Antibiotic Resistance Threats in the United States," U.S.
Department of Health and Human Services (HHS), April 23, 2013.

Antibiotics Aren't Always the Answer

Antibiotics do not fight infections caused by viruses like colds, flu,
most sore throats, bronchitis, and many sinus and ear infections.
Instead, symptom relief might be the best treatment option for viral
infections.

Get smart about when antibiotics are needed—to fight bacterial
infections. When you use antibiotics appropriately, you do the best
for your health, your family's health, and the health of those around
you. Taking antibiotics for viral infections, such as colds, flu, most sore
throats, bronchitis, and many sinus or ear infections:

- Will **not** cure the infection

- Will **not** keep other people from getting sick

- Will **not** help you or your child feel better

- May cause unnecessary and harmful side effects

- May contribute to antibiotic resistance, which is when bacteria are able to resist the effects of an antibiotic and continue to
  cause harm

Rest, fluids, and over-the-counter products may be your or your
child's best treatment option against viral infections. Remember–there
are potential risks when taking any prescription drug. Unneeded antibiotics may lead to harmful side effects and future antibiotic-resistant
infections.

What to Do

Just because your healthcare professional doesn't give you an antibiotic doesn't mean you aren't sick. Talk with your healthcare professional about the best treatment for your or your child's illness. To feel better when you or your child has a viral infection:

- Ask your healthcare professional about over-the-counter treatment options that may help reduce symptoms.

- Drink more fluids.

- Get plenty of rest.

- Use a cool-mist vaporizer or saline nasal spray to relieve congestion.

- Soothe your throat with crushed ice, sore throat spray, or lozenges. (Do not give lozenges to young children.)

- If you are diagnosed with the flu, there are flu antiviral drugs that can be used to treat flu illness. They are prescription drugs.

The Threat of Antibiotic Resistance

Antibiotic resistance is a worldwide problem. New forms of antibiotic resistance can cross international boundaries and spread between continents with ease. Many forms of resistance spread with remarkable speed. World health leaders have described antibiotic resistant microorganisms as "nightmare bacteria" that "pose a catastrophic threat" to people in every country in the world.

Each year in the United States, at least 2 million people acquire serious infections with bacteria that are resistant to one or more of the antibiotics designed to treat those infections. At least 23,000 people die each year as a direct result of these antibiotic-resistant infections. Many more die from other conditions that were complicated by an antibiotic resistant infection.

In addition, almost 250,000 people each year require hospital care for *Clostridium difficile (C. difficile)* infections. In most of these infections, the use of antibiotics was a major contributing factor leading to the illness. At least 14,000 people die each year in the United States from *C. difficile* infections. Many of these infections could have been prevented.

Antibiotic-resistant infections add considerable and avoidable costs to the already overburdened U.S. healthcare system. In most cases, antibiotic-resistant infections require prolonged and/or costlier treatments, extend hospital stays, necessitate additional doctor visits and healthcare use, and result in greater disability and death compared with infections that are easily treatable with antibiotics. The total economic cost of antibiotic resistance to the U.S. economy has been difficult to calculate. Estimates vary but have ranged as high as $20 billion in excess direct healthcare costs, with additional costs to society for lost productivity as high as $35 billion a year (2008 dollars).

The use of antibiotics is the single most important factor leading to antibiotic resistance around the world. Antibiotics are among the most commonly prescribed drugs used in human medicine. However, up to 50% of all the antibiotics prescribed for people are not needed or are not optimally effective as prescribed. Antibiotics are also commonly used in food animals to prevent, control, and treat disease, and to promote the growth

The other major factor in the growth of antibiotic resistance is spread of the resistant strains of bacteria from person to person, or from the non-human sources in the environment, including food.

- There are four core actions that will help fight these deadly infections:

  - preventing infections and preventing the spread of resistance

  - tracking resistant bacteria

  - improving the use of today's antibiotics

  - promoting the development of new antibiotics and developing new diagnostic tests for resistant bacteria

Bacteria will inevitably find ways of resisting the antibiotics we develop, which is why aggressive action is needed now to keep new resistance from developing and to prevent the resistance that already exists from spreading.

What Not to Do

- Do **not** demand antibiotics when your healthcare professional says they are not needed.

- Do **not** take an antibiotic for a viral infection.

- Do **not** take antibiotics prescribed for someone else. The antibiotic may not be right for your illness. Taking the wrong medicine may delay correct treatment and allow bacteria to grow.

If your healthcare professional prescribes an antibiotic for a bacterial infection:

- Do **not** skip doses.

- Do **not** stop taking the antibiotics early unless your healthcare professional tells you to do so.

- Do **not** save any of the antibiotics for the next time you or your child gets sick.

Illness	Usual Cause		Antibiotic Needed
	Viruses	Bacteria	
Cold/Runny Nose	✓		NO
Bronchitis/Chest Cold (in otherwise healthy children and adults)	✓		NO
Whooping Cough		✓	Yes
Flu	✓		NO
Strep Throat		✓	Yes
Sore Throat (except strep)	✓		NO
Fluid in the Middle Ear (otitis media with effusion)	✓		NO
Urinary Tract Infection		✓	Yes

Figure 67.1. *Antibiotics Aren't Always the Answer*

Section 67.3

Antiviral Drugs for Seasonal Flu

This section includes text excerpted from "What You Should Know About Flu Antiviral Drugs," Centers for Disease Control and Prevention (CDC), July 22, 2016.

Can the Flu Be Treated?

Yes. There are prescription medications called "antiviral drugs" that can be used to treat flu illness.

What Are Antiviral Drugs?

Antiviral drugs are prescription medicines (pills, liquid, an inhaled powder or an intravenous solution) that fight against the flu in your body. Antiviral drugs are not sold over-the-counter. You can only get them if you have a prescription from your doctor or healthcare provider. Antiviral drugs are different from antibiotics, which fight against bacterial infections.

What Should I Do If I Think I Have the Flu?

If you get the flu, antiviral drugs are a treatment option. Check with your doctor promptly if you are at high risk of serious flu complications. Flu symptoms can include fever, cough, sore throat, runny or stuffy nose, body aches, headache, chills and fatigue. Your doctor may prescribe antiviral drugs to treat your flu illness.

Should I Still Get a Flu Vaccine?

Yes. Antiviral drugs are not a substitute for getting a flu vaccine. While flu vaccine can vary in how well it works, a flu vaccine is the first and best way to prevent influenza. Antiviral drugs are a second line of defense to treat the flu if you get sick.

What Are the Benefits of Antiviral Drugs?

When used for treatment, antiviral drugs can lessen symptoms and shorten the time you are sick by 1 or 2 days. They also can prevent serious flu complications, like pneumonia. For people at high risk of serious flu complications, treatment with an antiviral drug can mean the difference between having milder illness instead of very serious illness that could result in a hospital stay.

What Are the Possible Side Effects of Antiviral Drugs?

Some side effects have been associated with the use of flu antiviral drugs, including nausea, vomiting, dizziness, runny or stuffy nose, cough, diarrhea, headache and some behavioral side effects. These are uncommon. Your doctor can give you more information about these drugs or you can check the Centers for Disease Control and Prevention (CDC) or the U.S. Food and Drug Administration (FDA) websites.

When Should Antiviral Drugs Be Taken for Treatment?

Studies show that flu antiviral drugs work best for treatment when they are started within 2 days of getting sick. However, starting them later can still be helpful, especially if the sick person is at high risk of serious flu complications or is very sick from the flu. Follow instructions for taking these drugs.

What Antiviral Drugs Are Recommended This Flu Season?

There are three FDA-approved influenza antiviral drugs recommended by CDC this season to treat influenza. The brand names for these are Tamiflu® (generic name oseltamivir), Relenza® (generic name zanamivir), and Rapivab® (generic name peramivir). Tamiflu® is available as a pill or liquid and Relenza® is a powder that is inhaled. (Relenza® is not for people with breathing problems like asthma or COPD, for example.) Rapivab® is given intravenously by a healthcare provider. There are no generic flu antiviral drugs.

How Long Should Antiviral Drugs Be Taken?

To treat the flu, Tamiflu® and Relenza® are usually prescribed for 5 days, although people hospitalized with the flu may need the medicine for longer than 5 days. Rapivab® is administered intravenously for 15 to 30 minutes.

Can Children Take Antiviral Drugs?

Yes. Children can take two of the approved antiviral drugs—oseltamivir and zanamivir. Oseltamivir (Tamiflu®) is recommended by the CDC and American Academy of Pediatrics (AAP) for the treatment of influenza in persons aged 2 weeks and older, and for the prevention of influenza in persons aged 3 months and older. Zanamivir (Relenza®) is recommended for the treatment of influenza in persons aged 7 years and older, and for the prevention of influenza in persons aged 5 years and older. Peramivir (Rapivab®) is recommended for use only in adults aged 18 and older.

Can Pregnant Women Take Antiviral Drugs?

Yes. Oral oseltamivir is preferred for treatment of pregnant women because it has the most studies available to suggest that it is safe and beneficial.

491

Who Should Take Antiviral Drugs?

It's very important that antiviral drugs are used early to treat hospitalized patients, people with severe flu illness, and people who are at high risk of serious flu complications based on their age or health. Other people also may be treated with antiviral drugs by their doctor. Most people who are otherwise healthy and get the flu do not need to be treated with antiviral drugs.

Following is a list of all the health and age factors that are known to increase a person's risk of getting serious complications from the flu:

- Asthma

- Neurological and neurodevelopmental conditions

- Blood disorders (such as sickle cell disease)

- Chronic lung disease (such as chronic obstructive pulmonary disease [COPD] and cystic fibrosis)

- Endocrine disorders (such as diabetes mellitus)

- Heart disease (such as congenital heart disease, congestive heart failure and coronary artery disease)

- Kidney disorders

- Liver disorders

- Metabolic disorders (such as inherited metabolic disorders and mitochondrial disorders)

- Morbid obesity (body mass index [BMI] of 40 or higher)

- People younger than 19 years of age on long-term aspirin therapy

- Weakened immune system due to disease or medication (such as people with HIV or AIDS, or cancer or those on chronic steroids)

Other people at high risk from the flu:

- Adults 65 years and older

- Children younger than 5 years old, but especially children younger than 2 years old

- Pregnant women and women up to 2 weeks after the end of pregnancy

- American Indians and Alaska Natives

Chapter 68

Antimicrobial (Drug) Resistance

Microbes, collectively, include bacteria, viruses, fungi, and parasites. For the past 70 years, antimicrobial drugs, such as antibiotics, have been successfully used to treat patients with bacterial and infectious diseases. Over time, however, many infectious organisms have adapted to the drugs designed to kill them, making the products less effective. To address this growing problem, National Institute of Allergy and Infectious Diseases (NIAID) is funding and conducting research on many aspects of antimicrobial (drug) resistance, including basic research on how microbes develop resistance, new and faster diagnostics, and clinical trials designed to find new vaccines and treatments effective against drug-resistant microbes.

What Is Antimicrobial (Drug) Resistance?

Microbes are constantly evolving enabling them to efficiently adapt to new environments. Antimicrobial resistance is the ability of microbes to grow in the presence of a chemical (drug) that would normally kill them or limit their growth

Antimicrobial resistance makes it harder to eliminate infections from the body as existing drugs become less effective. As a result, some

This chapter includes text excerpted from "Antimicrobial (Drug) Resistance," National Institute of Allergy and Infectious Diseases (NIAID), January 3, 2012. Reviewed August 2016.

infectious diseases are now more difficult to treat than they were just a few decades ago. As more microbes become resistant to antimicrobials, the protective value of these medicines is reduced. Overuse and misuse of antimicrobial medicines are among the factors that have contributed to the development of drug-resistant microbes.

Examples of Antimicrobial (Drug) Resistance

- Drug-resistant *Mycobacterium tuberculosis* (TB)
- Methicillin-resistant *Staphylococcus aureus* (MRSA)
- Vancomycin-resistant *Enterococci* (VRE)
- Multidrug-resistant *Neisseria gonorrhoeae* (Gonorrhea)
- Gram-negative Bacteria

Examples of Antimicrobials

- Tetracycline, an antibiotic that treats urinary tract infections
- Oseltamivir, also known as Tamiflu, an antiviral that treats the flu
- Terbinafine, also known as Lamisil, an antifungal that treats athlete's foot

Causes

Microbes, such as bacteria, viruses, fungi, and parasites, are living organisms that evolve over time. Their primary function is to reproduce, thrive, and spread quickly and efficiently. Therefore, microbes adapt to their environments and change in ways that ensure their survival. If something stops their ability to grow, such as an antimicrobial, genetic changes can occur that enable the microbe to survive. There are several ways this happens.

Natural (Biological) Causes

Selective Pressure

In the presence of an antimicrobial, microbes are either killed or if they carry resistance genes, survive. These survivors will replicate, and their progeny will quickly become the dominant type throughout the microbial population.

Mutation

Most microbes reproduce by dividing every few hours, allowing them to evolve rapidly and adapt quickly to new environmental conditions. During replication, mutations arise and some of these mutations may help an individual microbe survive exposure to an antimicrobial.

Gene Transfer

Microbes also may get genes from each other, including genes that make the microbe drug resistant.

Societal Pressures

The use of antimicrobials, even when used appropriately, creates a selective pressure for resistant organisms. However, there are additional societal pressures that act to accelerate the increase of antimicrobial resistance.

Inappropriate Use

Selection of resistant microorganisms is exacerbated by inappropriate use of antimicrobials. Sometimes healthcare providers will prescribe antimicrobials inappropriately, wishing to placate an insistent patient who has a viral infection or an as-yet undiagnosed condition.

Inadequate Diagnostics

More often, healthcare providers must use incomplete or imperfect information to diagnose an infection and thus prescribe an antimicrobial just-in-case or prescribe a broad-spectrum antimicrobial when a specific antibiotic might be better. These situations contribute to selective pressure and accelerate antimicrobial resistance.

Hospital Use

Critically ill patients are more susceptible to infections and, thus, often require the aid of antimicrobials. However, the heavier use of antimicrobials in these patients can worsen the problem by selecting for antimicrobial-resistant microorganisms. The extensive use of antimicrobials and close contact among sick patients creates a fertile environment for the spread of antimicrobial-resistant germs.

Agricultural Use

Scientists also believe that the practice of adding antibiotics to agricultural feed promotes drug resistance. More than half of the antibiotics produced in the United States are used for agricultural purposes. However, there is still much debate about whether drug-resistant microbes in animals pose a significant public health burden.

Diagnosis

Diagnostic tests are designed to determine which microbe is causing infection and to which antimicrobials the microbe might be resistant. This information would be used by a healthcare provider to choose an appropriate antimicrobial treatment. However, current diagnostic tests often take a few days or weeks to give results. This is because many of today's tests require the microbe to grow over a period of time before it can be identified.

Oftentimes, healthcare providers need to make treatment decisions before the results are known. While waiting for test results, healthcare providers may prescribe a broad-spectrum antimicrobial when a more specific treatment might be better. The common practice of treating unknown infections with broad-spectrum antimicrobials can accelerate the emergence of antimicrobial resistance.

Treatment

If you think you have an infection of any type—bacterial, viral or fungal—talk with your healthcare provider. Some infections will go away without medical intervention. Others will not and can become extremely serious. Ear infections are a good example. Some middle ear infections are caused by a virus and will get better without treatment. However, other middle ear infections caused by bacteria can cause perforated eardrums, or worse, if left untreated.

The decision to use antimicrobials should be left to your healthcare provider. In some cases, antimicrobials will not shorten the course of the disease, but they might reduce your chance of transmitting it to others, as is the case with pertussis (whooping cough).

Antibiotics are designed to kill or slow the growth of bacteria and some fungi. Antibiotics are commonly used to fight bacterial infections but cannot fight against infections caused by viruses.

Antibiotics are appropriate to use when:

- There is a known bacterial infection.

- The cause of the infection is unknown and bacteria are suspected. In that case, the consequences of not treating a condition could be devastating (e.g., in early meningitis).

Of note, the color of your sputum (saliva) does not indicate whether you need antibiotics. For example, most cases of bronchitis are caused by viruses. Therefore, a change in sputum color does not indicate a bacterial infection.

Prevention

To prevent antimicrobial resistance, you and your healthcare provider should discuss the appropriate medicine for your illness. Strictly follow prescription medicine directions, and never share or take medicine that was prescribed for someone else. Talk with your healthcare provider so that he or she has a clear understanding of your symptoms and can decide whether an antimicrobial drug, such as an antibiotic, is appropriate.

Do not save your antibiotic for the next time you get sick. Take the medicine exactly as directed by your healthcare provider. If your healthcare provider has prescribed more than the required dose, appropriately discard leftover medicines once you have completed the prescribed course of treatment.

Healthy lifestyle habits, including proper diet, exercise, and sleeping patterns as well as good hygiene, such as frequent hand washing, can help prevent illness, therefore also preventing the overuse or misuse of medications.

Chapter 69

Influenza Antiviral Drug Resistance

What Is Antiviral Resistance?

Antiviral resistance means that a virus has changed in such a way that antiviral drugs are less effective in treating or preventing illnesses with that virus. Influenza viruses can become resistant to influenza antiviral drugs. In the United States, there are three U.S. Food and Drug Administration (FDA)-approved neuraminidase inhibitor antiviral drugs recommended by Center for Disease Control and Prevention (CDC):

1. Oseltamivir (brand name Tamiflu®)

2. Zanamivir (Relenza®)

3. Peramivir (Rapivab®)

In the United States, most of the recently circulating influenza viruses have been susceptible to the neuraminidase inhibitor antiviral medications. There is another class of influenza antiviral drugs (amantadine and rimantadine) called the adamantanes that are not recommended for use in the United States at this time because of high levels of antiviral resistance to these drugs among circulating influenza viruses.

This chapter includes text excerpted from "Influenza Antiviral Drug Resistance," Center for Disease Control and Prevention (CDC), September 16, 2015.

How Does Antiviral Resistance Happen?

Influenza viruses are constantly changing; they can change from one season to the next and can even change within the course of one flu season. As a flu virus replicates (i.e., make copies of itself), the genetic makeup may change in a way that results in the virus becoming resistant to one or more of the antiviral drugs used to treat or prevent influenza. Influenza viruses can become resistant to antiviral drugs spontaneously or emerge during the course of antiviral treatment. Drug resistant viruses vary in their ability to transmit from a patient to contacts.

How Is Antiviral Resistance Detected?

CDC routinely collects flu viruses through a domestic and global surveillance system and test if they are resistant to any of the FDA-approved flu antiviral drugs. This information informs public health policy recommendations about the use of flu antiviral medications. Antiviral resistance testing involves several laboratory tests, including a specific functional assay, the neuraminidase inhibition (NI) assay, and molecular techniques (sequencing and pyrosequencing) to look for genetic changes that are associated with antiviral resistance.

What Is Oseltamivir Resistance?

Oseltamivir (trade name Tamiflu®) is an antiviral drug that is used to treat flu illness. "Oseltamivir resistance" refers to a flu virus that is resistant to the drug oseltamivir.

What Causes Oseltamivir Resistance?

Flu viruses are constantly changing. Changes that occur in circulating flu viruses typically involve the structures of the viruses' two primary surface proteins:

1. Neuraminidase (NA)

2. Hemagglutinin (HA)

Oseltamivir is known as a "NA inhibitor" because this antiviral drug binds to a flu virus' NA and inhibits the enzymatic activity of this protein. By inhibiting NA activity, oseltamivir prevents flu viruses from spreading from infected cells to other healthy cells.

However, if the NA proteins of flu virus change, oseltamivir can lose its ability to bind to and inhibit the function of the virus's NA proteins. This results in oseltamivir resistance (non-susceptibility). A particular genetic change known as the "H275Y" mutation is known to confer oseltamivir resistance in 2009 H1N1 flu viruses. (The H275Y mutation is a substitution of histidine for tyrosine at position 275 in the NA.) This substitution prevents oseltamivir from inhibiting NA activity and allows the mutated virus to spread to healthy cells, which results in the drug not working as well.

How Does CDC Improve Monitoring of Influenza Viruses for Antiviral Resistance?

CDC continually improves the ability to rapidly detect and monitor antiviral resistance through improvements in laboratory methods and by increasing the number of surveillance sites domestically and globally and increasing the number of laboratories that can test for antiviral resistance. Enhanced surveillance efforts have provided CDC with the capability to detect resistant viruses more quickly, and enabled CDC to monitor for changing trends over time.

How Did Influenza Antiviral Resistance Patterns Change during the Previous (2014–2015) Influenza Season?

Antiviral resistance patterns did not change in 2014–15 compared with the previous season. In both seasons, oseltamivir resistance was found in a small number of H1N1 viruses. Most of the influenza viruses tested during 2014–2015 continued to be susceptible to the antiviral drugs recommended for influenza by the Centers for Disease Control and Prevention (CDC) and the Advisory Committee on Immunization Practices (ACIP) (oseltamivir, zanamivir and peramivir) while resistance to the adamantanes class of antiviral drugs among A/H3N2 and A/H1N1 viruses remains widespread (influenza B viruses are not susceptible to adamantine drugs). Specifically, for the 2014–2015 season:

- 98.4% of the tested 2009 H1N1 viruses were susceptible to oseltamivir (Tamiflu®) and peramivir (Rapivab®), and 100% of the 2009 H1N1 viruses tested were susceptible to zanamivir (Relenza®).

- 100% of influenza A (H3N2) tested were susceptible to oseltamivir, zanamivir, and peramivir.

- 100% of influenza B viruses tested were susceptible to oseltamivir, zanamivir, and peramivir.

- High levels of resistance to the adamantanes (amantadine and rimantadine) persist among the influenza A viruses currently circulating. The adamantanes are not effective against influenza B viruses.

Because there were no dramatic changes in antiviral resistance patterns during 2014–2015 flu season, the 2015–2016 guidance on the use of influenza antiviral drugs remains unchanged.

What Antiviral Drugs Are Recommended for Use during the Flu Season?

Antiviral medications currently recommended include oseltamivir (Tamiflu®), zanamivir (Relenza®), and peramivir (Rapivab®). The vast majority of currently circulating influenza viruses are sensitive to these medications. Rare exceptions have been detected. Currently circulating flu viruses have high levels of resistance to the adamantane class of antiviral drugs (which includes amantadine and rimantadine), and therefore, these drugs are not recommended for use in the United States at this time.

What Can People Do to Protect Themselves against Antiviral Resistant Flu Viruses?

Getting a yearly seasonal flu vaccination is the first and most important step in preventing the flu. The vaccine protects against an influenza A (H1N1) virus, an influenza A (H3N2) virus, and one or two influenza B viruses (depending on the vaccine). CDC recommends that everyone six months of age and older get vaccinated each year. If you are in a group at high risk of serious flu-related complications and become ill with flu symptoms, call your doctor right away, you may benefit from early treatment. If you are not at high risk, if possible, stay home from work, school and errands when you are sick. This will help prevent you from spreading your illness to others.

What Implications Does Antiviral Resistance Have for the U.S. Antiviral Stockpile That Was Created as Part of the U.S. Pandemic Plan?

Antiviral drugs are one component of a multifaceted approach to pandemic preparedness planning and response. Oseltamivir is the drug recommended by the World Health Organization (WHO) as the primary influenza antiviral drug for the treatment of patients infected with novel influenza viruses. The U.S. influenza antiviral drug stockpile includes supplies of both of the NA inhibitor agents, oseltamivir and zanamivir. These medications are to be used in the event that a novel influenza A subtype virus, such as the avian influenza A (H5N1) virus, emerges and begins to spread easily among humans.

During the 2009 H1N1 pandemic, antiviral drugs were released from the Strategic National Stockpile (SNS) and used to treat infection with the 2009 influenza A (H1N1) virus. The stockpile is for public health emergencies in the United States, such as an influenza pandemic, not to provide medication for the treatment of seasonal influenza. Antiviral resistance among seasonal viruses does not predict resistance among pandemic influenza viruses.

CDC will continue ongoing surveillance and testing of influenza viruses for antiviral resistance among seasonal and novel influenza viruses, such as H5N1 viruses.

Chapter 70

Combating Antibiotic Resistance

Antibiotics are drugs used for treating infections caused by bacteria. Also known as antimicrobial drugs, antibiotics have saved countless lives. Misuse and overuse of these drugs, however, have contributed to a phenomenon known as antibiotic resistance. This resistance develops when potentially harmful bacteria change in a way that reduces or eliminates the effectiveness of antibiotics.

A Public Health Issue

Antibiotic resistance is a growing public health concern worldwide. When a person is infected with an antibiotic-resistant bacterium, not only is treatment of that patient more difficult, but the antibiotic-resistant bacterium may spread to other people. When antibiotics don't work, the result can be:

- longer illnesses

- more complicated illnesses

- more doctor visits

This chapter section contains text excerpted from the following sources: Text in this chapter begins with excerpts from "Combating Antibiotic Resistance," U.S. Food and Drug Administration (FDA), March 14, 2016; Text under the heading "Four Core Actions to Prevent Antibiotic Resistance" is excerpted from "Antibiotic Resistance Threats in the United States, 2013," Centers for Disease Control and Prevention (CDC), September 16, 2013.

- the use of stronger and more expensive drugs

- more deaths caused by bacterial infections

Examples of the types of bacteria that have become resistant to antibiotics include the species that cause skin infections, meningitis, sexually transmitted diseases and respiratory tract infections such as pneumonia.

In cooperation with other government agencies, the U.S. Food and Drug Administration (FDA) has launched several initiatives to address antibiotic resistance. The agency has issued drug labeling regulations, emphasizing the prudent use of antibiotics. The regulations encourage healthcare professionals to prescribe antibiotics only when clinically necessary, and to counsel patients about the proper use of such drugs and the importance of taking them as directed. FDA has also encouraged the development of new drugs, vaccines, and improved tests for infectious diseases.

Antibiotics Fight Bacteria, Not Viruses

Antibiotics are meant to be used against bacterial infections. For example, they are used to treat strep throat, which is caused by streptococcal bacteria, and skin infections caused by staphylococcal bacteria. Although antibiotics kill bacteria, they are not effective against viruses. Therefore, they will not be effective against viral infections such as colds, most coughs, many types of sore throat, and influenza (flu). Using antibiotics against viral infections:

- will not cure the infection

- will not keep other individuals from catching the virus

- will not help a person feel better

- may cause unnecessary, harmful side effects

- may contribute to the development of antibiotic-resistant bacteria

Patients and healthcare professionals alike can play an important role in combating antibiotic resistance. Patients should not demand antibiotics when a healthcare professional says the drugs are not needed. Healthcare professionals should prescribe antibiotics only for infections they believe to be caused by bacteria. As a patient, your best approach is to ask your healthcare professional whether an antibiotic is likely to be effective for your condition. Also, ask what else you can do to relieve your symptoms.

So how do you know if you have a bad cold or a bacterial infection?

Joseph Toerner, M.D., MPH, a medical officer in FDA's Center for Drug Evaluation and Research, says that the symptoms of a cold or flu generally lessen over the course of a week. But if you have a fever and other symptoms that persist and worsen with the passage of days, you may have a bacterial infection and should consult your healthcare provider.

Follow Directions for Proper Use

When you are prescribed an antibiotic to treat a bacterial infection, it's important to take the medication exactly as directed. Below are more tips to promote proper use of antibiotics:

Complete the full course of the drug. It's important to take all of the medication, even if you are feeling better. If treatment stops too soon, the drug may not kill all the bacteria. You may become sick again, and the remaining bacteria may become resistant to the antibiotic that you've taken.

Do not skip doses. Antibiotics are most effective when they are taken regularly.

Do not save antibiotics. You might think that you can save an antibiotic for the next time you get sick, but an antibiotic is meant for your particular infection at the time. Never take leftover medicine. Taking the wrong medicine can delay getting the appropriate treatment and may allow your condition to worsen.

Do not take antibiotics prescribed for someone else. These may not be appropriate for your illness, may delay correct treatment, and may allow your condition to worsen.

Talk with your healthcare professional. Ask questions, especially if you are uncertain about when an antibiotic is appropriate or how to take it.

It's important that you let your healthcare professional know of any troublesome side effects. Consumers and healthcare professionals can also report adverse events to FDA's MedWatch program at 800-FDA-1088 or online at MedWatch.

What FDA Is Doing

FDA is combating antibiotic resistance through activities that include:

Labeling regulations addressing proper use of antibiotics. Antibiotic labeling contains required statements in several places advising healthcare professionals that these drugs should be used only to treat infections that are believed to be caused by bacteria. Labeling also encourages healthcare professionals to counsel patients about proper use.

Partnering to promote public awareness. FDA is partnering with the Centers for Disease Control and Prevention (CDC) on "Get Smart: Know When Antibiotics Work," a campaign that offers Web pages, brochures, fact sheets, and other information sources aimed at helping the public learn about preventing antibiotic-resistant infections.

Encouraging the development of new antibiotics. FDA is actively engaged in developing guidance for industry on the types of clinical studies that could be performed to evaluate how an antibacterial drug works for the treatment of different types of infections.

Four Core Actions to Prevent Antibiotic Resistance

1. Preventing Infections, Preventing the Spread of Resistance

Avoiding infections in the first place reduces the amount of antibiotics that have to be used and reduces the likelihood that resistance will develop during therapy. There are many ways that drug-resistant infections can be prevented: immunization, safe food preparation, handwashing, and using antibiotics as directed and only when necessary. In addition, preventing infections also prevents the spread of resistant bacteria.

2. Tracking

Centers for Disease Control and Prevention (CDC) gathers data on antibiotic-resistant infections, causes of infections and whether there are particular reasons (risk factors) that caused some people to get a resistant infection. With that information, experts can develop specific strategies to prevent those infections and prevent the resistant bacteria from spreading.

3. Improving Antibiotic Prescribing / Stewardship

Perhaps the single most important action needed to greatly slow down the development and spread of antibiotic-resistant infections is to change the way antibiotics are used. Up to half of antibiotic use in humans and much of antibiotic use in animals is unnecessary and inappropriate and makes everyone less safe. Stopping even some of the inappropriate and unnecessary use of antibiotics in people and animals would help greatly in slowing down the spread of resistant bacteria. This commitment to always use antibiotics appropriately and safely—only when they are needed to treat disease, and to choose the right antibiotics and to administer them in the right way in every case—is known as antibiotic stewardship.

4. Developing New Drugs and Diagnostic Tests

Because antibiotic resistance occurs as part of a natural process in which bacteria evolve, it can be slowed but not stopped. Therefore, we will always need new antibiotics to keep up with resistant bacteria as well as new diagnostic tests to track the development of resistance.

Chapter 71

Surveillance of Antimicrobial Resistance Patterns and Rates

The Threat of Antibiotic Resistance

Antibiotic resistance is a worldwide problem. New forms of antibiotic resistance can cross international boundaries and spread between continents with ease. Many forms of resistance spread with remarkable speed. World health leaders have described antibiotic resistant microorganisms as "nightmare bacteria" that "pose a catastrophic threat" to people in every country in the world.

Statistics

Each year in the United States, at least 2 million people acquire serious infections with bacteria that are resistant to one or more of the antibiotics designed to treat those infections. At least 23,000 people

This chapter contains text excerpted from the following sources: Text beginning with the heading "The Threat of Antibiotic Resistance" is excerpted from "Antibiotic Resistance Threats," Centers for Disease Control and Prevention (CDC), September 16, 2013; Text under the heading "Biggest Threats" is excerpted from "Antibiotic / Antimicrobial Resistance," Centers for Disease Control and Prevention (CDC), August 26, 2015.

die each year as a direct result of these antibiotic-resistant infections. Many more die from other conditions that were complicated by an antibiotic resistant infection.

In addition, almost 250,000 people each year require hospital care for *Clostridium difficile* (*C. difficile*) infections. In most of these infections, the use of antibiotics was a major contributing factor leading to the illness. At least 14,000 people die each year in the United States from *C. difficile* infections. Many of these infections could have been prevented.

Antibiotic-resistant infections add considerable and avoidable costs to the already overburdened U.S. healthcare system. In most cases, antibiotic-resistant infections require prolonged and/or costlier treatments, extend hospital stays, necessitate additional doctor visits and healthcare use, and result in greater disability and death compared with infections that are easily treatable with antibiotics. The total economic cost of antibiotic resistance to the U.S. economy has been difficult to calculate. Estimates vary but have ranged as high as $20 billion in excess direct healthcare costs, with additional costs to society for lost productivity as high as $35 billion a year (2008 dollars).

Use of Antibiotics

The use of antibiotics is the single most important factor leading to antibiotic resistance around the world. Antibiotics are among the most commonly prescribed drugs used in human medicine. However, up to 50% of all the antibiotics prescribed for people are not needed or are not optimally effective as prescribed. Antibiotics are also commonly used in food animals to prevent, control, and treat disease, and to promote the growth of food-producing animals. The use of antibiotics for promoting growth is not necessary, and the practice should be phased out. Recent guidance from the U.S. Food and Drug Administration (FDA) describes a pathway toward this goal. It is difficult to directly compare the amount of drugs used in food animals with the amount used in humans, but there is evidence that more antibiotics are used in food production.

The other major factor in the growth of antibiotic resistance is spread of the resistant strains of bacteria from person to person, or from the non-human sources in the environment, including food.

Prevent Infections

There are four core actions that will help fight these deadly infections:

1. preventing infections and preventing the spread of resistance

2. tracking resistant bacteria

3. improving the use of today's antibiotics

4. promoting the development of new antibiotics and developing new diagnostic tests for resistant bacteria

Bacteria will inevitably find ways of resisting the antibiotics we develop, which is why aggressive action is needed now to keep new resistance from developing and to prevent the resistance that already exists from spreading.

Biggest Threats

In 2013, CDC published a report outlining the top 18 drug-resistant threats to the United States. These threats were categorized based on level of concern: urgent, serious, and concerning.

In general, threats assigned to the urgent and serious categories require more monitoring and prevention activities, whereas the threats in the concerning category require less. Regardless of category, threat-specific CDC activities are tailored to meet the epidemiology of the infectious agent and to address any gaps in the ability to detect resistance and to protect against infections.

Urgent Threats

Clostridium difficile (CDIFF)

Clostridium difficile (C. difficile) causes life-threatening diarrhea. These infections mostly occur in people who have had both recent medical care and antibiotics. Often, *C. difficile* infections occur in hospitalized or recently hospitalized patients.

A 2015 CDC study found that *C. difficile* caused almost half a million infections among patients in the United States in a single year. An estimated 15,000 deaths are directly attributable to *C. difficile* infections, making it a substantial cause of infectious disease death in the United States. We estimate that up to $3,800,000,000 in medical costs could be saved over 5 years.

Carbapenem-Resistant Enterobacteriaceae (CRE)

Untreatable and hard-to-treat infections from carbapenem-resistant Enterobacteriaceae (CRE) bacteria are on the rise among patients in medical facilities. CRE have become resistant to all or nearly all the antibiotics we have today. Almost half of hospital patients who get bloodstream infections from CRE bacteria die from the infection.

Neisseria gonorrhoeae

Neisseria gonorrhoeae causes gonorrhea, a sexually transmitted disease that can result in discharge and inflammation at the urethra, cervix, pharynx, or rectum.

Serious Threats

Multidrug-Resistant Acinetobacter

Acinetobacter is a type of gram-negative bacteria that is a cause of pneumonia or bloodstream infections among critically ill patients. Many of these bacteria have become very resistant to antibiotics.

Drug-Resistant Campylobacter

Campylobacter usually causes diarrhea (often bloody), fever, and abdominal cramps, and sometimes causes serious complications such as temporary paralysis.

Fluconazole-Resistant Candida

Candidiasis is a fungal infection caused by yeasts of the genus Candida. There are more than 20 species of Candida yeasts that can cause infection in humans, the most common of which is Candida albicans. Candida yeasts normally live on the skin and mucous membranes without causing infection. However, overgrowth of these microorganisms can cause symptoms to develop. Symptoms of candidiasis vary depending on the area of the body that is infected.

Candida is the fourth most common cause of healthcare-associated bloodstream infections in the United States. In some hospitals it is the most common cause. These infections tend to occur in the sickest patients.

Extended Spectrum Enterobacteriaceae (ESBL)

Extended-spectrum β-lactamase is an enzyme that allows bacteria to become resistant to a wide variety of penicillins and cephalosporins. Bacteria that contain this enzyme are known as ESBLs or ESBL-producing bacteria. ESBL-producing Enterobacteriaceae are resistant to strong antibiotics including extended spectrum cephalosporins.

Vancomycin-Resistant Enterococcus (VRE)

Enterococci cause a range of illnesses, mostly among patients receiving healthcare, but includes bloodstream infections, surgical site infections, and urinary tract infections.

Multidrug-Resistant Pseudomonas Aeruginosa

Pseudomonas aeruginosa is a common cause of healthcare-associated infections including pneumonia, bloodstream infections, urinary tract infections, and surgical site infections.

Drug-Resistant Non-Typhoidal Salmonella

Non-typhoidal Salmonella (serotypes other than Typhi, Paratyphi A, Paratyphi B, and Paratyphi C) usually causes diarrhea (sometimes bloody), fever, and abdominal cramps. Some infections spread to the blood and can have life-threatening complications.

Drug-Resistant Salmonella Serotype Typhi

Salmonella serotype Typhi causes typhoid fever, a potentially life-threatening disease. People with typhoid fever usually have a high fever, abdominal pain, and headache. Typhoid fever can lead to bowel perforation, shock, and death.

Drug-Resistant Shigella

Shigella usually causes diarrhea (sometimes bloody), fever, and abdominal pain. Sometimes it causes serious complications such as reactive arthritis. High-risk groups include young children, people with inadequate handwashing and hygiene habits, and men who have sex with men.

Methicillin-Resistant Staphylococcus aureus (MRSA)

Methicillin-resistant *Staphylococcus aureus* (MRSA) causes a range of illnesses, from skin and wound infections to pneumonia and bloodstream infections that can cause sepsis and death. Staph bacteria, including MRSA, are one of the most common causes of healthcare-associated infections.

Drug-Resistant Streptococcus Pneumoniae

Streptococcus pneumoniae (S. pneumoniae, or pneumococcus) is the leading cause of bacterial pneumonia and meningitis in the United States. It also is a major cause of bloodstream infections and ear and sinus infections.

Drug-Resistant Tuberculosis

Tuberculosis (TB) is among the most common infectious diseases and a frequent cause of death worldwide. TB is caused by the bacteria *Mycbacterium tuberculosis (M. tuberculosis)* and is spread mostly through the air. *M. tuberculosis* can affect any part of the body, but disease is found most often in the lungs. In most cases, TB is treatable and curable with the available first-line TB drugs; however, in some cases, *M. tuberculosis* can be resistant to one or more of the drugs used to treat it. Drug-resistant TB is more challenging to treat—it can be complex and requires more time and more expensive drugs that often have more side effects. Extensively drug-resistant TB (XDR TB) is resistant to most TB drugs; therefore the patients are left with treatment options that are much less effective. The major factors driving TB drug resistance are incomplete or wrong treatment, short drug supply, and lack of new drugs. In the United States most drug-resistant TB is found among persons born outside of the country.

Concerning Threats

Vancomycin-Resistant Staphylococcus Aureus

Staphylococcus aureus is a common type of bacteria that is found on the skin. During medical procedures when patients require catheters or ventilators or undergo surgical procedures, *Staphylococcus aureus* can enter the body and cause infections. When *Staphylococcus aureus* becomes resistant to vancomycin, there are few treatment options available because vancomycin-resistant *S. aureus* bacteria identified to date were also resistant to methicillin and other classes of antibiotics.

Erythromycin-Resistant Group A Streptococcus

Group A Streptococcus (GAS) causes many illnesses, including pharyngitis (strep throat), streptococcal toxic shock syndrome, necrotizing fasciitis ("flesh-eating" disease), scarlet fever, rheumatic fever, and skin infections such as impetigo.

Clindamycin-Resistant Group B Streptococcus

Group B Streptococcus (GBS) is a type of bacteria that can cause severe illness in people of all ages, ranging from bloodstream infections (sepsis) and pneumonia to meningitis and skin infections.

Part Five

Preventing
Contagious Diseases

Chapter 72

Handwashing Prevents the Spread of Germs

Keeping hands clean through improved hand hygiene is one of the most important steps we can take to avoid getting sick and spreading germs to others. Many diseases and conditions are spread by not washing hands with soap and clean, running water. If clean, running water is not accessible, as is common in many parts of the world, use soap and available water. If soap and water are unavailable, use an alcohol-based hand sanitizer that contains at least 60% alcohol to clean hands.

When Should You Wash Your Hands?

- Before, during, and after preparing food

- Before eating food

- Before and after caring for someone who is sick

- Before and after treating a cut or wound

- After using the toilet

This chapter contains text excerpted from the following sources: Text in the chapter begins with excerpts from "Handwashing: Clean Hands Save Lives," Centers for Disease Control and Prevention (CDC), September 4, 2015; Text beginning with the heading "How Germs Get onto Hands and Make People Sick" is excerpted from "Handwashing: Clean Hands Save Lives," Centers for Disease Control and Prevention (CDC), November 18, 2015.

- After changing diapers or cleaning up a child who has used the toilet
- After blowing your nose, coughing or sneezing
- After touching an animal, animal feed or animal waste
- After handling pet food or pet treats
- After touching garbage

How Should You Wash Your Hands?

- **Wet** your hands with clean, running water (warm or cold), turn off the tap, and apply soap.
- **Lather** your hands by rubbing them together with the soap. Be sure to lather the backs of your hands, between your fingers, and under your nails.
- **Scrub** your hands for at least 20 seconds. Need a timer? Hum the "Happy Birthday" song from beginning to end twice.
- **Rinse** your hands well under clean, running water.
- **Dry** your hands using a clean towel or air dry them.

What Should You Do If You Don't Have Soap and Clean, Running Water?

Washing hands with soap and water is the best way to reduce the number of germs on them in most situations. If soap and water are not available, use an alcohol-based hand sanitizer that contains at least 60% alcohol. Alcohol-based hand sanitizers can quickly reduce the number of germs on hands in some situations, but sanitizers do **not** eliminate all types of germs and might not remove harmful chemicals. **Hand sanitizers are not as effective when hands are visibly dirty or greasy.**

How do you use hand sanitizers?

- Apply the product to the palm of one hand (read the label to learn the correct amount).
- Rub your hands together.
- Rub the product over all surfaces of your hands and fingers until your hands are dry.

How Germs Get onto Hands and Make People Sick

Feces (poop) from people or animals is an important source of germs like *Salmonella, E. coli* O157, and norovirus that cause diarrhea, and it can spread some respiratory infections like adenovirus and hand-foot-mouth disease. These kinds of germs can get onto hands after people use the toilet or change a diaper, but also in less obvious ways, like after handling raw meats that have invisible amounts of animal poop on them. A single gram of human feces—which is about the weight of a paper clip—can contain one trillion germs. Germs can also get onto hands if people touch any object that has germs on it because someone coughed or sneezed on it or was touched by some other contaminated object. When these germs get onto hands and are not washed off, they can be passed from person to person and make people sick.

Washing Hands Prevents Illnesses and Spread of Infections to Others

Handwashing with soap removes germs from hands. This helps prevent infections because:

- People frequently touch their eyes, nose, and mouth without even realizing it. Germs can get into the body through the eyes, nose and mouth and make us sick.

- Germs from unwashed hands can get into foods and drinks while people prepare or consume them. Germs can multiply in some types of foods or drinks, under certain conditions, and make people sick.

- Germs from unwashed hands can be transferred to other objects, like handrails, table tops, or toys, and then transferred to another person's hands.

- Removing germs through handwashing therefore helps prevent diarrhea and respiratory infections and may even help prevent skin and eye infections.

Teaching people about hand washing helps them and their communities stay healthy. Handwashing education in the community:

- Reduces the number of people who get sick with diarrhea by 31%

- Reduces diarrheal illness in people with weakened immune systems by 58%

- Reduces respiratory illnesses, like colds, in the general population by 16–21%

Not Washing Hands Harms Children around the World

About 1.8 million children under the age of 5 die each year from diarrheal diseases and pneumonia, the top two killers of young children around the world.

- Handwashing with soap could protect about 1 out of every 3 young children who get sick with diarrhea and almost 1 out of 5 young children with respiratory infections like pneumonia.

- Although people around the world clean their hands with water, very few use soap to wash their hands. Washing hands with soap removes germs much more effectively.

- Handwashing education and access to soap in schools can help improve attendance.

- Good handwashing early in life may help improve child development in some settings.

Handwashing Helps Battle the Rise in Antibiotic Resistance

Preventing sickness reduces the amount of antibiotics people use and the likelihood that antibiotic resistance will develop. Handwashing can prevent about 30% of diarrhea-related sicknesses and about 20% of respiratory infections (e.g., colds). Antibiotics often are prescribed unnecessarily for these health issues. Reducing the number of these infections by washing hands frequently helps prevent the overuse of antibiotics—the single most important factor leading to antibiotic resistance around the world. Hand washing can also prevent people from getting sick with germs that are already resistant to antibiotics and that can be difficult to treat.

Chapter 73

Vaccines: What They Are and How They Work

How Vaccines Prevent Diseases[1]

The diseases that vaccines prevent can be dangerous or even deadly. Vaccines reduce the risk of infection by working with the body's natural defenses to help it safely develop immunity to disease.

When germs, such as bacteria or viruses, invade the body, they attack and multiply. This invasion is called an infection, and the infection is what causes illness. The immune system then has to fight the infection. Once it fights off the infection, the body is left with a supply of cells that help recognize and fight that disease in the future.

Vaccines help develop immunity by imitating an infection, but this "imitation" infection does not cause illness. It does, however, cause the immune system to develop the same response as it does to a real infection so the body can recognize and fight the vaccine-preventable disease in the future. Sometimes, after getting a vaccine, the imitation infection can cause minor symptoms, such as fever. Such minor symptoms are normal and should be expected as the body builds immunity.

This chapter contains text excerpted from documents published by two public domain sources. Text under headings marked 1 are excerpted from "For Parents: Vaccines for Your Children," Centers for Disease Control and Prevention (CDC), April 15, 2016; Text under headings marked 2 are excerpted from "Understanding How Vaccines Work," Centers for Disease Control and Prevention (CDC), February 2013.

As children get older, they require additional doses of some vaccines for best protection. Older kids also need to be protected against additional diseases they may encounter.

Vaccine Ingredients[1]

Vaccines contain ingredients, called antigens, which cause the body to develop immunity. Vaccines also contain very small amounts of other ingredients—all of which play necessary roles either in making the vaccine, or in ensuring that the vaccine is safe and effective. These types of ingredients are listed below.

Table 73.1. Ingredients and Purpose

Type of Ingredient	Examples	Purpose
Preservatives	Thimerosal (only in multi-dose vials of flu vaccine)	To prevent contamination
Adjuvants	Aluminum salts	To help stimulate the body's response to the antigens
Stabilizers	Sugars, gelatin	To keep the vaccine potent during transportation and storage
Residual cell culture materials	Egg protein	To grow enough of the virus or bacteria to make the vaccine
Residual inactivating ingredients	Formaldehyde	To kill viruses or inactivate toxins during the manufacturing process
Residual antibiotics	Neomycin	To prevent contamination by bacteria during the vaccine manufacturing process

Vaccines Require More than One Dose[2]

There are four reasons that babies—and even teens or adults for that matter—who receive a vaccine for the first time may need more than one dose:

1. For some vaccines (primarily inactivated vaccines), the first dose does not provide as much immunity as possible. So, more than one dose is needed to build more complete immunity. The vaccine that protects against the bacteria Hib, which causes meningitis, is a good example.

2. In other cases, such as the Diphtheria, Tetanus, and Pertussis (DTaP) vaccine, which protects against diphtheria, tetanus, and pertussis, the initial series of four shots that children receive as part of their infant immunizations helps them build immunity. After a while, however, that immunity begins to wear off. At that point, a "booster" dose is needed to bring immunity levels back up. This booster dose is needed at 4 years through 6 years old for DTaP. Another booster against these diseases is needed at 11 years or 12 years of age. This booster for older children—and teens and adults, too—is called Tetanus, Diphtheria, and Pertussis (Tdap).

3. For some vaccines (primarily live vaccines), studies have shown that more than one dose is needed for everyone to develop the best immune response. For example, after one dose of the Measles, Mumps, and Rubella (MMR) vaccine, some people may not develop enough antibodies to fight off infection. The second dose helps make sure that almost everyone is protected.

4. Finally, in the case of the flu vaccine, adults and children (older than 6 months) need to get a dose every year. Children 6 months through 8 years old who have never gotten the flu vaccine in the past or have only gotten one dose in past years need two doses the first year they are vaccinated against flu for best protection. Then, annual flu shots are needed because the disease-causing viruses may be different from year to year. Every year, the flu vaccine is designed to prevent the specific viruses that experts predict will be circulating.

Vaccine Side Effects/Risks[1]

Like any medication, vaccines can cause side effects. The most common side effects are mild. On the other hand, many vaccine-preventable disease symptoms can be serious, or even deadly. Even though many of these diseases are rare in this country, they still occur around the world and can be brought into the United States, putting unvaccinated children at risk.

The side effects associated with getting vaccines are almost always minor (such as redness and swelling where the shot was given) and go away within a few days. If your child experiences a reaction at the injection site, you can use a cool, wet cloth to reduce redness, soreness, and swelling.

Serious side effects following vaccination, such as severe allergic reaction, are very rare and doctors and clinic staff are trained to deal with them. Pay extra attention to your child for a few days after vaccination. If you see something that concerns you, call your child's doctor.

Ensuring Vaccine Safety[1]

The United States' long-standing vaccine safety system ensures that vaccines are as safe as possible. In fact, currently, the United States has the safest, most effective vaccine supply in its history. Safety monitoring begins with the U.S. Food and Drug Administration (FDA), who ensures the safety, effectiveness, and availability of vaccines for the United States. Before a vaccine is approved by the FDA for use by the public, results of studies on safety and effectiveness of the vaccine are evaluated by highly trained FDA scientists and doctors. FDA also inspects the sites where vaccines are made to make sure they follow strict manufacturing guidelines.

Although most common side effects of a vaccine are identified in studies before the vaccine is licensed, rare adverse events may not be detected in these studies. Therefore, the U.S. vaccine safety system continuously monitors for possible side effects after a vaccine is licensed. When millions of people receive a vaccine, less common side effects that were not identified earlier may occur.

If a link is found between a possible side effect and a vaccine, public health officials take appropriate action. The officials will weigh the benefits of the vaccine against its risks to determine if recommendations for using the vaccine should change.

The Bottom Line[2]

Some people believe that naturally acquired immunity—immunity from having the disease itself—is better than the immunity provided by vaccines. However, natural infections can cause severe complications and be deadly. This is true even for diseases that most people consider mild, like chickenpox. It is impossible to predict who will get serious infections that may lead to hospitalization.

Vaccines, like any medication, can cause side effects. The most common side effects are mild. However, many vaccine-preventable disease symptoms can be serious, or even deadly. Although many of these diseases are rare in this country, they do circulate around the world and can be brought into the United States, putting unvaccinated children at risk. Even with advances in healthcare, the diseases that vaccines prevent can still be very serious and vaccination is the best way to prevent them.

Chapter 74

Types of Vaccines and Vaccine Strategies

Different Types of Vaccines

Scientists take many approaches to designing vaccines against a microbe. These choices are typically based on fundamental information about the microbe, such as how it infects cells and how the immune system responds to it, as well as practical considerations, such as regions of the world where the vaccine would be used. The following are some of the options that researchers might pursue:

- Live, attenuated vaccines

- Inactivated vaccines

- Subunit vaccines

- Toxoid vaccines

- Conjugate vaccines

This chapter contains text excerpted from the following sources: Text under the heading "Different Types of Vaccines" is excerpted from "Vaccines," National Institute of Allergy and Infectious Diseases (NIAID), April 3, 2012. Reviewed August 2016; Text under the heading "Vaccine Strategies" is excerpted from "Understanding Vaccines," National Institute of Allergy and Infectious Diseases (NIAID), January 2008. Reviewed August 2016.

- DNA vaccines

- Recombinant vector vaccines

Live, Attenuated Vaccines

Live, attenuated vaccines contain a version of the living microbe that has been weakened in the lab so it can't cause disease. Because a live, attenuated vaccine is the closest thing to a natural infection, these vaccines are good "teachers" of the immune system: They elicit strong cellular and antibody responses and often confer lifelong immunity with only one or two doses.

Despite the advantages of live, attenuated vaccines, there are some downsides. It is the nature of living things to change, or mutate, and the organisms used in live, attenuated vaccines are no different. The remote possibility exists that an attenuated microbe in the vaccine could revert to a virulent form and cause disease. Also, not everyone can safely receive live, attenuated vaccines. For their own protection, people who have damaged or weakened immune systems—because they've undergone chemotherapy or have HIV, for example—cannot be given live vaccines.

Another limitation is that live, attenuated vaccines usually need to be refrigerated to stay potent. If the vaccine needs to be shipped overseas and stored by healthcare workers in developing countries that lack widespread refrigeration, a live vaccine may not be the best choice.

Live, attenuated vaccines are relatively easy to create for certain viruses. Vaccines against measles, mumps, and chickenpox, for example, are made by this method. Viruses are simple microbes containing a small number of genes, and scientists can therefore more readily control their characteristics. Viruses often are attenuated through a method of growing generations of them in cells in which they do not reproduce very well. This hostile environment takes the fight out of viruses: As they evolve to adapt to the new environment, they become weaker with respect to their natural host, human beings.

Live, attenuated vaccines are more difficult to create for bacteria. Bacteria have thousands of genes and thus are much harder to control. Scientists working on a live vaccine for a bacterium, however, might be able to use recombinant DNA technology to remove several key genes. This approach has been used to create a vaccine against the bacterium that causes cholera, *Vibrio cholerae*, although the live cholera vaccine has not been licensed in the United States.

Inactivated Vaccines

Scientists produce inactivated vaccines by killing the disease-causing microbe with chemicals, heat, or radiation. Such vaccines are more stable and safer than live vaccines: The dead microbes can't mutate back to their disease-causing state. Inactivated vaccines usually don't require refrigeration, and they can be easily stored and transported in a freeze-dried form, which makes them accessible to people in developing countries.

Most inactivated vaccines, however, stimulate a weaker immune system response than do live vaccines. So it would likely take several additional doses, or booster shots, to maintain a person's immunity. This could be a drawback in areas where people don't have regular access to healthcare and can't get booster shots on time.

Subunit Vaccines

Instead of the entire microbe, subunit vaccines include only the antigens that best stimulate the immune system. In some cases, these vaccines use epitopes—the very specific parts of the antigen that antibodies or T cells recognize and bind to. Because subunit vaccines contain only the essential antigens and not all the other molecules that make up the microbe, the chances of adverse reactions to the vaccine are lower.

Subunit vaccines can contain anywhere from 1 to 20 or more antigens. Of course, identifying which antigens best stimulate the immune system is a tricky, time-consuming process. Once scientists do that, however, they can make subunit vaccines in one of two ways:

They can grow the microbe in the laboratory and then use chemicals to break it apart and gather the important antigens.

They can manufacture the antigen molecules from the microbe using recombinant DNA technology. Vaccines produced this way are called "recombinant subunit vaccines."

A recombinant subunit vaccine has been made for the hepatitis B virus. Scientists inserted hepatitis B genes that code for important antigens into common baker's yeast. The yeast then produced the antigens, which the scientists collected and purified for use in the vaccine. Research is continuing on a recombinant subunit vaccine against hepatitis C virus.

Toxoid Vaccines

For bacteria that secrete toxins, or harmful chemicals, a toxoid vaccine might be the answer. These vaccines are used when a bacterial toxin is the main cause of illness. Scientists have found that they can inactivate toxins by treating them with formalin, a solution of formaldehyde and sterilized water. Such "detoxified" toxins, called toxoids, are safe for use in vaccines.

When the immune system receives a vaccine containing a harmless toxoid, it learns how to fight off the natural toxin. The immune system produces antibodies that lock onto and block the toxin. Vaccines against diphtheria and tetanus are examples of toxoid vaccines.

Conjugate Vaccines

If a bacterium possesses an outer coating of sugar molecules called polysaccharides, as many harmful bacteria do, researchers may try making a conjugate vaccine for it. Polysaccharide coatings disguise a bacterium's antigens so that the immature immune systems of infants and younger children can't recognize or respond to them. Conjugate vaccines, a special type of subunit vaccine, get around this problem.

When making a conjugate vaccine, scientists link antigens or toxoids from a microbe that an infant's immune system can recognize to the polysaccharides. The linkage helps the immature immune system react to polysaccharide coatings and defend against the disease-causing bacterium.

The vaccine that protects against *Haemophilus influenzae* type B (Hib) is a conjugate vaccine.

DNA Vaccines

Once the genes from a microbe have been analyzed, scientists could attempt to create a DNA vaccine against it.

Still in the experimental stages, these vaccines show great promise, and several types are being tested in humans. DNA vaccines take immunization to a new technological level. These vaccines dispense with both the whole organism and its parts and get right down to the essentials: the microbe's genetic material. In particular, DNA vaccines use the genes that code for those all-important antigens.

Researchers have found that when the genes for a microbe's antigens are introduced into the body, some cells will take up that DNA. The DNA then instructs those cells to make the antigen molecules. The cells secrete the antigens and display them on their surfaces. In other words, the body's own cells become vaccine-making factories, creating the antigens necessary to stimulate the immune system.

A DNA vaccine against a microbe would evoke a strong antibody response to the free-floating antigen secreted by cells, and the vaccine also would stimulate a strong cellular response against the microbial antigens displayed on cell surfaces. The DNA vaccine couldn't cause the disease because it wouldn't contain the microbe, just copies of a few of its genes. In addition, DNA vaccines are relatively easy and inexpensive to design and produce.

So-called naked DNA vaccines consist of DNA that is administered directly into the body. These vaccines can be administered with a needle and syringe or with a needle-less device that uses high-pressure gas to shoot microscopic gold particles coated with DNA directly into cells. Sometimes, the DNA is mixed with molecules that facilitate its uptake by the body's cells. Naked DNA vaccines being tested in humans include those against the viruses that cause influenza and herpes.

Recombinant Vector Vaccines

Recombinant vector vaccines are experimental vaccines similar to DNA vaccines, but they use an attenuated virus or bacterium to introduce microbial DNA to cells of the body. "Vector" refers to the virus or bacterium used as the carrier.

In nature, viruses latch on to cells and inject their genetic material into them. In the lab, scientists have taken advantage of this process. They have figured out how to take the roomy genomes of certain harmless or attenuated viruses and insert portions of the genetic material from other microbes into them. The carrier viruses then ferry that microbial DNA to cells. Recombinant vector vaccines closely mimic a natural infection and therefore do a good job of stimulating the immune system.

Attenuated bacteria also can be used as vectors. In this case, the inserted genetic material causes the bacteria to display the antigens of other microbes on its surface. In effect, the harmless bacterium mimics a harmful microbe, provoking an immune response.

Researchers are working on both bacterial and viral-based recombinant vector vaccines for HIV, rabies, and measles.

Vaccine Strategies

One promising, but still experimental, approach to vaccination is the prime-boost strategy. This strategy involves two vaccines. The first (frequently a DNA vaccine) is given to prepare ("prime") the immune system. Next, this response is boosted through the administration of a second vaccine (such as a viral-based vector vaccine). Several prime-boost HIV vaccine candidates are being tested in humans.

Some vaccines come in combinations. You might be familiar with the DTP (diphtheria, tetanus, pertussis) and the MMR (measles, mumps, rubella) vaccines that children in the United States receive.

Combination vaccines reduce visits to the doctor, saving time and money and sparing children extra needlesticks. Without combination vaccines, parents would have to bring their children in for each vaccination and all its boosters, and the chances would be greater that kids would miss their shots. Missed shots put children, as well as their communities, at risk.

Some people have wondered whether combination vaccines might overwhelm or weaken a child's immune system, but the immune system contains billions of circulating B and T cells capable of responding to millions of different antigens at once. Because the body constantly replenishes these cells, a healthy immune system cannot be "used up" or weakened by a vaccine. According to one published estimate, infants could easily handle 10,000 vaccines at once.

Adjuvants and Other Vaccine Ingredients

An **adjuvant** is an ingredient added to a vaccine to improve the immune response it produces. Currently, the only adjuvant licensed for human use in the United States is an "alum" adjuvant, which is composed of aluminum salts. Adjuvants do a variety of things; they can bind to the antigens in the vaccine, help keep antigens at the site of injection, and help deliver antigens to the lymph nodes, where immune responses to the antigens are initiated. The slowed release of antigens to tissue around the injection site and the improved delivery of antigens to the lymph nodes can produce a stronger antibody response than can the antigen alone. Alum adjuvants are also taken up by cells such as macrophages and help these cells better present antigens to lymphocytes.

Scientists are trying to develop new and better adjuvants. One oil-based adjuvant, MF59, has been used in seasonal influenza vaccines already available in Europe. Other adjuvants under study include tiny spheres made of fatty molecules that carry the vaccine's antigen, and inert nanobeads that can be coated with antigen.

In addition to adjuvants, vaccines may contain antibiotics to prevent bacterial contamination during manufacturing, preservatives to keep multidose vials of vaccine sterile after they are opened, or stabilizers to maintain a vaccine's potency at less-than-optimal temperatures.

Table 74.1. Some Vaccine Types and Diseases They Protect Against

Vaccine Type	Disease
Live, attenuated vaccines	Measles, mumps, rubella, polio (Sabin vaccine), yellow fever
Inactivated or "killed" vaccines	Cholera, flu, hepatitis A, Japanese "killed" vaccines encephalitis, plague, polio (Salk vaccine), rabies
Toxoid vaccine	Diphtheria, tetanus
Subunit vaccines	Hepatitis B, pertussis, pneumonia caused by *Streptococcus pneumoniae*
Conjugate vaccines	*Haemophilus influenzae* type b, pneumonia caused by *Streptococcus pneumoniae*
DNA vaccines	In clinical testing
Recombinant vector vaccines	In clinical testing

Table 74.2. Advantages and Disadvantages of Vaccines

Advantages	Disadvantages
• Produce a strong immune response • Often give lifelong immunity with one or two doses	• Remote possibility that the live microbe could mutate back to a virulent form • Must be refrigerated to stay potent
• Safer and more stable than live vaccines • Don't require refrigeration: more easily stored and transported	• Produce a weaker immune response than live vaccines • Usually require additional doses, or booster shots
• Teaches the immune system to fight off bacterial toxins	
• Targeted to very specific parts of the microbe • Fewer antigens, so lower chance of adverse reactions	• When developing a new vaccine, identifying the best antigens can be difficult and time consuming
• Allow infant immune systems to recognize certain bacteria	

Table 74.2. Continued

Advantages	Disadvantages
• Produce a strong antibody and cellular immune response • Relatively easy and inexpensive to produce	• Still in experimental stages
• Closely mimic a natural infection, stimulating a strong immune response	• Still in experimental stages

Chapter 75

Childhood Immunizations: Ten Vaccines for Fourteen Diseases

Vaccine-Preventable Diseases and Childhood Vaccines

Most medicines are given to cure an illness or to relieve its symptoms. Vaccines are different. They are given to prevent illness.

Vaccine-Preventable Diseases

Fourteen diseases can be prevented by routine childhood vaccines:

Diphtheria

- Caused by bacteria.

- Causes sore throat, fever, and chills.

- If not properly diagnosed and treated, it can produce a toxin that can cause heart failure or paralysis.

- About 1 person in 10 infected with diphtheria dies.

This chapter includes text excerpted from "Vaccine-Preventable Diseases and Childhood Vaccines," Centers for Disease Control and Prevention (CDC), October 26, 2015.

- Through the 1920s, about 150,000 people got diphtheria each year, and about 15,000 died.

Hepatitis A

- Caused by hepatitis A virus.

- Found mostly in bowel movements and spread by personal contact or through contaminated food or water.

- Causes liver disease—muscle and stomach pain, diarrhea or vomiting, loss of appetite, fatigue, yellow skin or eyes (jaundice).

- Children younger than about 6 years old might not have any symptoms.

- About 100 people die each year from liver failure caused by hepatitis A.

Hepatitis B

- Caused by hepatitis B virus.

- Spread through contact with blood or other body fluids.

- Causes liver disease–muscle and stomach pain, diarrhea or vomiting, loss of appetite, fatigue, yellow skin or eyes (jaundice).

- Some people recover and others become "chronically infected," which can lead to cirrhosis of the liver or liver cancer.

- Chronically infected people can infect others through, for example, unprotected sex or sharing needles.

- Babies of chronically infected mothers are usually infected at birth.

- About 3,000 to 5,000 people die each year.

Haemophilus Influenzae *Type B (Hib)*

- Caused by bacteria.

- If Hib bacteria enter the bloodstream they can cause meningitis, pneumonia, arthritis, and other problems.

- Before vaccine, Hib was the leading cause of bacterial meningitis in children younger than 5 (about 1 out of every 200 children in that age group).

- One child in 4 suffered permanent brain damage, and 1 in 20 died.

Influenza (Flu)

- Caused by influenza virus.
- Occurs mostly during the winter.
- Causes fever, sore throat, cough, headache, chills, muscle aches.
- Can lead to sinus infections, pneumonia, and inflammation of the heart.
- Hospitalization rates are high among children, especially babies under 1 year old.
- Flu causes more deaths each year than any other vaccine-preventable disease—mostly among the elderly, but it can also kill children.

Measles

- Caused by measles virus.
- Extremely contagious.
- Causes a rash all over the body, runny nose, fever, and cough.
- About 1 child in 10 also gets an ear infection, up to 1 in 20 gets pneumonia, 1 in 1,000 gets encephalitis.
- Before vaccine, almost all children got measles—about 48,000 were hospitalized each year, 7,000 had seizures, about 1,000 suffered permanent brain damage, and about 450 died.
- Measles still kills about a half million people a year around the world.
- About 1 person in 1,000 who gets measles will die.

Mumps

- Caused by mumps virus.
- Used to be a very common childhood disease.
- Usually a relatively mild disease—causes fever, headache, and inflammation of salivary glands.

- Mumps can lead to meningitis (about 1 child in 10), encephalitis or deafness (about 1 in 20,000) or death (about 1 in 10,000).

Pertussis (Whooping Cough)

- Caused by bacteria.
- Can look like a common cold at first.
- After one or two weeks, it can cause violent coughing spells that can interfere with eating, drinking or even breathing.
- Can lead to pneumonia, seizures, encephalopathy (brain infection), and death.

Pneumococcal Disease

- Caused by bacteria.
- Most common in winter and early spring.
- After Hib disease began to decline, pneumococcal disease became the most common cause of bacterial meningitis in children under 5.
- Can lead to ear infections, blood infections, and death.
- African Americans, some Native American tribes, children with sickle cell disease or with HIV infection and children without a working spleen are at higher risk.

Polio

- Caused by poliovirus.
- Can cause paralysis, leaving a person unable to walk or even breathe.
- About 1,200 polio victims in the United States were forced to live in 700-pound "iron lungs," which enabled them to breathe. Several of these people, first confined to an iron lung in the 1950s, still live in them today.
- Polio caused panic in the 1950s before vaccine—about 20,000 people were paralyzed each year.

Rotavirus

- Caused by a virus.

- Causes diarrhea and vomiting in young children—sometimes so severe it can lead to dehydration.

- Before vaccine, rotavirus caused more than 400,000 doctor visits, 200,000 emergency room visits, up to 70,000 hospitalizations, and 20 to 60 deaths each year.

Rubella (German Measles)

- Caused by a virus.

- Usually a mild disease, causing swollen glands in the neck, fever, rash on the face and neck, and sometimes arthritis-like symptoms.

- The greatest danger from rubella is to unborn babies. If a pregnant woman gets rubella, her unborn baby has about an 80% chance of "congenital rubella syndrome" (CRS), which can lead to deafness, blindness, mental impairment, or heart or brain damage. Miscarriages are also common.

- In 1964–65, before vaccine, a major rubella epidemic in the United States infected 12.5 million people and led to 20,000 cases of CRS.

Tetanus (Lockjaw)

- Caused by bacteria.

- Enters the body through cuts, burns, or other breaks in the skin–not spread from person to person.

- About 3 weeks after exposure, a child could become cranky, get a headache or have spasms in the jaw muscles.

- Tetanus can then produce a toxin that causes painful muscle cramps in the neck, arms, legs, and stomach—strong enough to break a child's bones.

- A child might have to spend several weeks in intensive care. One or two out of every 10 die.

Varicella (Chickenpox)

- Caused by varicella virus.

- Causes an itchy rash all over the body, fever, and drowsiness.

- Usually mild, but can cause skin infections and encephalitis. For every 100,000 infants younger than 1 year old who get chickenpox, about 4 die.

- If a pregnant woman gets chickenpox around the time of delivery, the baby can be infected, and 1 out of 3 will die if not treated quickly.

- Before vaccine, almost every child (about 4 million each year) got chickenpox.

Many of these diseases are spread from person to person through the air by coughing, sneezing, or just breathing. Exceptions are polio, hepatitis A, and rotavirus, which enter the body through the mouth; hepatitis B, which is transmitted through blood or body fluids; and tetanus, which enters the body through breaks in the skin. All of these diseases were much more common before vaccines.

Table 75.1. Annual Reported Cases 20th Century and Reported Cases 2013

Disease	Annual Reported Cases 20th Century (Pre-Vaccine)	Reported Cases 2013
Diphtheria	21053	0
Measles	530217	187
Tetanus	580	26
Mumps	162344	584
Rubella	47745	9

However, after declining for years, some of them—notably measles and pertussis—are again causing outbreaks in the United States, partly because some parents are not getting their children vaccinated.

Childhood Vaccines

Ten vaccines, which children receive between birth and 6 years of age can prevent these 14 diseases.

1. Hepatitis A (HepA)

2. Hepatitis B (HepB) vaccine

3. Hib (*Haemophilus influenzae* type b) vaccine

4. Influenza (flu) vaccine

5. PCV13 (pneumococcal disease) vaccine

6. Polio vaccine

7. Rotavirus (RV) vaccine

8. Varicella (chickenpox) vaccine

9. DTaP (Diphtheria, Tetanus, and Pertussis) vaccine

10. MMR (Measles, Mumps, and Rubella) vaccine

These vaccines are given by injection (shot), except for rotavirus, which is a liquid that is swallowed, and one type of flu vaccine, which is sprayed into the nose.

The Vaccine Schedule

All of these childhood vaccines are given in a series of 2 or more doses, at specific ages.

Table 75.2. The Vaccine Schedule

Age	Vaccine
at birth	HepB
2 months	HepB (1–2 mos) + DTaP + PCV 13 + Hib + Polio + RV
4 months	DTaP + PCV 13 + Hib + Polio + RV
6 months	HepB (6–18 mos) + DTaP + PCV 13 + Hib + Polio (6–18 mos) + RV
12 months	MMR (12–15 mos) + PCV13 (12–15 mos) + Hib (12–15 mos) + Varicella (12–15 mos) + HepA (12–23 mos)
15 months	DTaP (15–18 mos)

For some of these vaccines, a booster dose is also recommended at 4–6 years of age. A dose of flu vaccine is recommended every winter for children 6 months old or older. Several "combination" vaccines are available for children. These are vaccines that contain more than one vaccine in a single shot, which means fewer shots at one visit:

Table 75.3. Combination of Vaccines Available for Children

Vaccine Name	Contains
Pediarix®	DTaP, Polio, and HepB
Pentacel®	DTaP, Polio, and Hib

Table 75.3. Continued

Vaccine Name	Contains
Kinrix®	DTaP and Polio
Quadracel®	DTaP and Polio
ProQuad®	MMR and Varicella

Other Vaccines

There are other vaccines that might be recommended for older children or adolescents, or for young children in certain circumstances.

- **Rabies vaccine** might be recommended for a child who was bitten by an animal, or is traveling to a country where rabies is common. Children traveling abroad may need other vaccines, too. These could include **Japanese encephalitis, typhoid, meningococcal** or **yellow fever** vaccines.

- **Meningococcal vaccine** is also recommended for adolescents between 11 and 18 years of age, and for younger children with certain medical conditions, to protect them from infections that could cause bacterial meningitis.

- **Tdap** is a tetanus, diphtheria, pertussis vaccine that is similar to DTaP, but is formulated for adolescents and adults. It is recommended at the 11–12 year doctor's visit.

- **Human papillomavirus (HPV)** vaccine is also recommended at the 11–12 year visit. HPV is a virus that causes cervical cancer and other types of cancer.

Your healthcare provider can tell you more about these vaccines.

Chapter 76

Questions and Answers about Childhood Vaccines

Parents' Guide to Childhood Immunizations

How Do We Know Vaccines Aren't Causing Long-Term Health Problems?

Observing vaccinated children for many years to look for long-term health conditions would not be practical, and withholding an effective vaccine from children while long-term studies are being done wouldn't be ethical. A more practical approach is to look at health conditions themselves and at the factors that cause them. Scientists are already working to identify risk factors that can lead to conditions like cancer, stroke, heart disease, and autoimmune diseases such as lupus or rheumatoid arthritis.

Thousands of studies have already been done looking at hundreds of potential risk factors. If immunizations were identified as a risk factor in any of these studies, we would know about it. So far, they have not. We learn about a vaccine's safety during clinical trials before it is licensed, and monitor it continually as millions of doses are administered after it is licensed. We also know there is not a plausible biologic reason to believe vaccines would cause any serious long-term effects.

This chapter includes text excerpted from "For Parents: Vaccines for Your Children," Centers for Disease Control and Prevention (CDC), October 26, 2015.

Based on more than 50 years of experience with vaccines, we can say that the likelihood that a vaccine will cause unanticipated long-term problems is extremely low.

Why Do Children Need So Many Doses of Certain Vaccines?

The reason depends on whether the vaccine is inactivated (killed) or live. With an inactivated vaccine, each dose contains a fixed amount of disease antigen (virus or bacteria). Immunity is built in phases, with each dose boosting immunity to a protective level. Live vaccines are different in that they contain a small amount of antigen which reproduces and spreads throughout the body. One dose produces satisfactory immunity in most children. But a second dose is recommended, because not all children respond to the first one.

Aren't Some of the Ingredients in Vaccines Toxic?

Some vaccine ingredients could be toxic, but at much higher doses. Any substance—even water—can be toxic given a large enough dose. But at a very low dose, even a highly toxic substance can be safe. For example, many adults have one of the most toxic substances known to humanity, Botox, injected into their face to reduce wrinkles. We aren't always aware of it, but we are exposed to small amounts of these same "toxic" substances every day:

- **Mercury:** Babies are exposed to mercury in milk, including breast milk. Seafood also contains mercury.

- **Formaldehyde:** Formaldehyde is in automobile exhaust; in household products and furnishings such as carpets, upholstery, cosmetics, paint, and felt-tip markers; and in health products such as antihistamines, cough drops, and mouthwash.

- **Aluminum:** The average person takes in an estimated 30 to 50 mg of aluminum every day, mainly from foods, drinking water, and medicines. Not all vaccines contain aluminum, but those that do typically contain about .125 mg to .625 mg per dose or roughly 1% of that daily average.

Components of vaccines are all there for a reason. Some (like aluminum) help the vaccine work better. Others (like formaldehyde) were used during manufacturing and have been removed except for a tiny trace.

One final word—you can't believe everything you read about harmful ingredients in vaccines. For example, no vaccine contains or has ever contained, even a molecule of antifreeze, although you would never know that after reading any of a dozen websites claiming that they do.

Can a Child Get a Disease Even after Being Vaccinated?

It isn't very common, but it can happen. Depending on the vaccine, about 1% to 5% of children who are vaccinated fail to develop immunity. If these children are exposed to that disease, they could get sick. Sometimes giving an additional vaccine dose will stimulate an immune response in a child who didn't respond to 1 dose. For example, a single dose of measles vaccine protects about 95% of children, but after 2 doses, almost 100% are immune.

Sometimes a child is exposed to a disease just prior to being vaccinated, and gets sick before the vaccine has had time to work. Sometimes a child gets sick with something that is similar to a disease they have been vaccinated against. This often happens with flu. Many viruses cause symptoms that look like flu, and people even call some of them flu, even though they are really something else. Flu vaccine doesn't create immunity to these viruses.

Can a Child Actually Get the Disease from a Vaccine?

Almost never. With an inactivated (killed) vaccine, it isn't possible. Dead viruses or bacteria can't cause disease. With live vaccines, some children get what appears to be a mild case of disease (for example, what looks like a measles or chickenpox rash, but with only a few spots). This isn't harmful, and can actually show that the vaccine is working. A vaccine causing full-blown disease would be extremely unlikely. One exception was the live oral polio vaccine, which could very rarely mutate and actually cause a case of polio. This was a rare, but tragic, side effect of this otherwise effective vaccine. Oral polio vaccine is no longer used in the United States.

Can a Child Get a Disease Even after Being Vaccinated?

It isn't very common, but it can happen. About 1% to 5% of the time, depending on the vaccine, a child who is vaccinated fails to develop immunity. If these children are exposed to that disease they could get sick. Sometimes giving an additional vaccine dose will stimulate an

547

immune response in a child who didn't respond to one dose. For example, a single dose of measles vaccine protects about 95% of children, but after two doses almost 100% are immune.

Sometimes a child is exposed to a disease just prior to being vaccinated, and gets sick before the vaccine has time to work. Sometimes a child gets sick with something that is similar to a disease they have been vaccinated against. This often happens with flu. Many viruses cause symptoms that look like flu, and people even call some of them flu, even though they are really something else. Flu vaccine doesn't protect from these viruses.

Considering That Rates of Vaccine-Preventable Diseases Are Very Low, My Child Is Unlikely to Get One of These Diseases. Therefore, Isn't the Benefit of Vaccination Also Very Low?

That's a reasonable question. Statistically, the chances of any particular child getting measles, pertussis, or another vaccine-preventable disease might be low.

But you don't wear a seatbelt because you expect to be in a serious accident; you wear it because you want to be protected in the unlikely event that you are. If you're never in an accident, the benefit of wearing a seatbelt might be zero. But if you are, the consequences of not wearing it can be very high. It's the same with vaccines. Your child might never need the protection they offer, but you don't want him to be lacking that protection if he ever does need it.

Why Does the Government Require Children to Be Vaccinated to Attend School?

School immunization laws are not imposed by the federal government, but by the individual states. But that doesn't answer the question, which is often asked by people who see this as a violation of their individual rights.

Public health programs, such as immunization, are designed to protect the health of the public—that is, everybody. Remember that vaccines protect not only the person being vaccinated, but also people around them. Immunization laws exist not only to protect individual children, but to protect all children.

If vaccines were not mandatory, fewer people would get their children vaccinated–they would forget; they would put it off; they would feel they couldn't afford it; they wouldn't have time. This would lead to levels of immunity dropping below what are needed for herd immunity, which would, in turn, lead to outbreaks of disease.

So mandatory vaccination might not be a perfect solution, but it is a practical solution to a difficult problem. School immunization laws are like traffic laws. Laws forbidding us to drive as fast as we want on crowded streets or ignore traffic signals could also be seen as an infringement on individual rights. However, these laws are not so much to prevent drivers from harming themselves, which you could argue is their right, but to prevent them from harming other people, which is not.

Can Children Be Exempted from School Immunization Laws?

Under certain circumstances, yes. All states allow medical exemptions, so children who cannot safely receive certain vaccines are not required to get them. Most states also allow religious exemptions for children whose religion prohibits vaccination. Finally, some states allow philosophic exemptions for people who oppose vaccination on non-religious grounds. To protect themselves and others, unvaccinated students may be prohibited from attending classes if there is an outbreak of a vaccine-preventable disease at their school or in their community.

Vaccines Are Expensive. Is There a Way to Reduce the Cost?

You can go to a public clinic or health department rather than to a private physician. Vaccinations are generally cheaper there, and may be free except for an administration charge. There is also a national program called Vaccines for Children (or VFC), which allows qualified families to get free vaccinations for their children at participating doctors' offices.

Can't So Many Vaccines Overwhelm a Child's Immune System?

We may not know exactly how many germs a baby's immune system can handle at one time, but it is considerably more than they will ever get from vaccines. After all, this is the immune system's job. From the day a baby is born, her immune system has to deal with the thousands

549

of germs she is exposed to as part of daily life. As one doctor put it, "Worrying about too many vaccines is like worrying about a thimble of water getting you wet when you are swimming in an ocean."

Isn't Vaccination "Unnatural?"

No. Your child's immune system produces immunity following vaccination the same as it would following "natural" infection with a disease. The difference is that the child doesn't have to get sick first.

Chapter 77

Facts about Adolescent Immunization

For Preteens and Teens

Your social life is probably important to you. The last thing you want is for something to get in the way of hanging out with your friends, especially if it is a serious illness. Diseases like meningitis and whooping cough can not only threaten your social life, but more importantly, your health. The good news though is that there are vaccines to protect you from these diseases.

Did You Say SHOTS?

There are several reasons you need vaccines as you mature:

1. Some of the vaccines you got as a child wear off over time, so you need shots to keep you protected from serious diseases like tetanus, diphtheria, and pertussis (whooping cough).

This chapter contains text excerpted from the following sources: Text under the heading "For Preteens and Teens" is excerpted from "Preteen and Teen Vaccines," Centers For Disease Control and Prevention (CDC), May 11, 2016; Text under the heading "College and Young Adults" is excerpted from "College and Young Adults Age 19–24," vaccines.gov, U.S. Department of Health and Human Services (HHS), April 18, 2015.

2. As you get older, your risk of getting certain diseases like meningitis, septicemia, and HPV-related cancers increases. Specific vaccines, like HPV, should be given during your preteen (11–12) years because they work better at that age.

3. Vaccines not only protect you from serious diseases, but also your siblings, your friends, and the people that care for you like your parents or grandparents.

You probably see a doctor or other healthcare professional for physicals before participating in sports, camping events, travelling, applying to college, and so on. All of these check-ups are a perfect time to ask about vaccines.

What Vaccines Do I Need?

-   One shot of Tdap vaccine to protect against tetanus, diphtheria, and pertussis (whooping cough).

-   Two shots of meningococcal vaccine to protect against meningococcal disease. The two most severe and common forms of meningococcal disease are meningitis, an infection of the fluid and lining around the brain and spinal cord, and septicemia, a bloodstream infection.

-   Three shots of human papillomavirus (HPV) vaccine to protect against HPV infection and cancers caused by HPV. HPV infection can cause cervical, vaginal, and vulvar cancer in girls and penile cancer in boys. HPV can also cause anal cancer, throat cancer and genital warts in both boys and girls.

Plus, everyone should get a flu vaccine every year to protect against seasonal influenza. You also need catch-up vaccines if you weren't fully vaccinated as a child. Catch-up vaccines you might need include measles, mumps, rubella (MMR), hep B, polio, and varicella (chickenpox). If you are travelling or have a chronic health condition like diabetes, heart disease or asthma, you may need other vaccines as well. Ask your healthcare professional during your next visit if you need additional vaccines.

After You Get the Shots

1. Stay seated for 15 minutes after the shot to prevent fainting.

2. Your arm will probably be a little sore/tender, red or swollen where the shot was given—which is a common reaction. A cool wet cloth on the spot might help.

3. Take a non-aspirin pain reliever if the pain in your arm persists.

If you have any questions about vaccines, ask your doctor or nurse, and talk to your parents.

College and Young Adults

Most vaccines are given early in childhood or early adolescence, but college students and young adults need certain immunizations, too. These vaccines are specifically recommended for young adults ages 19 through 24:

- **Meningococcal conjugate vaccine (MenACWY)** helps protect against bacterial meningitis and may be required for certain college students (requirements vary by state).

    - First-year college students living in residence halls are recommended to be vaccinated with meningococcal conjugate vaccine. If they received this vaccine before their 16th birthday, they should get a booster dose before going to college for maximum protection.

    - The risk for meningococcal disease among non-first-year college students is similar to that for the general population. However, MenACWY is safe and effective and therefore can be provided to non-first-year college students.

- **Tdap vaccine** protects against tetanus, diphtheria, and pertussis, or whooping cough.

    - A single dose of Tdap is routinely recommended for preteens and teens (preferably at age 11–12 years); however, adults 19 or older who did not receive Tdap as a preteen or teen should receive a single dose of Tdap.

    - Tdap is especially important for pregnant women and those in close contact with infants. Pregnant women should receive a dose of Tdap during each pregnancy, preferably at 27 through 36 weeks to maximize that amount of protective antibodies passed to the baby, but the vaccine can be safely given at any time during pregnancy. New mothers who have never gotten Tdap should get a dose as soon as possible after delivery.

    - Tdap can be given no matter when Td (tetanus and diphtheria vaccine) was last received. HPV vaccine protects against

553

the human papillomavirus (HPV), which causes most cases of cervical and anal cancers, as well as genital warts.

- **HPV vaccination** is recommended for teens and young adults who did not start or finish the HPV vaccine series at age 11 or 12 years.

  - Young women under age 27 and young men under age 22 should be vaccinated.

  - Young men between the ages of 22 and 27 may be vaccinated and should discuss this with their doctor or nurse. Young men between the ages of 22 and 27 who have compromised immune systems or have sex with other men should also be vaccinated.

  - Even if it has been many years since a first or second dose of HPV vaccine, young adults should still complete the HPV vaccination series. The HPV vaccine series does not need to be restarted if there is a long gap in between doses.

- **Seasonal flu vaccine** protects against the three or four flu viruses that research indicates will be most common during the upcoming season.

  - The flu can cause severe illness that may require hospital care, even in healthy adults.

  - In general, the flu vaccine works best among young healthy adults and older children.

  - Flu vaccination can reduce flu illnesses, doctors' visits, and missed work and school due to flu, as well as prevent flu-related hospitalizations and deaths.

If you are leaving the country, you may need certain vaccines before you travel.

- Learn what vaccines your state college or university may require.

- If you are entering or enlisting in the Armed Services, you may be required to receive certain vaccines.

Chapter 78

Adult Immunization Recommendations

Adult Immunization Schedule

Recommended Immunization Schedule for Adults Aged 19 Years or Older, by Vaccine and Age Group

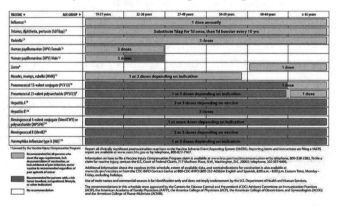

Figure 78.1. *Recommended Immunization Schedule for Adults Aged 19 Years or Older, by Vaccine and Age Group*

This chapter includes text excerpted from "Adult Immunization Schedule," Centers for Disease Control and Prevention (CDC), February 1, 2016.

555

Vaccines That Might Be Indicated for Adults Aged 19 Years or Older Based on Medical and Other Indications

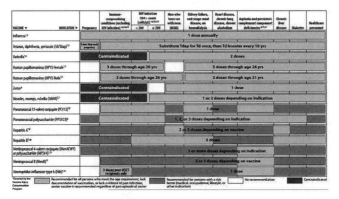

Figure 78.2. *Vaccines That Might Be Indicated for Adults Aged 19 Years or Older Based on Medical and Other Indications*

Recommended Adult Immunization Schedule for Adults Aged 19 Years or Older

1. Additional Information

- Additional guidance for the use of the vaccines described in this supplement can be found in the ACIP Recommendations.

- Information on vaccination recommendations when vaccination status is unknown and other general immunization information can be found in the General Recommendations on Immunization.

- Information on travel vaccine (e.g., for hepatitis A and B, meningococcal, and other vaccines) can be found in travel vaccine requirements and recommendations.

- Additional information and resources regarding pregnant women can be found in vaccination of pregnant women.

2. Influenza Vaccination

- Annual vaccination against influenza is recommended for all persons aged ≥6 months.

- Persons aged ≥6 months, including pregnant women, can receive the inactivated influenza vaccine (IIV). An age-appropriate IIV formulation should be used.

- Intradermal IIV is an option for persons aged 18 through 64 years.

- High-dose IIV is an option for persons aged ≥65 years.

- Live attenuated influenza vaccine (LAIV [FluMist]) is an option for healthy, nonpregnant persons aged 2 through 49 years.

- Recombinant influenza vaccine (RIV [Flublok]) is approved for persons aged ≥18 years.

- RIV, which does not contain any egg protein, may be administered to persons aged ≥18 years with egg allergy of any severity; IIV may be used with additional safety measures for persons with hives-only allergy to eggs.

- Healthcare personnel who care for severely immunocompromised persons who require care in a protected environment should receive IIV or RIV; healthcare personnel who receive LAIV should avoid providing care for severely immunosuppressed persons for 7 days after vaccination.

3. Tetanus, Diphtheria, and Acellular Pertussis (Td / Tdap) Vaccination

- Administer 1 dose of Tdap vaccine to pregnant women during each pregnancy (preferably during 27–36 weeks' gestation) regardless of interval since prior Td or Tdap vaccination.

- Persons aged ≥11 years who have not received Tdap vaccine or for whom vaccine status is unknown should receive a dose of Tdap followed by tetanus and diphtheria toxoids (Td) booster doses every 10 years thereafter. Tdap can be administered regardless of interval since the most recent tetanus or diphtheria—toxoid containing vaccine.

- Adults with an unknown or incomplete history of completing a 3-dose primary vaccination series with Td-containing vaccines should begin or complete a primary vaccination series including a Tdap dose.

- For unvaccinated adults, administer the first 2 doses at least 4 weeks apart and the third dose 6–12 months after the second.

- For incompletely vaccinated (i.e., less than 3 doses) adults, administer remaining doses.

- Refer to the ACIP statement for recommendations for administering Td/Tdap as prophylaxis in wound management

4. Varicella Vaccination

- All adults without evidence of immunity to varicella (as defined below) should receive 2 doses of single-antigen varicella vaccine or a second dose if they have received only 1 dose.

- Vaccination should be emphasized for those who have close contact with persons at high risk for severe disease (e.g., healthcare personnel and family contacts of persons with immunocompromising conditions) or are at high risk for exposure or transmission (e.g., teachers; child care employees; residents and staff members of institutional settings, including correctional institutions; college students; military personnel; adolescents and adults living in households with children; nonpregnant women of childbearing age; and international travelers).

- Pregnant women should be assessed for evidence of varicella immunity. Women who do not have evidence of immunity should receive the first dose of varicella vaccine upon completion or termination of pregnancy and before discharge from the healthcare facility. The second dose should be administered 4–8 weeks after the first dose.

- Evidence of immunity to varicella in adults includes any of the following:

  - documentation of 2 doses of varicella vaccine at least 4 weeks apart;

  - United States—born before 1980, except healthcare personnel and pregnant women;

  - history of varicella based on diagnosis or verification of varicella disease by a healthcare provider;

  - history of herpes zoster based on diagnosis or verification of herpes zoster disease by a healthcare provider; or

  - laboratory evidence of immunity or laboratory confirmation of disease.

5. Human Papillomavirus (HPV) Vaccination

- Three HPV vaccines are licensed for use in females (bivalent HPV vaccine [2vHPV], quadrivalent HPV vaccine [4vHPV], and 9-valent HPV vaccine [9vHPV]) and two HPV vaccines are licensed for use in males (4vHPV and 9vHPV).

- For females, 2vHPV, 4vHPV, or 9vHPV is recommended in a 3-dose series for routine vaccination at age 11 or 12 years and for those aged 13 through 26 years, if not previously vaccinated.

- For males, 4vHPV or 9vHPV is recommended in a 3-dose series for routine vaccination at age 11 or 12 years and for those aged 13 through 21 years, if not previously vaccinated. Males aged 22 through 26 years may be vaccinated.

- HPV vaccination is recommended for men who have sex with men through age 26 years who did not get any or all doses when they were younger.

- Vaccination is recommended for immunocompromised persons (including those with HIV infection) through age 26 years for those who did not get any or all doses when they were younger.

- A complete HPV vaccination series consists of 3 doses. The second dose should be administered 4–8 weeks (minimum interval of 4 weeks) after the first dose; the third dose should be administered 24 weeks after the first dose and 16 weeks after the second dose (minimum interval of at least 12 weeks).

- HPV vaccines are not recommended for use in pregnant women. However, pregnancy testing is not needed before vaccination. If a woman is found to be pregnant after initiating the vaccination series, no intervention is needed; the remainder of the 3-dose series should be delayed until completion or termination of pregnancy.

6. Zoster Vaccination

- A single dose of zoster vaccine is recommended for adults aged ≥60 years regardless of whether they report a prior episode of herpes zoster. Although the vaccine is licensed by the U.S. Food and Drug Administration (FDA) for use among and can be administered to persons aged ≥50 years, ACIP recommends that vaccination begin at age 60 years.

- Persons aged ≥60 years with chronic medical conditions may be vaccinated unless their condition constitutes a contraindication, such as pregnancy or severe immunodeficiency.

559

7. Measles, Mumps, Rubella (MMR) Vaccination

- Adults born before 1957 are generally considered immune to measles and mumps. All adults born in 1957 or later should have documentation of 1 or more doses of MMR vaccine unless they have a medical contraindication to the vaccine or laboratory evidence of immunity to each of the three diseases. Documentation of provider-diagnosed disease is not considered acceptable evidence of immunity for measles, mumps, or rubella.

Measles Component:

- A routine second dose of MMR vaccine, administered a minimum of 28 days after the first dose, is recommended for adults who:

  - are students in postsecondary educational institutions,

  - work in a healthcare facility, or

  - plan to travel internationally.

- Persons who received inactivated (killed) measles vaccine or measles vaccine of unknown type during 1963–1967 should be revaccinated with 2 doses of MMR vaccine.

Mumps Component:

- A routine second dose of MMR vaccine, administered a minimum of 28 days after the first dose, is recommended for adults who:

  - are students in a postsecondary educational institution,

  - work in a healthcare facility, or

  - plan to travel internationally.

- Persons vaccinated before 1979 with either killed mumps vaccine or mumps vaccine of unknown type who are at high risk for mumps infection (e.g., persons who are working in a healthcare facility) should be considered for revaccination with 2 doses of MMR vaccine.

Rubella Component:

- For women of childbearing age, regardless of birth year, rubella immunity should be determined. If there is no evidence of immunity, women who are not pregnant should be vaccinated. Pregnant women who do not have evidence of immunity should receive MMR vaccine upon completion or termination of pregnancy and before discharge from the healthcare facility.

Healthcare Personnel Born before 1957:

- For unvaccinated healthcare personnel born before 1957 who lack laboratory evidence of measles, mumps, and/or rubella immunity or laboratory confirmation of disease, healthcare facilities should consider vaccinating personnel with 2 doses of MMR vaccine at the appropriate interval for measles and mumps or 1 dose of MMR vaccine for rubella.

8. Pneumococcal Vaccination

- General information

  - Adults are recommended to receive 1 dose of 13-valent pneumococcal conjugate vaccine (PCV13) and 1, 2 or 3 doses (depending on indication) of 23-valent pneumococcal polysaccharide vaccine (PPSV23).

  - PCV13 should be administered at least 1 year after PPSV23.

  - PPSV23 should be administered at least 1 year after PCV13, except among adults with immunocompromising conditions, anatomical or functional asplenia, cerebrospinal fluid leak, or cochlear implant, for whom the interval should be at least 8 weeks; the interval between PPSV23 doses should be at least 5 years.

  - No additional dose of PPSV23 is indicated for adults vaccinated with PPSV23 at age ≥65 years.

  - When both PCV13 and PPSV23 are indicated, PCV13 should be administered first; PCV13 and PPSV23 should not be administered during the same visit.

  - When indicated, PCV13 and PPSV23 should be administered to adults whose pneumococcal vaccination history is incomplete or unknown.

- Adults aged ≥65 years (immunocompetent) who:

  - have not received PCV13 or PPSV23: administer PCV13 followed by PPSV23 at least 1 year after PCV13.

- have not received PCV13 but have received a dose of PPSV23 at age ≥65 years: administer PCV13 at least 1 year after PPSV23.

- have not received PCV13 but have received 1 or more doses of PPSV23 at age <65 years: administer PCV13 at least 1 year after the most recent dose of PPSV23. Administer a dose of PPSV23 at least 1 year after PCV13 and at least 5 years after the most recent dose of PPSV23.

- have received PCV13 but not PPSV23 at age <65 years: administer PPSV23 at least 1 year after PCV13.

- have received PCV13 and 1 or more doses of PPSV23 at age <65 years: administer PPSV23 at least 1 year after PCV13 and at least 5 years after the most recent dose of PPSV23.

- Adults aged ≥19 years with immunocompromising conditions or anatomical or functional asplenia (defined below) who:

  - have not received PCV13 or PPSV23: administer PCV13 followed by PPSV23 at least 8 weeks after PCV13. Administer a second dose of PPSV23 at least 5 years after the first dose of PPSV23.

  - have not received PCV13 but have received 1 dose of PPSV23: administer PCV13 at least 1 year after the PPSV23. Administer a second dose of PPSV23 at least 8 weeks after PCV13 and at least 5 years after the first dose of PPSV23.

  - have not received PCV13 but have received 2 doses of PPSV23: administer PCV13 at least 1 year after the most recent dose of PPSV23.

  - have received PCV13 but not PPSV23: administer PPSV23 at least 8 weeks after PCV13. Administer a second dose of PPSV23 at least 5 years after the first dose of PPSV23.

  - have received PCV13 and 1 dose of PPSV23: administer a second dose of PPSV23 at least 8 weeks after PCV13 and at least 5 years after the first dose of PPSV23.

  - If the most recent dose of PPSV23 was administered at age <65 years, at age ≥65 years, administer a dose of PPSV23 at least 8 weeks after PCV13 and at least 5 years after the last dose of PPSV23.

  - Immunocompromising conditions that are indications for pneumococcal vaccination are: congenital or acquired immunodeficiency (including B-or T-lymphocyte deficiency, complement deficiencies, and phagocytic disorders excluding chronic granulomatous disease), HIV infection, chronic renal failure, nephrotic syndrome, leukemia, lymphoma, Hodgkin disease, generalized malignancy, multiple myeloma, solid organ transplant, and iatrogenic immunosuppression (including long-term systemic corticosteroids and radiation therapy).

- Anatomical or functional asplenia that are indications for pneumococcal vaccination are: sickle cell disease and other hemoglobinopathies, congenital or acquired asplenia, splenic dysfunction, and splenectomy. Administer pneumococcal vaccines at least 2 weeks before immunosuppressive therapy or an elective splenectomy, and as soon as possible to adults who are newly diagnosed with asymptomatic or symptomatic HIV infection.

- Adults aged ≥19 years with cerebrospinal fluid leaks or cochlear implants: administer PCV13 followed by PPSV23 at least 8 weeks after PCV13; no additional dose of PPSV23 is indicated if aged <65 years. If PPSV23 was administered at age <65 years, at age ≥65 years, administer another dose of PPSV23 at least 5 years after the last dose of PPSV23.

- Adults aged 19 through 64 years with chronic heart disease (including congestive heart failure and cardiomyopathies, excluding hypertension), chronic lung disease (including chronic obstructive lung disease, emphysema, and asthma), chronic liver disease (including cirrhosis), alcoholism, or diabetes mellitus, or who smoke cigarettes: administer PPSV23. At age ≥65 years, administer PCV13 at least 1 year after PPSV23, followed by another dose of PPSV23 at least 1 year after PCV13 and at least 5 years after the last dose of PPSV23.

- Routine pneumococcal vaccination is not recommended for American Indian/Alaska Native or other adults unless they have the indications as above; however, public health authorities may consider recommending the use of pneumococcal vaccines for American Indians/Alaska Natives or other adults who live in areas with increased risk for invasive pneumococcal disease.

9. Hepatitis A Vaccination

- Vaccinate any person seeking protection from hepatitis A virus (HAV) infection and persons with any of the following indications:

- men who have sex with men;

- persons who use injection or non injection illicit drugs;

- persons working with HAV-infected primates or with HAV in a research laboratory setting;

- persons with chronic liver disease and persons who receive clotting factor concentrates;

- persons traveling to or working in countries that have high or intermediate endemicity of hepatitis A and

- unvaccinated persons who anticipate close personal contact (e.g., household or regular babysitting) with an international adoptee during the first 60 days after arrival in the United States from a country with high or intermediate endemicity for hepatitis A. The first dose of the 2-dose hepatitis A vaccine series should be administered as soon as adoption is planned, ideally 2 or more weeks before the arrival of the adoptee.

- Single-antigen vaccine formulations should be administered in a 2-dose schedule at either 0 and 6–12 months (Havrix), or 0 and 6–18 months (Vaqta). If the combined hepatitis A and hepatitis B vaccine (Twinrix) is used, administer 3 doses at 0, 1, and 6 months; alternatively, a 4-dose schedule may be used, administered on days 0, 7, and 21–30, followed by a booster dose at 12 months.

10. Hepatitis B Vaccination

- Vaccinate any person seeking protection from hepatitis B virus (HBV) infection and persons with any of the following indications:

  - sexually active persons who are not in a long-term, mutually monogamous relationship (e.g., persons with more than 1 sex partner during the previous 6 months); persons seeking evaluation or treatment for a sexually transmitted disease (STD); current or recent injection drug users; and men who have sex with men;

  - healthcare personnel and public safety workers who are potentially exposed to blood or other infectious body fluids;

  - persons who are aged <60 years with diabetes as soon as feasible after diagnosis; persons with diabetes who are aged

≥60 years at the discretion of the treating clinician based on the likelihood of acquiring HBV infection, including the risk posed by an increased need for assisted blood glucose monitoring in long-term care facilities, the likelihood of experiencing chronic sequelae if infected with HBV, and the likelihood of immune response to vaccination;

- persons with end-stage renal disease (including patients receiving hemodialysis), persons with HIV infection, and persons with chronic liver disease;

- household contacts and sex partners of hepatitis B surface antigen-positive persons, clients and staff members of institutions for persons with developmental disabilities, and international travelers to regions with high or intermediate levels of endemic HBV infection and

- all adults in the following settings: STD treatment facilities, HIV testing and treatment facilities, facilities providing drug abuse treatment and prevention services, healthcare settings targeting services to injection drug users or men who have sex with men, correctional facilities, end-stage renal disease programs and facilities for chronic hemodialysis patients, and institutions and nonresidential day care facilities for persons with developmental disabilities.

- Administer missing doses to complete a 3-dose series of hepatitis B vaccine to those persons not vaccinated or not completely vaccinated. The second dose should be administered at least 1 month after the first dose; the third dose should be administered at least 2 months after the second dose (and at least 4 months after the first dose). If the combined hepatitis A and hepatitis B vaccine (Twinrix) is used, give 3 doses at 0, 1, and 6 months; alternatively, a 4-dose Twinrix schedule may be used, administered on days 0, 7, and 21–30, followed by a booster dose at 12 months.

- Adult patients receiving hemodialysis or with other immuno-compromising conditions should receive 1 dose of 40 mcg/mL (Recombivax HB) administered on a 3-dose schedule at 0, 1, and 6 months or 2 doses of 20 mcg/mL (Engerix-B) administered simultaneously on a 4-dose schedule at 0, 1, 2, and 6 months.

11. Meningococcal Vaccination

- General Information

- Serogroup A, C, W, and Y meningococcal vaccine is available as a conjugate (MenACWY [Menactra, Menveo]) or a polysaccharide (MPSV4 [Menomune]) vaccine.

- Serogroup B meningococcal (MenB) vaccine is available as a 2-dose series of MenB-4C vaccine (Bexsero) administered at least 1 month apart or a 3-dose series of MenB-FHbp (Trumenba) vaccine administered at 0, 2, and 6 months; the two MenB vaccines are not interchangeable, i.e., the same MenB vaccine product must be used for all doses.

- MenACWY vaccine is preferred for adults with serogroup A, C, W, and Y meningococcal vaccine indications who are aged ≤55 years, and for adults aged ≥56 years: 1. who were vaccinated previously with MenACWY vaccine and are recommended for revaccination or 2. for whom multiple doses of vaccine are anticipated; MPSV4 vaccine is preferred for adults aged ≥56 years who have not received MenACWY vaccine previously and who require a single dose only (e.g., persons at risk because of an outbreak).

- Revaccination with MenACWY vaccine every 5 years is recommended for adults previously vaccinated with MenACWY or MPSV4 vaccine who remain at increased risk for infection (e.g., adults with anatomical or functional asplenia or persistent complement component deficiencies, or microbiologists who are routinely exposed to isolates of *Neisseria meningitidis*).

- MenB vaccine is approved for use in persons aged 10 through 25 years; however, because there is no theoretical difference in safety for persons aged >25 years compared to those aged 10 through 25 years, MenB vaccine is recommended for routine use in persons aged ≥10 years who are at increased risk for serogroup B meningococcal disease.

- There is no recommendation for MenB revaccination at this time.

- MenB vaccine may be administered concomitantly with MenACWY vaccine but at a different anatomic site, if feasible.

- HIV infection is not an indication for routine vaccination with MenACWY or MenB vaccine; if an HIV-infected person of any age is to be vaccinated, administer 2 doses of MenACWY vaccine at least 2 months apart.

566

- Adults with anatomical or functional asplenia or persistent complement component deficiencies: administer 2 doses of Men-ACWY vaccine at least 2 months apart and revaccinate every 5 years. Also administer a series of MenB vaccine.

- Microbiologists who are routinely exposed to isolates of *Neisseria meningitidis*: administer a single dose of MenACWY vaccine; revaccinate with MenACWY vaccine every 5 years if remain at increased risk for infection. Also administer a series of MenB vaccine.

- Persons at risk because of a meningococcal disease outbreak: if the outbreak is attributable to serogroup A, C, W or Y, administer a single dose of MenACWY vaccine; if the outbreak is attributable to serogroup B, administer a series of MenB vaccine.

- Persons who travel to or live in countries in which meningococcal disease is hyperendemic or epidemic: administer a single dose of MenACWY vaccine and revaccinate with MenACWY vaccine every 5 years if the increased risk for infection remains MenB vaccine is not recommended because meningococcal disease in these countries is generally not caused by serogroup B.

- Military recruits: administer a single dose of MenACWY vaccine.

- First-year college students aged ≤21 years who live in residence halls: administer a single dose of MenACWY vaccine if they have not received a dose on or after their 16th birthday.

- Young adults aged 16 through 23 years (preferred age range is 16 through 18 years): may be vaccinated with a series of MenB vaccine to provide short-term protection against most strains of serogroup B meningococcal disease.

12. Haemophilus Influenzae *Type B (Hib) Vaccination*

- One dose of Hib vaccine should be administered to persons who have anatomical or functional asplenia or sickle cell disease or are undergoing elective splenectomy if they have not previously received Hib vaccine. Hib vaccination 14 or more days before splenectomy is suggested.

- Recipients of a hematopoietic stem cell transplant (HSCT) should be vaccinated with a 3-dose regimen 6–12 months after a successful transplant, regardless of vaccination history; at least 4 weeks should separate doses.

- Hib vaccine is not recommended for adults with HIV infection since their risk for Hib infection is low.

13. Immunocompromising Conditions

- Inactivated vaccines (e.g., pneumococcal, meningococcal, and inactivated influenza vaccine) generally are acceptable and live vaccines generally should be avoided in persons with immune deficiencies or immunocompromising conditions.

Chapter 79

Problems with Vaccinations

Common Vaccine Safety Concerns

Each of us is our own best health advocate. Many times, our loved ones depend on us for information and protection too. With so much information—and sometimes incorrect information—available today, learning the facts before making health decisions is very important. These pages will help answer common questions about vaccine safety.

- Vaccine Adjuvants (Additives)
- Autism and Vaccines
- Fainting (Syncope)
- Febrile Seizures after Childhood Vaccinations
- Guillain-Barré Syndrome (GBS)
- Sudden Infant Death Syndrome (SIDS)
- Thimerosal (Preservative used in Some Flu Vaccines)
- Multiple Vaccines and the Immune System
- Vaccines During Pregnancy
- Vaccine Recalls
- Historical Vaccine Safety Concerns

This chapter includes text excerpted from "Possible Side-Effects from Vaccines," Centers for Disease Control and Prevention (CDC), July 9, 2015.

Vaccine Adjuvants (Additives)

What Is an Adjuvant and Why Are Adjuvants Added to Vaccines?

An adjuvant is an ingredient of a vaccine that helps create a stronger immune response in the patient's body. In other words, adjuvants help vaccines work better. Some vaccines made from weakened or dead germs contain naturally occurring adjuvants and help the body produce a strong protective immune response. However, most vaccines developed today include just small components of germs, such as their proteins, rather than the entire virus or bacteria. These vaccines often must be made with adjuvants to ensure the body produces an immune response strong enough to protect the patient from the germ he or she is being vaccinated against.

Two adjuvants, aluminum and monophosphoryl lipid A, are used in some U.S. vaccines.

Aluminum gels or aluminum salts are vaccine ingredients that have been used in vaccines since the 1930s. Small amounts of aluminum are added to help the body build stronger immunity against the germ in the vaccine. Aluminum is one of the most common metals found in nature and is present in air, food, and water. The amount of aluminum present in vaccines is low and is regulated by the U.S. Food and Drug Administration (FDA).

Monophosphoryl lipid A has been used since 2009 in one vaccine in the United States, Cervarix. This immune-boosting substance was isolated from the surface of bacteria. It has been tested for safety in tens of thousands of people and found to be safe.

Adjuvants have been used safely in vaccines for many decades.

Aluminum salts, such as aluminum hydroxide, aluminum phosphate, and aluminum potassium sulfate have been used safely in vaccines for more than 70 years. Aluminum salts were initially used in the 1930s, 1940s, and 1950s with diphtheria and tetanus vaccines after it was found that this addition strengthened the body's immune response to these vaccines. Monophosphoryl lipid A is a type of adjuvant that was developed more recently, as experts continue to increase their knowledge of how to stimulate certain specific elements of the body's immune response to vaccines.

Adjuvants improve the body's response to vaccination.

Vaccine adjuvants improve the body's immune response and often allow for smaller amounts of an inactivated virus or bacteria to be used in a vaccine.

Only some vaccines contain adjuvants.

Aluminum is present in U.S. childhood vaccines that prevent hepatitis A, hepatitis B, diphtheria-tetanus-pertussis (DTaP, Tdap), *Haemophilus influenzae* type b (Hib), human papillomavirus (HPV) and pneumococcus infection. Monophosphoryl lipid A is included in one human papillomavirus (HPV) vaccine, Cervarix. One licensed pandemic influenza vaccine contains an adjuvant called AS03. It is included in the U.S. pandemic influenza vaccine stockpile, but it is not available to the general public. In some vaccines, the weakened or inactivated virus stimulates a strong immune response so no additional adjuvant is needed for it to be effective to protect against infections. In the United States, vaccines against measles, mumps, rubella, chickenpox, rotavirus, polio, and seasonal influenza vaccines do not contain added adjuvants.

Autism and Vaccines

There is no link between vaccines and autism.

Some people have had concerns that ASD might be linked to the vaccines children receive, but studies have shown that there is no link between receiving vaccines and developing ASD. In 2011, an Institute of Medicine (IOM) report on eight vaccines given to children and adults found that with rare exceptions, these vaccines are very safe.

A 2013 CDC study added to the research showing that vaccines do not cause ASD. The study looked at the number of antigens (substances in vaccines that cause the body's immune system to produce disease-fighting antibodies) from vaccines during the first two years of life. The results showed that the total amount of antigen from vaccines received was the same between children with ASD and those that did not have ASD.

Vaccine ingredients do not cause autism.

One vaccine ingredient that has been studied specifically is thimerosal, a mercury-based preservative used to prevent contamination of multidose vials of vaccines. Research shows that thimerosal does not cause ASD. In fact, a 2004 scientific review by the IOM concluded that "the evidence favors rejection of a causal relationship between thimerosal–containing vaccines and autism." Since 2003, there have been nine CDC-funded or conducted studies that have found no link between thimerosal-containing vaccines and ASD, as well as no link between the measles, mumps, and rubella (MMR) vaccine and ASD in children.

Between 1999 and 2001, thimerosal was removed or reduced to trace amounts in all childhood vaccines except for some flu vaccines. This was done as part of a broader national effort to reduce all types of mercury exposure in children before studies were conducted that determined that thimerosal was not harmful. It was done as a precaution. Currently, the only childhood vaccines that contain thimerosal are flu vaccines packaged in multidose vials. Thimerosal-free alternatives are also available for flu vaccine

Besides thimerosal, some people have had concerns about other vaccine ingredients in relation to ASD as well. However, no links have been found between any vaccine ingredients and ASD.

Fainting (Syncope)

Fainting can happen after many types of vaccinations.

Fainting can be triggered by many types of medical procedures. In fact, CDC has received reports of people fainting after nearly all vaccines. Fainting after getting a vaccine is most commonly reported after three vaccines given to adolescents: HPV, MCV4, and Tdap. Because the ingredients of these three vaccines are different, yet fainting is seen with all of them, scientists think that fainting is due to the vaccination process and not to the vaccines themselves. However, there is not yet a definite answer about whether an ingredient of the vaccines is responsible for the fainting or if adolescents are simply more likely than children or adults to experience fainting.

About 3% of men and 3.5% of women report fainting at least once during their lifetimes, but it is not known just how often fainting happens after vaccination. Because fainting usually has no lasting effects, it is hard to study using medical records-based systems. However, the Vaccine Adverse Event Reporting System (VAERS), receives many reports of syncope each year, and many more are likely to go unreported.

Fainting can be common among adolescents after vaccination.

Reports from the Vaccine Adverse Event Reporting System (VAERS) shows that fainting after vaccinations is common in adolescents. One study of VAERS reports found that 62% of syncope reports were among adolescents 11 to 18 years old. However, because syncope may not always be reported, VAERS data cannot be used to determine how often fainting happens after vaccination.

Falls after fainting can cause injuries.

Fainting itself is generally not serious, but harm from related falls or other accidents can cause injury. The main concern is head injury.

In a study of syncope-related VAERS reports, 7% of the fainting reports were coded as serious; 12% of these involved head injuries. Although fainting itself might or might not be preventable, it is important to prevent injuries when people do faint.

Fainting and related injuries after immunization can be prevented.

Giving patients a beverage, a snack, or some reassurance about the procedure has been shown to prevent some fainting. Studies are being done to look more into these strategies. However, many falls due to fainting can be prevented by having the patient sit or lie down. For this reason, experts recommend having patients sit in a chair or lay down when they receive a vaccination. In addition, patients should be observed for 15 minutes after vaccination.

If a patient does faint after a vaccination, she or he should be observed by medical personnel until she or he regains consciousness so that further treatment needs can be determined. If fainting happens outside the medical setting and the patient does not recover immediately, contact local emergency medical services. Patients who faint after vaccination generally recover within a few minutes.

Febrile Seizures after Childhood Vaccinations

What Is a Febrile Seizure?

Sometimes, fevers can cause a child to experience spasms or jerky movements called seizures. Seizures caused by fever are called "febrile seizures." They are most common with fevers of 102°F (38.9°C) or higher, but they can also happen at lower body temperatures or when a fever is going down. Most febrile seizures last for less than one or two minutes.

Febrile seizures can be frightening, but nearly all children who have a febrile seizure recover quickly. Febrile seizures do not cause any permanent harm and do not have any lasting effects.

Febrile seizures can happen with any condition that causes a fever.

Fevers can be caused by common childhood illnesses like colds, the flu, an ear infection, or roseola. Vaccines can sometimes cause fevers, but febrile seizures are uncommon after vaccination.

Infants and young children are most at risk for febrile seizures.

Up to 5% of young children will have a febrile seizure at some time in their life. Febrile seizures happen in children between the ages of

6 months and 5 years, with most occurring between 14–18 months of age. About 1 out of every 3 children who have a febrile seizure will have at least one more during childhood. **There is a small increased risk for febrile seizures after MMR and MMRV vaccines.**

Studies have shown a small increased risk for febrile seizures during the 5 to 12 days after a child has received their first vaccination with the measles, mumps, rubella (MMR) vaccine. The risk is slightly higher with the measles, mumps, rubella, varicella (MMRV) combination vaccine, but the risk is still small. Studies have not shown an increased risk for febrile seizures after the separate varicella (chickenpox) vaccine.

There is a small increased risk for febrile seizures when influenza (flu) vaccine is given at the same doctor visit as either the PCV13 vaccine or the DTaP vaccine.

A CDC study has shown a small increased risk for febrile seizures during the 24 hours after a child receives the inactivated influenza vaccine (IIV) at the same time as the pneumococcal 13-valent conjugate (PCV13) vaccine or the diphtheria, tetanus, acellular pertussis (DTaP) vaccine. IIV was not associated with an increased risk of febrile seizures when it was given on a different day from the other two vaccines. Studies have not shown an increased risk for febrile seizures after the diphtheria, tetanus, acellular pertussis (DTaP) vaccine, except when it is given at the same time as the IIV vaccine. There may still be a small increase in the risk of febrile seizure when PCV13 is given by itself.

The risk of febrile seizure with any combination of these vaccines is small and CDC's Advisory Committee on Immunization Practices (ACIP) does not recommend getting any of these vaccines on separate days.

Vaccines can also help prevent febrile seizures.

Vaccinating children at the recommended age may prevent some febrile seizures by protecting children against measles, mumps, rubella, chickenpox, influenza, pneumococcal infections and other diseases that can cause fever and febrile seizures.

CDC and FDA closely monitor the safety of all vaccines.

CDC and the U.S. Food and Drug Administration (FDA) are committed to ensuring that vaccines provided to the public are safe and effective. Once vaccines are licensed in the United States, CDC and FDA monitor the safety of these vaccines through several systems. If any vaccine is found to cause health problems, the vaccine may be withdrawn and no longer given to the public.

Guillain-Barré Syndrome (GBS)

GBS is rare.

Anyone can develop GBS; however, it is more common among older adults. The rate of GBS increases with age, and people older than 50 years are at greatest risk for developing GBS. Each year, between 3,000 and 6,000 people in the United States get GBS, regardless of vaccination. To study whether a new vaccine might be causing GBS, CDC would compare this usual rate of GBS to the observed rate of GBS while the new vaccine was being given. This helps to determine whether a vaccine could be causing more cases.

GBS may have several causes.

While it is not known what causes all cases of GBS, it is known that about two-thirds of people who get GBS do so several days or weeks after they have been sick with diarrhea or a lung or sinus illness. Infection with the bacteria Campylobacter jejuni is one of the most common risk factors for GBS. People also can develop GBS after having the flu or other infections such as cytomegalovirus and Epstein Barr virus. On very rare occasions, people develop GBS in the days or weeks after getting a vaccination.

In 1976, there was a small increased risk of GBS after swine flu vaccination.

The Institute of Medicine (IOM) conducted a scientific review of this issue in 2003 and found that people who received the 1976 swine influenza vaccine had an increased risk for developing GBS. The increased risk was approximately one additional case of GBS for every 100,000 people who got the swine flu vaccine. Scientists have several theories about the cause, but the exact reason for this link remains unknown.

The link between GBS and flu vaccination in other years is unclear, and if there is any risk for GBS after seasonal flu vaccines it is very small, about one in a million. Studies suggest that it is more likely that a person will get GBS after getting the flu than after vaccination. It is important to keep in mind that severe illness and death are associated with flu, and getting vaccinated is the best way to prevent flu infection and its complications.

Vaccine safety monitoring systems are used to investigate cases of GBS that start after vaccination.

Tracking vaccine safety is a high priority for CDC. Several systems are in place to monitor vaccine safety. One of these systems is the Vaccine Adverse Event Reporting System (VAERS).

CDC and the U.S. Food and Drug Administration (FDA) co-manage VAERS, which serves as an early warning system to collect voluntary reports about possible health problems that people experience following vaccinations. Anyone can report a suspected health problem after vaccination to VAERS. CDC and FDA scientists regularly review all reports to detect new, unusual, or rare health events that could be linked to vaccines.

Sudden Infant Death Syndrome (SIDS)

Vaccines do not cause SIDS.

Multiple research studies have been conducted to look for possible links between vaccines and SIDS. Results from these studies and continued monitoring show that vaccines do not cause SIDS.

Some studies include:

- A study looked at the ages and seasons of infant deaths after vaccinations reported to the Vaccine Adverse Event Reporting System (VAERS). This study examined VAERS reports following DTP and hepatitis B vaccination found no link between SIDS and these vaccines.

- A 2003 Institute of Medicine (IOM) report "Immunization Safety Review: Vaccination and Sudden Unexpected Death in Infancy." The committee reviewed scientific evidence focusing on sudden unexpected death in infancy and looked for possible relationships between SIDS and vaccines. Based on all the research findings they reviewed, the committee concluded that vaccines did not cause SIDS.

- Additional work on defining SIDS and reviewing the literature by the Brighton Collaboration, an international network of vaccine safety experts.

SIDS deaths declined due to recommendations to put infants on their backs to sleep.

As a result of the American Academy of Pediatrics' 1992 recommendation to place healthy babies on their backs to sleep, and the success of the National Institute of Child Health and Human Development's Back to Sleep campaign in 1994, SIDS deaths have declined considerably.

Thimerosal (Preservative Used in Some Flu Vaccines)

Thimerosal contains ethylmercury.

Mercury is a naturally occurring element found in the earth's crust, air, soil, and water. Two types of mercury to which people may be exposed—methylmercury and ethylmercury—are very different.

Methylmercury is the type of mercury found in certain kinds of fish. At high exposure levels methylmercury can be toxic to people. In the United States, federal guidelines keep as much methylmercury as possible out of the environment and food, but over a lifetime, everyone is exposed to some methylmercury.

Thimerosal contains ethylmercury, which is cleared from the human body more quickly than methylmercury, and is therefore less likely to cause any harm.

Thimerosal prevents the growth of bacteria in vaccines.

Thimerosal is added to vials of vaccine that contain more than one dose (multi-dose vials) to prevent growth of germs, like bacteria and fungi. Introduction of bacteria and fungi has the potential to occur when a syringe needle enters a vial as a vaccine is being prepared for administration. Contamination by germs in a vaccine could cause severe local reactions, serious illness or death. In some vaccines, preservatives, including thimerosal, are added during the manufacturing process to prevent germ growth.

The human body eliminates thimerosal easily.

Thimerosal does not stay in the body a long time so it does not build up and reach harmful levels. When thimerosal enters the body, it breaks down to ethylmercury and thiosalicylate, which are readily eliminated.

Thimerosal has been shown to be safe when used in vaccines.

Thimerosal use in medical products has a record of being very safe. Data from many studies show no evidence of harm caused by the low doses of thimerosal in vaccines.

There are some side effects of thimerosal in vaccines.

The most common side-effects are minor reactions like redness and swelling at the injection site. Although rare, some people may be allergic to thimerosal.

Scientific research does not show a connection between thimerosal and autism.

Research does not show any link between thimerosal in vaccines and autism, a neurodevelopmental disorder. Many well conducted studies have concluded that thimerosal in vaccines does not contribute to the development of autism. Even after thimerosal was removed from almost all childhood vaccines, autism rates continued to increase, which is the opposite of what would be expected if thimerosal caused autism.

Thimerosal was taken out of childhood vaccines in the United States in 2001.

Measles, mumps, and rubella (MMR) vaccines do not and never did contain thimerosal. Varicella (chickenpox), inactivated polio (IPV), and pneumococcal conjugate vaccines have also never contained thimerosal.

Influenza (flu) vaccines are currently available in both thimerosal-containing (for multi-dose vaccine vials) and thimerosal-free versions.

Multiple Vaccines and the Immune System

Early vaccination is important to prevent diseases.

Children are given shots (vaccines) at a young age because this is when they are at highest risk of getting sick or dying if they get these diseases. Newborn babies are immune to some diseases because they have antibodies they get from their mothers, usually before they are born. However, this immunity lasts a few months. Most babies do not get protective antibodies against diphtheria, whooping cough, polio, tetanus, hepatitis B, or Hib from their mothers. This is why it's important to vaccinate a child before she or he is exposed to a disease.

Vaccines contain weakened or killed versions of the germs that cause a disease. These elements of vaccines, and other molecules and micro-organisms that stimulate the immune system, are called "antigens." Babies are exposed to thousands of germs and other antigens in the environment from the time they are born. When a baby is born, his or her immune system is ready to respond to the many antigens in the environment and the selected antigens in vaccines.

Different childhood vaccines can be given at the same time.

Many vaccines are recommended early in life to protect young children from dangerous infectious diseases. In order to reduce the number of shots a child receives in a doctor's visit, some vaccines are offered as combination vaccines. A combination vaccine is two or more different vaccines that have been combined into a single shot. Combination vaccines have been in use in the United States since the mid-1940s. Examples of combination vaccines are: DTap (diphtheria-tetanus-pertussis), trivalent IPV (three strains of inactivated polio vaccine), MMR (measles-mumps-rubella), DTap-Hib, and Hib-Hep B.

Often, more than one shot will be given during the same doctor's visit, usually in separate limbs (e.g., one in each arm). For example, a baby might get DTaP in one arm or leg and IPV in another arm or leg during the same visit.

Giving a child several vaccines during the same visit offers two advantages.

First, children should be given their vaccines as quickly as possible to give them protection during the vulnerable early months of their lives. Second, giving several shots at the same time means fewer office visits. This saves parents time and money, and can be less traumatic for the child.

Getting multiple vaccines at the same time has been shown to be safe.

Scientific data show that getting several vaccines at the same time does not cause any chronic health problems. A number of studies have been done to look at the effects of giving various combinations of vaccines, and when every new vaccine is licensed, it has been tested along with the vaccines already recommended for a particular aged child. The recommended vaccines have been shown to be as effective in combination as they are individually. Sometimes, certain combinations of vaccines given together can cause fever, and occasionally febrile seizures; these are temporary and do not cause any lasting damage. Based on this information, both the Advisory Committee on Immunization Practices and the American Academy of Pediatrics recommend getting all routine childhood vaccines on time.

CDC's recommended childhood vaccine schedule ensures children get the best protection during the many different stages in growth and development.

From the moment babies are born, they are exposed to numerous bacteria and viruses on a daily basis. Eating food introduces new bacteria into the body; numerous bacteria live in the mouth and nose; and an infant places his or her hands or other objects in his or her mouth hundreds of times every hour, exposing the immune system to still more germs. When a child has a cold, he or she is exposed to up to 10 antigens, and exposure to "strep throat" is about 25 to 50 antigens. Each vaccine in the childhood vaccination schedule has between 1-69 antigens. A child who receives all the recommended vaccines in the 2014 childhood immunization schedule may be exposed to up to 315 antigens through vaccination by the age of 2.

In fact, a 1994 report from the Institute of Medicine, Adverse Events Associated with Childhood Vaccines, states: "In the face of these normal events, it seems unlikely that the number of separate antigens contained in childhood vaccines would represent an appreciable added burden on the immune system that would be immunosuppressive."

Vaccines during Pregnancy

Are Vaccines Safe during Pregnancy?

Some vaccines are safe and recommended for pregnant women. These vaccines help keep pregnant women and their developing babies healthy.

Which Vaccines Should I Receive If I Am Pregnant?

If you are pregnant or planning a pregnancy, the specific vaccines you need are determined by your age, lifestyle, medical conditions, travel, and previous vaccinations.

Can a Vaccine Harm My Developing Baby?

Some vaccines, especially vaccines made using live strains of a virus, should not be given to pregnant women because they may be harmful to the baby. The recommendations for which vaccines to get during pregnancy, and in which trimester, are developed with highest concern for the safety of both mothers and babies in mind.

Are Vaccines Safe If I Am Breastfeeding?

Yes. It is safe for a woman to receive routine vaccines right after giving birth, even while she is breastfeeding.

What If I Receive a Vaccine and Then Learn That I Am Pregnant?

Some vaccines are not recommended during pregnancy, such as:

- Human papillomavirus (HPV)
- Measles, mumps, and rubella (MMR)
- Some kinds of flu vaccines
- Varicella (chicken pox)

If you receive any of these vaccines and then find out that you are pregnant, talk to your doctor. In most cases, there is no cause for concern.

Vaccine Recalls

Many types of products including cars, toys, and food products are sometimes recalled for short times or withdrawn permanently from the market because they don't work properly or pose a safety risk. Although every vaccine goes through years of testing before being used, vaccines or vaccine lots (specific batches) can also be withdrawn or recalled.

Why Would a Vaccine, or Certain Batches of a Vaccine, Be Withdrawn or Recalled?

There have been only a few vaccine recalls or withdrawals due to concerns about either how well the vaccine was working or about its safety. Several vaccine lots have been recalled in recent years because of a possible safety concern before anyone reported any injury. Rather, the manufacturer's quality testing noticed some irregularity in some vaccine vials. In these cases, the safety of these vaccines was monitored continuously before and after they were in use. CDC analyzed reports to the Vaccine Adverse Event Reporting System (VAERS) to search for any side effects that might have been caused by the irregularity, and found none. Any time such an irregularity is found in a vaccine lot which could make it unsafe, the manufacturer, in collaboration with the U.S. Food and Drug Administration (FDA), will recall it immediately. Information on recalled lots of is available by year from FDA.

How Is a Vaccine Recalled?

Vaccine recalls or withdrawals are almost always initiated voluntarily by the vaccine manufacturer. The FDA rarely issues a recall, and if safety is a concern, the recall is immediate. The manufacturer contacts vaccine distributors and healthcare facilities who might have purchased the vaccine to inform them of the suspected problem. Whenever a vaccine lot is to be recalled, FDA's role is to oversee a manufacturer's strategy and help ensure the recall goes well.

How Is a Vaccine Recall Communicated?

You would most likely hear from your doctor if a vaccine given to you or your child is recalled. When a recalled product has been widely distributed, the news media often reports on the recall. Not all recalls are announced in the media, but all recalls are listed in FDA's weekly Enforcement Reports. See a list of vaccines that have been recalled in the past few years on CDC's Recalled Vaccines page.

What Do I Do If a Vaccine Is Recalled?

In many cases, the person who is vaccinated will not need to do anything after a vaccine is recalled. When a vaccine recall is due to low vaccine potency or strength, vaccines from the lot might not produce an immune response that is strong enough to protect against disease. People who were vaccinated with a vaccine from that lot might need to be vaccinated again to ensure they are protected against the disease.

When a recall is related to a possible safety concern noted by the manufacturer, people who were vaccinated should be aware of their reaction to the vaccine, and talk to their doctor if they have any concerns that they may be having a reaction.

Historical Vaccine Safety Concerns

There is solid medical and scientific evidence that the benefits of vaccines far outweigh the risks. Despite this, there have been concerns about the safety of vaccines for as long as they have been available in the United States. This section will explain past vaccine safety concerns, how they have been resolved, and what we have learned.

Cutter Incident—1955

In 1955, some batches of polio vaccine given to the public contained live polio virus, even though they had passed required safety testing. Over 250 cases of polio were attributed to vaccines produced by one company: Cutter Laboratories. This case, which came to be known as the Cutter Incident, resulted in many cases of paralysis. The vaccine was recalled as soon as cases of polio were detected.

The Cutter Incident was a defining moment in the history of vaccine manufacturing and government oversight of vaccines, and led to the creation of a better system of regulating vaccines. After the government improved this process and increased oversight, polio vaccinations resumed in the fall of 1955.

At the time, there was no system in place to compensate people who might have been harmed by a vaccine. Today we have the National Vaccine Injury Compensation Program (VICP), which uses scientific evidence to determine whether a vaccine might be the cause of an illness or injury, and provides compensation to individuals found to have been harmed by a vaccine. The VICP remains a model method for ensuring that all persons harmed by vaccines are compensated quickly and fairly, while also protecting companies that make lifesaving products from financially unsustainable liability claims through the tort system.

Simian Virus 40 (SV40)—1955–1963

Some of the polio vaccine administered from 1955 to 1963 was contaminated with a virus called simian virus 40 (SV40). The virus came from the monkey kidney cells used to produce the vaccines. Once the contamination was discovered in the Salk inactivated polio vaccine in use at that time, the U.S. government established requirements for vaccine testing to verify that all new batches of the polio vaccine were free of SV40. Because of research done with SV40 in animal models, there was some concern that the virus could cause cancer. However, evidence suggests that SV40 has not caused cancer in humans.

Swine Flu Vaccine and Guillain-Barré Syndrome—1976

In 1976 there was a small increased risk of a serious neurological disorder called Guillain-Barré Syndrome (GBS) following vaccination with a swine flu vaccine. The increased risk was approximately 1 additional case of GBS for every 100,000 people who got the swine flu vaccine. When over 40 million people were vaccinated against swine flu, federal health officials decided that the possibility of an association of GBS with the vaccine, however small, necessitated stopping immunization until the issue could be explored.

The Institute of Medicine (IOM) conducted a thorough scientific review of this issue in 2003 and concluded that people who received the 1976 swine influenza vaccine had an increased risk for developing GBS. Scientists have multiple theories on why this increased risk may have occurred, but the exact reason for this association remains unknown.

Today, CDC continually monitors the safety of seasonal and pandemic flu vaccines, and any possible safety problems are discussed by the Advisory Committee on Immunization Practices. Vaccination is the best way to prevent flu infection and its complications, and having safe and effective flu vaccines is extremely important.

Hepatitis B Vaccine and Multiple Sclerosis—1998

In 1998, some research caused concern that hepatitis B vaccination might be linked with multiple sclerosis (MS), a progressive nerve disease. However, this link has not been found in the large body of research that has been done since that time. In 2002, the Institute of Medicine thoroughly reviewed all available evidence and published a report. In this thorough review, the IOM committee concluded that there is no link between hepatitis B vaccination and MS.

Rotavirus Vaccine and Intussusception—1998–1999

In 1998, the FDA approved RotaShield vaccine, the first vaccine to prevent rotavirus gastroenteritis. Shortly after it was licensed, some infants developed intussusception (rare type of bowel obstruction that occurs when the bowel folds in on itself) after being vaccinated. At first, it was not clear if the vaccine or some other factor was causing the bowel obstructions. CDC quickly recommended that use of the vaccine be suspended and immediately started two emergency investigations to find out if receiving RotaShield vaccine was causing some of the cases of intussusception.

The results of the investigations showed that RotaShield vaccine caused intussusception in some healthy infants younger than 12 months of age who normally would be at low risk for this condition.

The Advisory Committee on Immunization Practices (ACIP) withdrew its recommendation to vaccinate infants with RotaShield® vaccine, and the manufacturer voluntarily withdrew RotaShield from the market in October 1999.

Guillain-Barré Syndrome and Meningococcal Vaccine—2005–2008

There were concerns that the meningococcal vaccine Menactra caused a serious neurological disorder called Guillain-Barré Syndrome (GBS). Between 2005 and 2008, there were a number of youth who reported GBS after receiving Menactra. However, to investigate whether GBS was caused by the vaccine or was coincidental with vaccination, two large studies were conducted, with a combined total of over 2 million vaccinated adolescents. The results of these studies showed that there was no link between Menactra and GBS.

Hib Vaccine Recall—2007

In 2007, Merck & Company, Inc. voluntarily recalled 1.2 million doses of *Haemophilus influenzae* type b (Hib) vaccines due to concerns about potential contamination with bacteria called B. cereus. The recall was a precaution, and after careful review, no evidence of B. cereus infection was found in recipients of recalled Hib vaccines.

H1N1 Influenza Vaccine and Narcolepsy—2009–2010

An increased risk of narcolepsy (a chronic sleep disorder) was found following vaccination with Pandemrix, a monovalent 2009 H1N1 influenza vaccine that was used in several European countries during the H1N1 influenza pandemic. This risk was initially found in Finland, and then some other European countries also detected an association. Pandemrix is manufactured by GlaxoSmithKline in Europe and was specifically produced for pandemic 2009 H1N1 influenza. Pandemrix was never licensed for use in the United States.

In 2014, CDC published a study on the association between 2009 H1N1 influenza vaccines, 2010/2011 seasonal influenza vaccines, and narcolepsy. The study found that vaccination was not associated with an increased risk for narcolepsy.

Porcine Circovirus in Rotavirus Vaccines—2010

Porcine circovirus (PCV) is a common virus found in pigs. In 2010, it was discovered that both rotavirus vaccines licensed in the U.S.- Rotarix and RotaTeq- contained PCV type 1. PCV1 is not known to cause disease in animals or humans. In fact, PCV is common in healthy pigs, and humans are routinely exposed to the virus by eating pork. Safety monitoring of both vaccines has not shown any reason for concern about PCV.

HPV Vaccine Recall—2013

In 2013, Merck & Company, Inc. recalled one batch of Gardasil, a human papillomavirus (HPV) vaccine. The recall was a precaution following an error in the manufacturing process. The company had concerns that a small number of vials might have contained glass particles due to breakage. No health problems were reported relating to this recall other than known side effects that can result from any vaccination, like arm redness and soreness where the shot was given.

Chapter 80

Vaccine Adverse Event Reporting System (VAERS)

What Is VAERS?

The Vaccine Adverse Event Reporting System (VAERS) is a national vaccine safety surveillance program run by Centers for Disease Control and Prevention (CDC) and the U.S. Food and Drug Administration (FDA). VAERS serves as an early warning system to detect possible safety issues with U.S. vaccines by collecting information about adverse events (possible side effects or health problems) that occur after vaccination. VAERS was created in 1990 in response to the National Childhood Vaccine Injury Act. If any health problem happens after vaccination, anyone-doctors, nurses, vaccine manufacturers, and any member of the general public-can submit a report to VAERS.

How VAERS Is Used

VAERS is used to detect possible safety problems—called "signals"—that may be related to vaccination. If a vaccine safety signal is identified through VAERS, scientists may conduct further studies to find out if the signal represents an actual risk.

This chapter includes text excerpted from "Vaccine Safety," Centers for Disease Control and Prevention (CDC), August 28, 2015.

The main goals of VAERS are to:

- Detect new, unusual or rare adverse events that happen after vaccination

- Monitor increases in known side effects, like arm soreness where a shot was given

- Identify potential patient risk factors for particular types of health problems related to vaccines

- Assess the safety of newly licensed vaccines

- Watch for unexpected or unusual patterns in adverse event reports

- Serve as a monitoring system in public health emergencies

How to Report Adverse Events to VAERS

There are two ways to submit a report to VAERS:

- **Report Online**

  Complete a VAERS form online at: http://vaers.hhs.gov/

- **Report by Fax**

  Fax a completed VAERS Form to (877) 721-0366.

- **Report by Mail**

  Mail a completed VAERS Form to VAERS, P.O. Box 1100, Rockville, MD 20849–1100.

What to Report to VAERS

Anyone who gives or receives a licensed vaccine in the United States is encouraged to report any significant health problem that occurs after vaccination. An adverse event can be reported even if it is uncertain or unlikely that the vaccine caused it. Reporting to VAERS helps scientists at CDC and FDA better understand the safety of vaccines.

The Reportable Events Table (RET) lists conditions that are believed to be caused by vaccines. It is used by the National Vaccine Injury Compensation Program, which is operated by the U.S Health Resources and Services Administration. Healthcare providers are required by law to report any conditions on the RET to VAERS, and are strongly encouraged to report clinically significant or unexpected events following vaccination.

What Happens after a VAERS Report Is Submitted

Each VAERS report is assigned a VAERS identification number. This number can be used to provide additional information to VAERS if necessary. CDC or FDA scientists follow up on selected cases of serious adverse events immediately by obtaining medical records to better understand the event. Then, letters are sent one year after vaccination to check the recovery status of the patient for all serious reports that listed recovery status as "not recovered" on the initial report.

The Vaccine Injury Compensation Program (VICP), administered by the Health Resources and Services Administration, compensates people whose injuries may have been caused by certain vaccines. The VICP is separate from VAERS, and reporting an event to VAERS does not file a claim for compensation to the VICP.

What We Can Learn from VAERS Data

Approximately 30,000 VAERS reports are filed each year. About 85–90% of the reports describe mild side effects such as fever, arm soreness, and crying or mild irritability. The remaining reports are classified as serious, which means that the adverse event resulted in permanent disability, hospitalization, life-threatening illness, or death. While these problems happen after vaccination, they are rarely caused by the vaccine.

The VAERS form collects information about:

- The type of vaccine received

- The timing of the vaccination

- The onset of the adverse event

- Current illnesses or medication

- Past history of adverse events following vaccination

- Demographic information

FDA and CDC use VAERS data to monitor vaccine safety and conduct research studies.

Strengths and Limitations of VAERS Data

When evaluating VAERS data, it is important to understand the strengths and limitations. VAERS data contain both coincidental events and those truly caused by vaccines.

Table 80.1. Strengths and Limitations of VAERS Data

Strengths	Limitations
VAERS collects national data from all U.S. states and territories.	It is generally not possible to find out from VAERS data if a vaccine caused the adverse event.
VAERS accepts reports from anyone.	Reports submitted to VAERS often lack details and sometimes contain errors.
The VAERS form collects information about the vaccine, the person vaccinated, and the adverse event.	Serious adverse events are more likely to be reported than mild side effects.
Data are publicly available.	Rate of reports may increase in response to media attention and increased public awareness.
VAERS can be used as an early warning system to identify rare adverse events.	It is not possible to use VAERS data to calculate how often an adverse event occurs in a population.
It is possible to follow-up with patients to obtain health records, when necessary.	

Chapter 81

Vaccination Records

Records and Requirements

Keeping up-to-date immunization records for your family, especially your children, is important. You will need your children's immunization records to register them for school, child care, athletic teams, and summer camps or to travel.

Recording Immunizations

Good record—keeping begins with good record-taking. When you need official copies of immunizations records to enroll your child in child care, school, and summer camps or for international travel, they will be much easier to get if you have accurate, up-to-date personal records.

You can get an immunization tracking card from your child's doctor or from your state health department to keep record of your child's vaccines. Or, you can use Centers for Disease Control and Prevention (CDC)'s Immunization Tracker to record your children's immunizations, developmental milestones, and growth from birth through 6

This chapter contains text excerpted from the following sources: Text beginning with the heading "Records and Requirements" is excerpted from "For Parents: Vaccines for Your Children," Centers for Disease Control and Prevention (CDC), April 15, 2016; Text beginning with the heading "Keeping Your Vaccine Records up to Date" is excerpted from "Vaccine Information for Adults," Centers for Disease Control and Prevention (CDC), May 2, 2016.

years old. You can also ask your doctor to record the vaccines your child has received in your state's immunization registry.

Keep your child's immunization record in a safe place where you can easily locate it. Bring the record to each of your child's doctor visits. Ask the doctor or nurse to record the vaccine given, date, and dosage on your child's immunization record. You should also note where your child got the shot—knowing at which doctor's office or clinic your child received a vaccine will help you get official records when you need them.

Finding Official Immunization Records

CDC does not have immunization record information. If you need official copies of immunization records for your child, or if you need to update your personal records, there are several places you can look:

- Check with your child's doctor or public health clinic. However, doctor's offices and clinics may only keep immunization records for a few years.

- Check with your state's health department. You can request a copy of your child's immunization record. Or, you can find out if your child's immunization record is in an immunization registry or Immunization Information System (IIS). An IIS is a computer system that your doctor or public health clinic may use to keep track of immunizations your child has received. Most states have an IIS; contact the IIS in the state where your child received their last shots to see if records exist.

- Check with your child's school. Some schools keep on file the immunization records of children who attended. However, these records generally are kept for only a year or two after the student graduates, transfers to another school, or leaves the school system. After a student leaves the school system, records are sent to storage and may not be accessible unless the record is stored in an IIS.

- Check with college medical or student health services for your college-age child. Many colleges provide vaccinations, especially those required for enrollment. Contact your college's medical services or student health department for further information.

If your child's vaccination records cannot be located or are incomplete, your child should be considered susceptible to disease and be vaccinated (or revaccinated) against vaccine-preventable diseases. Children can have their blood tested for antibodies to determine their immunity to certain diseases. However, these tests may not always be accurate, so the doctor may not be sure your child is truly protected. In some cases, doctors may prefer to re vaccinate your child for best protection. It is safe for your child to be vaccinated, even if they he or she may have already received that vaccine. Talk to your child's doctor to determine what vaccines are needed to protect against diseases.

Immunization Records for Adoption and Foster Care

You should ask your adoption coordinator for your child's immunization records. An internationally adopted child should be considered susceptible to disease and be vaccinated (or revaccinated) against vaccine-preventable diseases if vaccination records:

- cannot be located

- are incomplete

- cannot be understood

- if you or your child's doctor thinks they are inaccurate

Immunization Requirements for Child Care and School

The CDC does not set immunization requirements for schools or childcare centers. Instead, each state decides which immunizations are required for your child's enrollment and attendance at a childcare facility or school in that state. Immunization requirements and allowable exemptions may vary by state, and they may be updated and changed regularly.

- Talk to a staff member to learn what vaccines are required at the school or childcare facility in which you would like to enroll your child. They will be able to provide you with specific information about their requirements.

Keeping Your Vaccine Records up to Date

Your vaccination record (sometimes called your immunization record) provides a history of all the vaccines you received as a child and adult. This record may be required for certain jobs, travel abroad or school registration.

How to Locate Your Vaccination Records

Unfortunately, there is no national organization that maintains vaccination records. The CDC does not have this information. The records that exist are the ones you or your parents were given when the vaccines were administered and the ones in the medical record of the doctor or clinic where the vaccines were given. If you need official copies of vaccination records, or if you need to update your personal records, there are several places you can look:

- Ask parents or other caregivers if they have records of your childhood immunizations.

- Try looking through baby books or other saved documents from your childhood.

- Check with your high school and/or college health services for dates of any immunizations. Keep in mind that generally records are kept only for 1–2 years after students leave the system.

- Check with previous employers (including the military) that may have required immunizations.

- Check with your doctor or public health clinic. Keep in mind that vaccination records are maintained at doctor's office for a limited number of years.

- Contact your state's health department. Some states have registries (Immunization Information Systems) that include adult vaccines.

What to Do If You Can't Find Your Records

If you can't find your personal records or records from the doctor, you may need to get some of the vaccines again. While this is not ideal, it is safe to repeat vaccines. The doctor can also sometimes do blood tests to see if you are immune to certain vaccine-preventable diseases.

Tools to Record Your Vaccinations

Today we move, travel, and change healthcare providers more than we did in previous generations. Finding old immunization information can be difficult and time—consuming. Therefore, it is critical that you keep an accurate and up-to-date record of the vaccinations you have received. Keeping an immunization record and storing it with other important documents (or in a safe place) will save you time and unnecessary hassle.

Ask your doctor, pharmacist or other vaccine provider for an immunization record form. Bring this record with you to health visits, and ask your vaccine provider to sign and date the form for each vaccine you receive. That way, you can be sure that the immunization information is current and correct. If your vaccine provider participates in an immunization registry, ask that your vaccines be documented there as well.

Chapter 82

Vaccine Misinformation May Have Tragic Consequences

Vaccines

Vaccines are generally made from weakened strains of disease-causing microbes that are not virulent enough to cause an infection. When they are introduced to the body, the immune system learns to produce cells that can defeat the infection, thus making the body capable of resisting the disease in the future.

The Success of Vaccination

Immunization programs have been very successful at controlling infectious diseases. More than 200 years ago, British physician Edward Jenner pioneered the smallpox vaccine. Smallpox has since been eradicated worldwide, and it is estimated that five million lives are saved annually as a result of the smallpox vaccine. This achievement should be compelling evidence that vaccines work, and do so astonishingly well.

In total, the United Nations International Children's Emergency Fund (UNICEF) estimates that immunization saves approximately nine million lives annually the world over. In addition to smallpox, vaccination has brought under control such diseases as diphtheria, tetanus, yellow fever, whooping cough, polio, and measles.

"Vaccine Misinformation May Have Tragic Consequences," © 2017 Omnigraphics. Reviewed August 2016.

Misinformation about Vaccines

A report by the Centers for Disease Control and Prevention (CDC) estimated that 77 percent of U.S. children between 19 and 35 months of age were being fully immunized with the recommended vaccinations. Reasons for the remaining 33 percent being either not immunized or under-immunized include limited healthcare access, financial barriers, and misconceptions about vaccinations and vaccine safety.

Misinformation about vaccines has existed as long as vaccines themselves. Parents who delay or refuse vaccination because of misinformation can place their own children, as well as other children, at risk of contracting preventable diseases.

The anti-vaccine debate increased in intensity with the publication of a study by Dr. Andrew Wakefield in the scientific journal *Lancet* in 1998, which concluded that autism was linked to the measles, mumps, and rubella vaccine (MMR). This led to ripples in the medical community and spread panic among some parents, celebrities, and politicians, with a resultant drop in vaccination rates. The study was later declared a fraud, and Wakefield was stripped of his medical license.

Why Would Parents Willingly Put Their Children at Risk of Vaccine-Preventable Diseases?

- The absence of societal fear is one factor. For centuries, people lived in terror of communicable diseases, but immunization resulted in lower incidences of such illnesses, and subsequent generations have not been exposed to such diseases as polio, rubella, and diphtheria. The absence of disease visibility has resulted in a lack of community fear, so in a sense the immunization program has become a victim of its own success. But, fortunately, the majority of parents have continued to realize that vaccination is essential for the safety of their children and the benefit of community health.

- The timing of vaccinations makes them scapegoats for various disorders that may occur around the same time as immunization. Children of vaccination age are often subject to a number of minor illnesses, but just because a disorder is detected at the time of vaccination does not necessarily indicate that vaccination caused the disorder. Additionally, fever is a common side effect of vaccination, but life-threatening reactions are very rare, and most medical professionals advise that this and other minor side effects should not be a deterrent to the protection offered by immunization.

- Uninformed people may disseminate misinformation. Parents rely on multiple resources for information about vaccines, including web sites, family members, friends, and celebrities, some of whom could be seriously misinformed.

- A person often perceives risk based on his or her limited experiences and knowledge. Someone who has come across the child of a family member or friend who had an adverse reaction to vaccination might perceive it as overly risky. People also tend to tolerate natural risks (infectious diseases) more easily than man-made risks (vaccination side effects). Risks that have clear benefits associated with them are generally tolerated better than risks with benefits that are not immediate or not understood well.

Vaccination in the United States

All 50 U.S. states mandate that children be vaccinated against certain diseases before they enter school. Children who have health conditions that could be exacerbated by vaccination can seek to be exempted. And, except for Mississippi, all states allow religious exemptions, while exemptions based on personal and moral beliefs are allowed in 20 states.

The Consequences of Misinformation

Vaccination rates are still high in the United States, but requests for exemptions have increased. Since the chances of contracting a vaccine-preventable infection is quite small in the United States, what is the risk?

The danger lies in clusters of communities in which like-minded anti-vaccination parents live. In 1991, a measles outbreak occurred in Philadelphia in schools run by fundamentalist churches. About 350 children attending these schools were not immunized, and the infection spread to 1,500 children, leading to nine fatalities.

Pockets of unvaccinated children exist around the nation, particularly in the states of California, Utah, Oregon, and Washington. Vaccine exemptions are particularly high in Washington, where some elementary schools have an exemption rate of 43 percent. Nevertheless, overall vaccination rates in these states remain relatively high.

Measles was declared to have been eliminated in the United States in the year 2000. But in 2015, a measles outbreak occurred at Disneyland in California. It turned into a large-scale outbreak that spread to 13 states across the country and affected 147 people. The disease was determined to have been primarily carried by unvaccinated children whose parents put them and other children at risk by taking them to a crowded public place.

That the outbreak was contained serves as testament to the success of vaccination programs. It also demonstrates that science by itself cannot totally overcome the detrimental effects of virulent misinformation. The risks of immunization are very negligible, while the advantages are great and the repercussions of not vaccinating are extremely high. Vaccines are backed by more than a century of scientific research and safeguards. They are rigorously tested, and effective systems ensure potency, purity, and safety.

Children need to be protected against preventable diseases by ensuring vaccination. And this seems to be possible only if we inoculate ourselves with facts.

References

1. Patel, Kavita and Hart, Rio. "What the Anti-Vaxxers Are Getting Dangerously Wrong," Brookings, February 6, 2015.

2. Myers, Martin G and Pineda, Diego. "Misinformation about Vaccines," AutismTruths, n.d.

3. Parker, Laura. "The Anti-Vaccine Generation: How Movement Against Shots Got Its Start," National Geographic, February 6, 2015.

4. "Vaccinating Ourselves Against Misinformation," Union of Concerned Scientists, February, 2015.

Chapter 83

What Would Happen If We Stopped Vaccinations?

Before the middle of the last century, diseases like whooping cough, polio, measles, *Haemophilus influenzae*, and rubella struck hundreds of thousands of infants, children, and adults in the United States. Thousands died every year from them. As vaccines were developed and became widely used, rates of these diseases declined until today most of them are nearly gone from our country.

- Nearly everyone in the United States got measles before there was a vaccine, and hundreds died from it each year. Today, most doctors have never seen a case of measles.

- More than 15,000 Americans died from diphtheria in 1921, before there was a vaccine. Only one case of diphtheria has been reported to Centers for Disease Control and Prevention (CDC) since 2004.

- An epidemic of rubella (German measles) in 1964–65 infected 12½ million Americans, killed 2,000 babies, and caused 11,000 miscarriages. In 2012, 9 cases of rubella were reported to CDC.

Given successes like these, it might seem reasonable to ask, "Why should we keep vaccinating against diseases that we will probably never see?" Here is why:

This chapter includes text excerpted from "Vaccines and Immunization," Centers for Disease Control and Prevention (CDC), May 19, 2014.

Vaccines Don't Just Protect Yourself

Most vaccine—preventable diseases are spread from person to person. If one person in a community gets an infectious disease, he can spread it to others who are not immune. But a person who is immune to a disease because she has been vaccinated can't get that disease and can't spread it to others. The more people who are vaccinated, the fewer opportunities a disease has to spread.

If one or two cases of disease are introduced into a community where most people are not vaccinated, outbreaks will occur. In 2013, for example, several measles outbreaks occurred around the country, including large outbreaks in New York City and Texas—mainly among groups with low vaccination rates. If vaccination rates dropped to low levels nationally, diseases could become as common as they were before vaccines.

Diseases Haven't Disappeared

The United States has very low rates of vaccine-preventable diseases, but this isn't true everywhere in the world. Only one disease—smallpox—has been totally erased from the planet. Polio no longer occurs in the United States, but it is still paralyzing children in several African countries. More than 350,000 cases of measles were reported from around the world in 2011, with outbreaks in the Pacific, Asia, Africa, and Europe. In that same year, 90% of measles cases in the United States were associated with cases imported from another country. Only the fact that most Americans are vaccinated against measles prevented these clusters of cases from becoming epidemics.

Disease rates are low in the United States today. But if we let ourselves become vulnerable by not vaccinating, a case that could touch off an outbreak of some disease that is currently under control is just a plane ride away.

A Final Example: What Could Happen

We know that a disease that is apparently under control can suddenly return, because we have seen it happen, in countries like Japan, Australia, and Sweden. Here is an example from Japan. In 1974, about 80% of Japanese children were getting pertussis (whooping cough) vaccine. That year there were only 393 cases of whooping cough in the entire country, and not a single pertussis-related death. Then immunization rates began to drop, until only about 10% of children were being vaccinated. In 1979, more than 13,000 people got whooping cough and 41 died. When routine vaccination was resumed, the disease numbers dropped again.

The chances of your child getting a case of measles or chickenpox or whooping cough might be quite low today. But vaccinations are not just for protecting ourselves, and are not just for today. They also protect the people around us (some of whom may be unable to get certain vaccines, or might have failed to respond to a vaccine, or might be susceptible for other reasons). And they also protect our children's children and their children by keeping diseases that we have almost defeated from making a comeback.

What Would Happen If We Stopped Vaccinations?

We could soon find ourselves battling epidemics of diseases we thought we had conquered decades ago.

Chapter 84

Preventing Transmission of Infections in Hospitals and Nursing Homes

Chapter Contents

Section 84.1

Tips for Surgery Patients to Prevent Antibiotic Resistance

This section includes text excerpted from "Mission Critical: Preventing Antibiotic Resistance," Center for Disease Control and Prevention(CDC), April 28, 2014.

What Can We Do to Prevent Antibiotic Resistance in Healthcare Settings?

Patients, healthcare providers, healthcare facility administrators, and policy makers must work together to employ effective strategies for improving antibiotic use-ultimately improving medical care and saving lives.

Patients Can:

- Ask if tests will be done to make sure the right antibiotic is prescribed.

- Take antibiotics exactly as the doctor prescribes. Do not skip doses. Complete the prescribed course of treatment, even when you start feeling better.

- Only take antibiotics prescribed for you; do not share or use leftover antibiotics. Antibiotics treat specific types of infections. Taking the wrong medicine may delay correct treatment and allow bacteria to multiply.

- Do not save antibiotics for the next illness. Discard any leftover medication once the prescribed course of treatment is completed.

- Do not ask for antibiotics when your doctor thinks you do not need them. Remember antibiotics have side effects.

- Prevent infections by practicing good hand hygiene and getting recommended vaccines.

Healthcare Providers Can:

- Prescribe antibiotics correctly-get cultures, start the right drug promptly at the right dose for the right duration. Reassess the prescription within 48 hours based on tests and patient exam.

- Document the dose, duration and indication for every antibiotic prescription.

- Stay aware of antibiotic resistance patterns in your facility.

- Participate in and lead efforts within your hospital to improve prescribing practices.

- Follow hand hygiene and other infection control measures with every patient.

Healthcare Facility Administrators and Payers Can:

To protect patients and preserve the power of antibiotics, hospital CEOs/medical officers can:

- Adopt an antibiotic stewardship program that includes, at a minimum, this checklist:

    1. Leadership commitment: Dedicate necessary human, financial, and IT resources.

    2. Accountability: Appoint a single leader responsible for program outcomes. Physicians have proven successful in this role.

    3. Drug expertise: Appoint a single pharmacist leader to support improved prescribing.

    4. Action: Take at least one prescribing improvement action, such as requiring reassessment within 48 hours to check drug choice, dose, and duration.

    5. Tracking: Monitor prescribing and antibiotic resistance patterns.

    6. Reporting: Regularly report to staff prescribing and resistance patterns, and steps to improve.

    7. Education: Offer education about antibiotic resistance and improving prescribing practices.

Work with other healthcare facilities to prevent infections, transmission, and resistance.

Preventing Antibiotic Resistance

Can you imagine a day when antibiotics don't work anymore? It's concerning to think that the antibiotics that we depend upon for everything from skin and ear infections to life-threatening bloodstream infections could no longer work. Unfortunately, the threat of untreatable infections is very real.

Antibiotic resistance occurs when germs outsmart drugs. In today's healthcare and community settings, we are already seeing germs stronger than the drugs we have to treat them. This is an extremely scary situation for patients and healthcare workers alike.

So, What Is Fueling Antibiotic Resistance, You May Ask?

We're finding that the widespread overuse and incorrect prescribing practices are significant problems. In addition to driving drug resistance, these poor practices introduce unnecessary side effects, allergic reactions, and serious diarrheal infections caused by *Clostridium difficile*. These complications of antibiotic therapy can have serious outcomes, even death.

According to Center for Disease Control and Prevention(CDC)'s National Healthcare Safety Network, a growing number of healthcare-associated infections are caused by bacteria that are resistant to multiple antibiotics. These include: MRSA, vancomycin-resistant *Enterococcus*, extended-spectrum cephalosporin-resistant *K. pneumonia* (and *K. oxytoca*), *E. coli* and *Enterobacter* spp., carbapenem-resistant *P. aeruginosa*, carbapenem-resistant *K. pneumonia*(and *K. oxytoca*), *E. coli*, and *Enterobacter* spp.

Section 84.2

Prevention and Control of Influenza in Hospitals

This section includes text excerpted from "Prevention Strategies for Seasonal Influenza in Healthcare Settings," Center for Disease Control and Prevention(CDC), January 9, 2013.

Influenza is primarily a community-based infection that is transmitted in households and community settings. Each year, 5% to 20% of U.S. residents acquire an influenza virus infection, and many will seek medical care in ambulatory healthcare settings (e.g., pediatricians' offices, urgent-care clinics). In addition, more than 200,000 persons, on average, are hospitalized each year for influenza-related complications. Healthcare-associated influenza infections can occur in any healthcare setting and are most common when influenza is also circulating in the community. Therefore, the influenza prevention measures outlined in this guidance should be implemented in all healthcare settings. Supplemental measures may need to be implemented during influenza season if outbreaks of healthcare-associated influenza occur within certain facilities, such as long-term care facilities and hospitals.

Influenza Modes of Transmission

Traditionally, influenza viruses have been thought to spread from person to person primarily through large-particle respiratory droplet transmission (e.g., when an infected person coughs or sneezes near a susceptible person). Transmission via large-particle droplets requires close contact between source and recipient persons, because droplets generally travel only short distances (approximately 6 feet or less) through the air. Indirect contact transmission via hand transfer of influenza virus from virus-contaminated surfaces or objects to mucosal surfaces of the face (e.g., nose, mouth) may also occur. Airborne transmission via small particle aerosols in the vicinity of the infectious

609

individual may also occur; however, the relative contribution of the different modes of influenza transmission is unclear. Airborne transmission over longer distances, such as from one patient room to another has not been documented and is thought not to occur. All respiratory secretions and bodily fluids, including diarrheal stools, of patients with influenza are considered to be potentially infectious; however, the risk may vary by strain. Detection of influenza virus in blood or stool in influenza infected patients is very uncommon.

Fundamental Elements to Prevent Influenza Transmission

Preventing transmission of influenza virus and other infectious agents within healthcare settings requires a multi-faceted approach. Spread of influenza virus can occur among patients, HCP, and visitors; in addition, HCP may acquire influenza from persons in their household or community. The core prevention strategies include:

- administration of influenza vaccine

- implementation of respiratory hygiene and cough etiquette

- appropriate management of ill HCP

- adherence to infection control precautions for all patient-care activities and aerosol-generating procedures

- implementing environmental and engineering infection control measures

Successful implementation of many, if not all, of these strategies is dependent on the presence of clear administrative policies and organizational leadership that promote and facilitate adherence to these recommendations among the various people within the healthcare setting, including patients, visitors, and HCP. These administrative measures are included within each recommendation where appropriate. Furthermore, this guidance should be implemented in the context of a comprehensive infection prevention program to prevent transmission of all infectious agents among patients and HCP.

Recommendations

1. Promote and Administer Seasonal Influenza Vaccine

Annual vaccination is the most important measure to prevent seasonal influenza infection. Achieving high influenza vaccination rates of HCP and patients is a critical step in preventing healthcare transmission of influenza from HCP to patients and from patients to HCP. According to current national guidelines, unless contraindicated, vaccinate all people aged 6 months and older, including HCP, patients and residents of long-term care facilities.

Systematic strategies employed by some institutions to improve HCP vaccination rates have included providing incentives, providing vaccine at no cost to HCP, improving access (e.g., offering vaccination at work and during work hours), requiring personnel to sign declination forms to acknowledge that they have been educated about the benefits and risks of vaccination, and mandating influenza vaccination for all HCP without contraindication. Many of these approaches have been shown to increase vaccination rates; tracking influenza vaccination coverage among HCP can be an important component of a systematic approach to protecting patients and HCP. Regardless of the strategy used, strong organizational leadership and an infrastructure for clear and timely communication and education, and for program implementation, have been common elements in successful programs.

2. Take Steps to Minimize Potential Exposures

A range of administrative policies and practices can be used to minimize influenza exposures before arrival, upon arrival, and throughout the duration of the visit to the healthcare setting. Measures include screening and triage of symptomatic patients and implementation of respiratory hygiene and cough etiquette. Respiratory hygiene and cough etiquette are measures designed to minimize potential exposures of all respiratory pathogens, including influenza virus, in healthcare settings and should be adhered to by everyone—patients, visitors, and HCP—upon entry and continued for the entire duration of stay in healthcare settings.

Before Arrival to a Healthcare Setting

- When scheduling appointments, instruct patients and persons who accompany them to inform HCP upon arrival if they have symptoms of any respiratory infection (e.g., cough, runny nose, fever) and to take appropriate preventive actions (e.g., wear a facemask upon entry, follow triage procedure).

- During periods of increased influenza activity:

  - Take steps to minimize elective visits by patients with suspected or confirmed influenza. For example, consider

611

establishing procedures to minimize visits by patients seeking care for mild influenza-like illness who are not at increased risk for complications from influenza (e.g., provide telephone consultation to patients with mild respiratory illness to determine if there is a medical need to visit the facility).

Upon Entry and during Visit to a Healthcare Setting

- Take steps to ensure all persons with symptoms of a respiratory infection adhere to respiratory hygiene, cough etiquette, hand hygiene, and triage procedures throughout the duration of the visit. These might include:

  - Posting visual alerts (e.g., signs, posters) at the entrance and in strategic places (e.g., waiting areas, elevators, cafeterias) to provide patients and HCP with instructions (in appropriate languages) about respiratory hygiene and cough etiquette, especially during periods when influenza virus is circulating in the community. Instructions should include:

    - How to use facemasks or tissues to cover nose and mouth when coughing or sneezing and to dispose of contaminated items in waste receptacles.

    - How and when to perform hand hygiene.

  - Implementing procedures during patient registration that facilitate adherence to appropriate precautions (e.g., at the time of patient check-in, inquire about presence of symptoms of a respiratory infection, and if present, provide instructions).

- Provide facemasks to patients with signs and symptoms of respiratory infection.

- Provide supplies to perform hand hygiene to all patients upon arrival to facility (e.g., at entrances of facility, waiting rooms, at patient check-in) and throughout the entire duration of the visit to the healthcare setting.

- Provide space and encourage persons with symptoms of respiratory infections to sit as far away from others as possible. If available, facilities may wish to place these patients in a separate area while waiting for care.

- During periods of increased community influenza activity, facilities should consider setting up triage stations that facilitate rapid screening of patients for symptoms of influenza and separation from other patients.

3. Monitor and Manage Ill Healthcare Personnel

HCP who develop fever and respiratory symptoms should be:

- Instructed not to report to work, or if at work, to stop patient-care activities, don a facemask, and promptly notify their supervisor and infection control personnel/occupational health before leaving work.

- Reminded that adherence to respiratory hygiene and cough etiquette after returning to work is always important. If symptoms such as cough and sneezing are still present, HCP should wear a facemask during patient-care activities. The importance of performing frequent hand hygiene (especially before and after each patient contact and contact with respiratory secretions) should be reinforced.

- Excluded from work until at least 24 hours after they no longer have a fever (without the use of fever-reducing medicines such as acetaminophen). Those with ongoing respiratory symptoms should be considered for evaluation by occupational health to determine appropriateness of contact with patients.

- Considered for temporary reassignment or exclusion from work for 7 days from symptom onset or until the resolution of symptoms, whichever is longer, if returning to care for patients in a Protective Environment (PE) such as hematopoietic stem cell transplant patients (HSCT).

  - Patients in these environments are severely immunocompromised, and infection with influenza virus can lead to severe disease. Furthermore, once infected, these patients can have prolonged viral shedding despite antiviral treatment and expose other patients to influenza virus infection. Prolonged shedding also increases the chance of developing and spreading antiviral-resistant influenza strains; clusters of influenza antiviral resistance cases have been found among severely immunocompromised persons exposed to a common source or healthcare setting.

- HCP with influenza or many other infections may not have fever or may have fever alone as an initial symptom or sign. Thus, it can be very difficult to distinguish influenza from many other causes, especially early in a person's illness. HCP with fever alone should follow workplace policy for HCP with fever until a more specific cause of fever is identified or until fever resolves.

HCP Who Develop Acute Respiratory Symptoms without Fever May Still Have Influenza Infection and Should Be:

- Considered for evaluation by occupational health to determine appropriateness of contact with patients. HCP suspected of having influenza may benefit from influenza antiviral treatment.

- Reminded that adherence to respiratory hygiene and cough etiquette after returning to work is always important. If symptoms such as cough and sneezing are still present, HCP should wear a facemask during patient care activities. The importance of performing frequent hand hygiene (especially before and after each patient contact) should be reinforced.

- Allowed to continue or return to work unless assigned to care for patients requiring a PE such as HSCT; these HCP should be considered for temporary reassignment or considered for exclusion from work for 7 days from symptom onset or until the resolution of all non-cough symptoms, whichever is longer.

Facilities and Organizations Providing Healthcare Services Should:

- Develop sick leave policies for HCP that are non-punitive, flexible and consistent with public health guidance to allow and encourage HCP with suspected or confirmed influenza to stay home.

  - Policies and procedures should enhance exclusion of HCPs who develop a fever and respiratory symptoms from work for at least 24 hours after they no longer have a fever, without the use of fever-reducing medicines.

- Ensure that all HCP, including staff who are not directly employed by the healthcare facility but provide essential daily services, are aware of the sick leave policies.

- Employee health services should establish procedures for tracking absences; reviewing job tasks and ensuring that personnel known to be at higher risk for exposure to those with suspected or confirmed influenza are given priority for vaccination; ensuring that employees have prompt access, including via telephone to medical consultation and, if necessary, early treatment; and promptly identifying individuals with possible influenza. HCP should self-assess for symptoms of febrile respiratory illness. In most cases, decisions about work restrictions and assignments for personnel with respiratory illness should be guided by clinical signs and symptoms rather than by laboratory testing for influenza because laboratory testing may result in delays in diagnosis, false negative test results or both.

4. Adhere to Standard Precautions

During the care of any patient, all HCP in every healthcare setting should adhere to standard precautions, which are the foundation for preventing transmission of infectious agents in all healthcare settings. Standard precautions assume that every person is potentially infected or colonized with a pathogen that could be transmitted in the healthcare setting. Elements of standard precautions that apply to patients with respiratory infections, including those caused by the influenza virus, are summarized below.

Hand Hygiene

- HCP should perform hand hygiene frequently, including before and after all patient contact, contact with potentially infectious material, and before putting on and upon removal of personal protective equipment, including gloves. Hand hygiene in healthcare settings can be performed by washing with soap and water or using alcohol-based hand rubs. If hands are visibly soiled, use soap and water, not alcohol—based hand rubs.

- Healthcare facilities should ensure that supplies for performing hand hygiene are available.

Gloves

- Wear gloves for any contact with potentially infectious material. Remove gloves after contact, followed by hand hygiene. Do not wear the same pair of gloves for care of more than one patient. Do not wash gloves for the purpose of reuse.

Gowns

- Wear gowns for any patient-care activity when contact with blood, body fluids, secretions (including respiratory), or excretions is anticipated. Remove gown and perform hand hygiene before leaving the patient's environment. Do not wear the same gown for care of more than one patient.

615

5. Adhere to Droplet Precautions

- Droplet precautions should be implemented for patients with suspected or confirmed influenza for 7 days after illness onset or until 24 hours after the resolution of fever and respiratory symptoms, whichever is longer, while a patient is in a healthcare facility. In some cases, facilities may choose to apply droplet precautions for longer periods based on clinical judgment, such as in the case of young children or severely immunocompromised patients, who may shed influenza virus for longer periods of time.

- Place patients with suspected or confirmed influenza in a private room or area. When a single patient room is not available, consultation with infection control personnel is recommended to assess the risks associated with other patient placement options (e.g., cohorting [i.e., grouping patients infected with the same infectious agents together to confine their care to one area and prevent contact with susceptible patients], keeping the patient with an existing roommate).

- HCP should don a facemask when entering the room of a patient with suspected or confirmed influenza. Remove the facemask when leaving the patient's room, dispose of the facemask in a waste container, and perform hand hygiene.

  - If some facilities and organizations opt to provide employees with alternative personal protective equipment, this equipment should provide the same protection of the nose and mouth from splashes and sprays provided by facemasks (e.g., face shields and N95 respirators or powered air purifying respirators).

- If a patient under droplet precautions requires movement or transport outside of the room.

  - Have the patient wear a facemask, if possible, and follow respiratory hygiene and cough etiquette and hand hygiene.

  - Communicate information about patients with suspected, probable, or confirmed influenza to appropriate personnel before transferring them to other departments in the facility (e.g., radiology, laboratory) or to other facilities.

- Patients under droplet precautions should be discharged from medical care when clinically appropriate, not based on the period of potential virus shedding or recommended duration of droplet precautions. Before discharge, communicate the patient's diagnosis and current precautions with post-hospital care providers (e.g., home-healthcare agencies, long-term care facilities) as well as transporting personnel.

6. Use Caution When Performing Aerosol-Generating Procedures

Some procedures performed on patients with suspected or confirmed influenza infection may be more likely to generate higher concentrations of infectious respiratory aerosols than coughing, sneezing, talking, or breathing. These procedures potentially put HCP at an increased risk for influenza exposure. Although there are limited data available on influenza transmission related to such aerosols, many authorities recommend that additional precautions be used when such procedures are performed. These include some procedures that are usually planned ahead of time, such as bronchoscopy, sputum induction, elective intubation and extubation, and autopsies; and some procedures that often occur in unplanned, emergent settings and can be life-saving, such as cardiopulmonary resuscitation, emergent intubation and open suctioning of airways. Ideally, a combination of measures should be used to reduce exposures from these aerosol-generating procedures when performed on patients with suspected or confirmed influenza. However, it is appropriate to take feasibility into account, especially in challenging emergent situations, where timeliness in performing a procedure can be critical to achieving a good patient outcome. Precautions for aerosol-generating procedures include:

- Only performing these procedures on patients with suspected or confirmed influenza if they are medically necessary and cannot be postponed.

- Limiting the number of HCP present during the procedure to only those essential for patient care and support. As is the case for all HCP, ensure that HCP whose duties require them to perform or be present during these procedures are offered influenza vaccination.

- Conducting the procedures in an airborne infection isolation room (AIIR) when feasible. This will not be feasible for unplanned, emergent procedures, unless the patient is already in an AIIR. Such rooms are designed to reduce the concentration of infectious aerosols and prevent their escape into adjacent areas using controlled air exchanges and directional airflow. They are single patient rooms at negative pressure relative to the surrounding areas, and with a minimum of 6 air changes per hour (12 air changes per hour are recommended for new construction or renovation). Air from these rooms should be exhausted directly to the outside or be filtered through a high-efficiency particulate air (HEPA) filter before recirculation. Room doors should be kept closed except when entering or leaving the room, and entry and exit should be minimized during and shortly after the procedure. Facilities should monitor and document the proper negative-pressure function of these rooms.

- Considering use of portable HEPA filtration units to further reduce the concentration of contaminants in the air. Some of these units can connect to local exhaust ventilation systems (e.g., hoods, booths, tents) or have inlet designs that allow close placement to the patient to assist with source control; however, these units do not eliminate the need for respiratory protection for individuals entering the room because they may not entrain all of the room air. Information on air flow/air entrainment performance should be evaluated for such devices.

- HCP should adhere to standard precautions, including wearing gloves, a gown, and either a face shield that fully covers the front and sides of the face or goggles.

- HCP should wear respiratory protection equivalent to a fitted N95 filtering facepiece respirator or equivalent N95 respirator (e.g., powered air purifying respirator, elastomeric) during aerosol-generating procedures. When respiratory protection is required in an occupational setting, respirators must be used in the context of a comprehensive respiratory protection program that includes fit-testing and training as required under OSHA's Respiratory Protection standard.

- Unprotected HCP should not be allowed in a room where an aerosol-generating procedure has been conducted until sufficient time has elapsed to remove potentially infectious particles.

- Conduct environmental surface cleaning following procedures.

7. Manage Visitor Access and Movement within the Facility

Limit visitors for patients in isolation for influenza to persons who are necessary for the patient's emotional well-being and care. Visitors who have been in contact with the patient before and during hospitalization are a possible source of influenza for other patients, visitors, and staff.

For persons with acute respiratory symptoms, facilities should develop visitor restriction policies that consider location of patient being visited (e.g., oncology units) and circumstances, such as end-of-life situations, where exemptions to the restriction may be considered at the discretion of the facility. Regardless of restriction policy, all visitors should follow precautions listed in the respiratory hygiene and cough etiquette section.

Visits to patients in isolation for influenza should be scheduled and controlled to allow for:

- Screening visitors for symptoms of acute respiratory illness before entering the hospital.

- Facilities should provide instruction, before visitors enter patients' rooms, on hand hygiene, limiting surfaces touched, and use of personal protective equipment (PPE) according to current facility policy while in the patient's room.

- Visitors should not be present during aerosol-generating procedures.

- Visitors should be instructed to limit their movement within the facility.

- If consistent with facility policy, visitors can be advised to contact their healthcare provider for information about influenza vaccination.

8. Monitor Influenza Activity

Healthcare settings should establish mechanisms and policies by which HCP are promptly alerted about increased influenza activity in the community or if an outbreak occurs within the facility and when collection of clinical specimens for viral culture may help to inform public health efforts. Close communication and collaboration with local and state health authorities is recommended. Policies should include designations of specific persons within the healthcare facility who are responsible for communication with public health officials and dissemination of information to HCP.

9. Implement Environmental Infection Control

Standard cleaning and disinfection procedures (e.g., using cleaners and water to preclean surfaces prior to applying disinfectants to frequently touched surfaces or objects for indicated contact times) are adequate for influenza virus environmental control in all settings within the healthcare facility, including those patient-care areas in which aerosol-generating procedures are performed. Management of laundry, food service utensils, and medical waste should also be performed in accordance with standard procedures. There are no data suggesting these items are associated with influenza virus transmission when these items are properly managed. Laundry and food service utensils should first be cleaned, then sanitized as appropriate. Some medical waste may be designated as regulated or biohazardous waste and require special handling and disposal methods approved by the State authorities.

10. Implement Engineering Controls

Consider designing and installing engineering controls to reduce or eliminate exposures by shielding HCP and other patients from infected individuals. Examples of engineering controls include installing physical barriers such as partitions in triage areas or curtains that are drawn between patients in shared areas. Engineering controls may also be important to reduce exposures related to specific procedures such as using closed suctioning systems for airways suction in intubated patients. Another important engineering control is ensuring that appropriate air-handling systems are installed and maintained in healthcare facilities.

11. Train and Educate Healthcare Personnel

Healthcare administrators should ensure that all HCP receive job- or task-specific education and training on preventing transmission of infectious agents, including influenza, associated with healthcare during orientation to the healthcare setting. This information should be updated periodically during ongoing education and training programs. Competency should be documented initially and repeatedly, as appropriate, for the specific staff positions. A system should be in place to ensure that HCP employed by outside employers meet these education and training requirements through programs offered by the outside employer or by participation in the healthcare facility's program.

- Key aspects of influenza and its prevention that should be emphasized to all HCP include:
  - Influenza signs, symptoms, complications, and risk factors for complications. HCP should be made aware that, if they

have conditions that place them at higher risk of complications, they should inform their healthcare provider immediately if they become ill with an influenza-like illness so they can receive early treatment if indicated.

- Central role of administrative controls such as vaccination, respiratory hygiene and cough etiquette, sick policies, and precautions during aerosol-generating procedures.

- Appropriate use of personal protective equipment including respirator fit testing and fit checks.

- Use of engineering controls and work practices including infection control procedures to reduce exposure.

12. Administer Antiviral Treatment and Chemoprophylaxis of Patients and Healthcare Personnel When Appropriate

Both HCP and patients should be reminded that persons treated with influenza antiviral medications continue to shed influenza virus while on treatment. Thus, hand hygiene, respiratory hygiene and cough etiquette practices should continue while on treatment.

13. Considerations for Healthcare Personnel at Higher Risk for Complications of Influenza

HCP at higher risk for complications from influenza infection include pregnant women and women up to 2 weeks postpartum, persons 65 years old and older, and persons with chronic diseases such as asthma, heart disease, diabetes, diseases that suppress the immune system, certain other chronic medical conditions, and morbid obesity. Vaccination and early treatment with antiviral medications are very important for HCP at higher risk for influenza complications because they can decrease the risk of hospitalizations and deaths. HCP at higher risk for complications should check with their healthcare provider if they become ill so that they can receive early treatment.

Some HCP may identify themselves as being at higher risk of complications, and express concerns about their risks. These concerns should be discussed and the importance of careful adherence to these guidelines should be emphasized. Work accommodations to avoid potentially high-risk exposure scenarios, such as performing or assisting with aerosol-generating procedures on patients with suspected or confirmed influenza, may be considered in some settings, particularly for HCP with more severe or unstable underlying disease.

Chapter 85

Quarantine and Isolation to Control the Spread of Contagious Diseases

When someone is known to be ill with a contagious disease, they are placed in isolation and receive special care, with precautions taken to protect uninfected people from exposure to the disease.

When someone has been exposed to a contagious disease and it is not yet known if they have caught it, they may be quarantined or separated from others who have not been exposed to the disease. For example, they may be asked to remain at home to prevent further potential spread of the illness. They also receive special care and observation for any early signs of the illness.

How Long Can Quarantine and Isolation Last? What Is Done to Help the People Who Experience Isolation or Quarantine?

The list of diseases for which quarantine or isolation is authorized is specified in an Executive Order of the President. This list currently includes cholera, diphtheria, infectious tuberculosis, plague,

This chapter includes text excerpted from "Understand Quarantine and Isolation: Questions and Answers," Centers for Disease Control and Prevention (CDC), January 31, 2014.

smallpox, yellow fever, viral hemorrhagic fevers (Lassa, Marburg, Ebola, Crimean—Congo, South American, and others not yet isolated or named), Severe Acute Respiratory Syndrome (SARS), and influenza caused by novel or reemergent influenza viruses that are causing, or have the potential to cause, a pandemic.

Isolation

Isolation would last for the period of communicability of the illness, which varies by disease and the availability of specific treatment. Usually it occurs at a hospital or other healthcare facility or in the person's home. Typically, the ill person will have his or her own room and those who care for him or her will wear protective clothing and take other precautions, depending on the level of personal protection needed for the specific illness.

In most cases, isolation is voluntary; however, federal, state and local governments have the authority to require isolation of sick people to protect the public.

Quarantine

Modern quarantine lasts only as long as necessary to protect the public by:

1. Providing public healthcare (such as immunization or drug treatment, as required)

2. Ensuring that quarantined persons do not infect others if they have been exposed to a contagious disease

Modern quarantine is more likely to involve limited numbers of exposed persons in small areas than to involve large numbers of persons in whole neighborhoods or cities. Quarantined individuals will be sheltered, fed, and cared for at home, in a designated emergency facility, or in a specialized hospital, depending on the disease and the available resources. They will also be among the first to receive all available medical interventions to prevent and control disease, including:

- Vaccination

- Antibiotics

- Early and rapid diagnostic testing and symptom monitoring

- Early treatment if symptoms appear

The duration and scope of quarantine measures would vary, depending on their purpose and what is known about the incubation period (how long it takes for symptoms to develop after exposure) of the disease—causing agent.

Examples

A few hours for assessment. Passengers on airplanes, trains or boats believed to be infected with or exposed to a dangerous contagious disease might be delayed for a few hours while health authorities determine the risk they pose to public health. Some passengers may be asked to provide contact information and then released while others who are ill are transported to where they can receive medical attention. There have been a few instances where state and local public health authorities have imposed a brief quarantine at a public gathering, such as a shelter, while investigating if one or more people may be ill.

Enough time to provide preventive treatment or other intervention. If public health authorities determine that a passenger or passengers on airplanes, trains or boats are sick with a dangerous contagious disease, the other passengers may be quarantined in a designated facility where they may receive preventive treatment and have their health monitored.

For the duration of the incubation period. If public health officials determine that one or more passenger on airplanes, trains or boats are infected with a contagious disease and that passengers sitting nearby may have had close contact with the infected passenger(s), those at risk might be quarantined in a designated facility, observed for signs of illness and cared for under isolation conditions if they become ill.

When Would Quarantine and Isolation Be Used and by Whom?

If people in a certain area were potentially exposed to a contagious disease, this is what would happen: State and local health authorities would let people know that they may have been exposed and would direct them to get medical attention, undergo diagnostic tests, and stay at home, limiting their contact with people who have not been exposed to the disease. Only rarely would federal, state, or local health authorities issue an "order" for quarantine and isolation.

However, both quarantine and isolation may be compelled on a mandatory basis through legal authority as well as conducted on a voluntary basis. States have the authority to declare and enforce quarantine and isolation within their borders. This authority varies widely, depending on state laws. It derives from the authority of state governments granted by the United States Constitution to enact laws and promote regulations to safeguard the health and welfare of people within state borders.

Further, at the national level, the Centers for Disease Control and Prevention (CDC) may detain, medically examine or conditionally release persons suspected of having certain contagious diseases. This authority applies to individuals arriving from foreign countries, including Canada and Mexico, on airplanes, trains, automobiles, boats or by foot. It also applies to individuals traveling from one state to another or in the event of "inadequate local control."

The CDC regularly uses its authority to monitor passengers arriving in the United States for contagious diseases. In modern times, most quarantine measures have been imposed on a small scale, typically involving small numbers of travelers (airline or cruise ship passengers) who have curable diseases, such as infectious tuberculosis or cholera. No instances of large-scale quarantine have occurred in the United States since the "Spanish Flu" pandemic of 1918–1919.

Based on years of experience working with state and local partners, the CDC anticipates that the need to use its federal authority to involuntarily quarantine a person would occur only in rare situations—for example, if a person posed a threat to public health and refused to cooperate with a voluntary request.

Part Six

Additional Help and Information

Chapter 86

Glossary of Terms Related to Contagious Diseases

acute: A short-term, intense health effect.

adjuvant: A substance sometimes included in a vaccine formulation to enhance the immune-stimulating properties of the vaccine.

adverse events: Undesirable experiences occurring after immunization that may or may not be related to the vaccine.

anaphylaxis: An immediate and severe allergic reaction to a substance (e.g., food or drugs).

antibiotics: Medicines that damage or kill bacteria and are used to treat some bacterial diseases.

antibodies: Molecules (also called immunoglobulins) produced by a B cell in response to an antigen. When an antibody attaches to an antigen, it destroys the antigen.

antigen: A substance or molecule that is recognized by the immune system. The molecule can come from foreign materials such as bacteria or viruses.

antitoxin: Antibodies capable of destroying toxins generated by microorganisms including viruses and bacteria.

This glossary contains terms excerpted from documents produced by several sources deemed reliable.

artificially acquired immunity: Immunity provided by vaccines, as opposed to naturally acquired immunity, which is acquired from exposure to a disease-causing organism.

asthma: A chronic medical condition where the bronchial tubes (in the lungs) become easily irritated.

asymptomatic infection: The presence of an infection without symptoms.

attenuated vaccine: A vaccine in which live virus is weakened through chemical or physical processes in order to produce an immune response without causing the severe effects of the disease.

B cells: Small white blood cells crucial to the immune defenses. Also known as B lymphocytes.

bone marrow: Soft tissue located within bones that produce all blood cells, including the ones that fight infection.

booster shot: Supplementary dose of a vaccine, usually smaller than the first dose, that is given to maintain immunity.

cell: The smallest unit of life.

chronic health condition: A health related state that lasts for a long period of time (e.g., cancer, asthma).

communicable disease: An infectious disease that is contagious and which can be transmitted from one source to another by infectious bacteria or viral organisms.

conjugate vaccine: A vaccine in which proteins that are easily recognizable to the immune system are linked to the molecules that form the outer coat of disease-causing bacteria to promote an immune response.

contagious disease: A very communicable disease capable of spreading rapidly from one person to another by contact or close proximity.

contraindication: A condition in a recipient which is likely to result in a life-threatening problem if a vaccine were given.

diphtheria: A bacterial disease marked by the formation of a false membrane, especially in the throat, which can cause death.

disease: A state in which a function or part of the body is no longer in a healthy condition.

DNA (deoxyribonucleic acid): A complex molecule found in the cell nucleus that contains an organism's genetic information.

DNA vaccine or naked DNA vaccine: A vaccine that uses a microbe's genetic material, rather than the whole organism or its parts, to stimulate an immune response.

encephalitis: Inflammation of the brain caused by a virus. Encephalitis can result in permanent brain damage or death.

encephalopathy: A general term describing brain dysfunction.

endemic: The continual, low-level presence of disease in a community.

epidemic: A disease outbreak that affects many people in a region at the same time.

exposure: Contact with infectious agents (bacteria or viruses) in a manner that promotes transmission and increases the likelihood of disease.

genes: Units of genetic material (DNA) that carry the directions a cell uses to perform a specific function.

genetic material: Molecules of DNA (deoxyribonucleic acid) or RNA (ribonucleic acid) that carry the directions that cells or viruses use to perform a specific function, such as making a particular protein molecule.

genomes: All of an organism's genetic material. A genome is organized into specific functional units called genes.

herd immunity or community immunity: The resistance to a particular disease gained by a community when a critical number of people are vaccinated against that disease.

herpes zoster: A disease characterized by painful skin lesions that occur mainly on the trunk (back and stomach) of the body but which can also develop on the face and in the mouth. Also known as the shingles.

hives: The eruption of red marks on the skin that are usually accompanied by itching.

hyposensitivity: A condition in which the body has a weakened or delayed reaction to a substance.

immune globulin: A protein found in the blood that fights infection. Also known as gamma globulin.

immune response: Reaction of the immune system to foreign invaders such as microbes.

immune system: A complex network of specialized cells, tissues, and organs that defends the body against attacks by disease-causing microbes.

immunity: Protection from germs.

inactivated vaccine or killed vaccine: A vaccine made from a whole virus or bacteria inactivated with chemicals or heat.

incubation period: The time from contact with infectious agents (bacteria or viruses) to onset of disease.

infection: A state in which disease-causing microbes have invaded or multiplied in body tissues.

infectious agents: Organisms capable of spreading disease (e.g., bacteria or viruses).

intussusception: A type of bowel blockage that happens when one portion of the bowel slides into the next, much like the pieces of a telescope.

jaundice: Yellowing of the skin and eyes. This condition is often a symptom of hepatitis infection.

lesion: An abnormal change in the structure of an organ, due to injury or disease.

live, attenuated vaccine: A vaccine made from microbes that have been weakened in the laboratory so that they can't cause disease.

lupus: A disease characterized by inflammation of the connective tissue (which supports and connects all parts of the body).

lymph node: A small bean-shaped organ of the immune system, distributed widely throughout the body and linked by lymphatic vessels.

lymphocyte: A white blood cell central to the immune system's response to foreign microbes. B cells and T cells are lymphocytes.

macrophage: A large and versatile immune cell that devours and kills invading microbes and other intruders.

memory cells: A subset of T cells and B cells that have been exposed to antigens and can then respond more readily and rapidly when the immune system encounters the same antigens again.

meningoencephalitis: Inflammation of the brain and meninges (membranes) that involves the encephalon (area inside the skull) and spinal column.

molecule: A building block of a cell. Some examples are proteins, fats, and carbohydrates.

mutate: To change a gene or unit of hereditary material that results in a new inheritable characteristic.

naturally acquired immunity: Immunity produced by antibodies passed from mother to fetus (passive), or by the body's own antibody and cellular immune response to a disease-causing organism (active).

orchitis: A complication of mumps infection occurring in males (who are beyond puberty).

otitis media: A viral or bacterial infection that leads to inflammation of the middle ear.

outbreak: Sudden appearance of a disease in a specific geographic area (e.g., neighborhood or community) or population (e.g., adolescents).

pandemic: An epidemic occurring over a very large geographic area.

parasites: Plants or animals that live, grow, and feed on or within another living organism.

pathogens: Organisms (e.g., bacteria, viruses, parasites and fungi) that cause disease in human beings.

petechiae: A tiny reddish or purplish spot on the skin or mucous membrane, commonly part of infectious diseases such as typhoid fever.

placebo: A substance or treatment that has no effect on human beings.

pneumonia: Inflammation of the lungs characterized by fever, chills, muscle stiffness, chest pain, cough, shortness of breath, rapid heart rate and difficulty breathing.

polysaccharide: A long, chain-like molecule made up of a linked sugar molecule. The outer coats of some bacteria are made of polysaccharides.

potency: A measure of strength.

quarantine: The isolation of a person or animal who has a disease (or is suspected of having a disease) in order to prevent further spread of the disease.

recombinant: Of or resulting from new combinations of genetic material or cells

Reye syndrome: Encephalopathy (general brain disorder) in children following an acute illness such as influenza or chickenpox. Symptoms include vomiting, agitation and lethargy. This condition may result in coma or death.

serology: Measurement of antibodies, and other immunological properties, in the blood serum.

severe combined immune Deficiency (SCID): Included in a group of rare, life-threatening disorders caused by at least 15 different single gene defects that result in profound deficiencies in T- and B- lymphocyte function.

strain: A specific version of an organism. Many diseases, including HIV/AIDS and hepatitis, have multiple strains.

subunit vaccine: A vaccine that uses one or more components of a disease-causing organism, rather than the whole, to stimulate an immune response.

T cell or T lymphocyte: A white blood cell that directs or participates in immune defenses.

tetanus: Toxin-producing bacterial disease marked by painful muscle spasms.

thimerosal: Thimerosal is a mercury-containing preservative used in some vaccines and other products since the 1930's.

tissue: A group of similar cells joined to perform the same function.

titer: The detection of antibodies in blood through a laboratory test.

toxin: Agent produced by plants and bacteria, normally very damaging to cells.

toxoid or inactivated toxin: A toxin, such as those produced by certain bacteria, that has been treated by chemical means, heat or irradiation and is no longer capable of causing disease.

toxoid vaccine: A vaccine containing a toxoid, used to protect against toxins produced by certain bacteria.

vaccine: A product that produces immunity therefore protecting the body from the disease. Vaccines are administered through needle injections, by mouth and by aerosol.

virulence: The relative capacity of a pathogen to overcome body defenses.

virus: A tiny organism that multiplies within cells and causes disease such as chickenpox, measles, mumps, rubella, pertussis and hepatitis. Viruses are not affected by antibiotics, the drugs used to kill bacteria.

Chapter 87

Directory of Organizations That Provide Information about Contagious Diseases

Government Agencies That Provide Information about Contagious Diseases

Agency for Healthcare Research and Quality (AHRQ)
540 Gaither Rd. Ste. 2000
Rockville, MD 20850
Toll-Free: 800-358-9295
Phone: 301-427-1364
Fax: 301-427-1430
Website: www.ahrq.gov
E-mail: richard.kronick@ahrq.hhs.gov

CDC Division of STD Prevention (DSTDP)
1600 Clifton Rd.
Atlanta, GA 30333
Toll-Free: 800-CDC-INFO
(800-232-4636)
Toll-Free TTY: 888-232-6348
Website: www.cdc.gov/std
E-mail: dstd@cdc.gov

Resources in this chapter were compiled from several sources deemed reliable; all contact information was verified and updated in August 2016.

CDC Division of Viral Hepatitis

1600 Clifton Rd.
Atlanta, GA 30333
Toll-Free: 800-CDC-INFO
(800-232-4636)
Phone: 404-718-8596 (M–F, 8:00 am–5:00 pm)
Toll-Free TTY: 888-232-6348
Fax: 404-718-8588
Website: www.cdc.gov/hepatitis
E-mail: info@cdcnpin.org

CDC National Prevention Information Network (NPIN)

P.O. Box 6003
Rockville, MD 20849
Toll-Free: 800-458-5231
Toll-Free TTY: 800-243-7012
Toll-Free Fax: 888-282-7681
Website: www.cdcnpin.org
E-mail: info@cdcnpin.org

CDC Vaccines and Immunizations

1600 Clifton Rd.
Atlanta, GA 30333
Toll-Free: 800-CDC-INFO
(800-232-4636)
Toll-Free TTY: 888-232-6348
Website: www.cdc.gov/vaccines
E-mail: info@cdcnpin.org

Centers for Disease Control and Prevention (CDC)

1600 Clifton Rd.
Atlanta, GA 30333
Toll-Free: 800-CDC-INFO
(800-232-4636)
Toll-Free TTY: 888-232-6348
Fax: 770-488-4760
Website: www.cdc.gov
E-mail: cdcinfo@cdc.gov

Eunice Kennedy Shriver National Institute of Child Health and Human Development (NICHD)

Information Resource Center
P.O. Box 3006
Rockville, MD 20847
Toll-Free: 800-370-2943
Toll-Free TTY: 888-320-6942
Fax: 301-984-1473
Website: www.nichd.nih.gov
E-mail: nichdinformation
ResourceCenter@mail.nih.gov

FDA MedWatch

5600 Fishers Ln.
Rockville, MD 20857
Toll-Free: 800-332-1088
Toll-Free Fax: 800-332-0178
Website: www.fda.gov/Safety/
MedWatch/default.htm
E-mail: webmail@oc.fda.gov

Federal Trade Commission (FTC)

Consumer Response Center
600 Pennsylvania Ave. N.W.
Washington, DC 20580
Toll-Free: 877-FTC-HELP
(877-382-4357)
Toll-Free TDD/TTY:
866-653-4261
Website: www.ftc.gov
E-mail: antitrust@ftc.gov

Health Resources and Services Administration (HRSA)
Information Center
P.O. Box 2910
Merrifield, VA 22116
Toll-Free: 888-275-4772
Toll-Free TTY: 877-489-4772
Fax: 703-821-2098
Website: www.hrsa.gov
E-mail: ask@hrsa.gov

Healthfinder®
National Health Information
Center (NHIC)
P.O. Box 1133
Washington, DC 20013
Fax: 301-984-4256
Website: www.healthfinder.gov
E-mail: healthfinder@nhic.org

MedlinePlus
National Library of Medicine
(NLM)
8600 Rockville Pike
Bethesda, MD 20894
Toll-Free: 888-346-3656
Website: www.medlineplus.gov

National Cancer Institute (NCI)
NCI Public Inquiries Office
6116 Executive Blvd. Rm. 3036A
Bethesda, MD 20892
Toll-Free: 800-4-CANCER
(800-422-6237)
Toll-Free TTY: 800-332-8615
Website: www.cancer.gov
E-mail: cancergovstaff@mail.nih.gov

National Center for Complementary and Alternative Medicine (NCCAM)
P.O. Box 7923
Gaithersburg
Bethesda, MD 20892
Toll-Free: 888-644-6226
Phone: 301-519-3153
Toll-Free TTY: 866-464-3615
Fax: 866-464-3616
Website: nccam.nih.gov
E-mail: info@nccam.nih.gov

National Diabetes Information Clearinghouse (NDIC)
1 Information Way
Bethesda, MD 20892-3560
Toll-Free: 800-860-8747
Phone: 301-654-3327
Fax: 703-738-4929
Website: diabetes.niddk.nih.gov
E-mail: healthinfo@niddk.nih.gov

National Health Information Center (NHIC)
P.O. Box 1133
Washington, DC 20013
Toll-Free: 800-336-4797
Phone: 301-565-4167
Fax: 301-984-4256
Website: www.health.gov/NHIC
E-mail: nhic@hhs.gov

National Heart, Lung, and Blood Institute (NHLBI)
P.O. Box 30105
Bethesda, MD 20824
Phone: 301-592-8573
TTY: 240-629-3255
Fax: 240-629-3246
Website: www.nhlbi.nih.gov
E-mail: nhlbiinfo@nhlbi.nih.gov

National Institute of Allergy and Infectious Diseases (NIAID)
6610 Rockledge Dr. MSC 6612
Bethesda, MD 20892
Toll-Free: 866-284-4107
Phone: 301-496-5717
Toll-Free TDD: 800-877-8339
Fax: 301-402-3573
Website: www3.niaid.nih.gov
E-mail: cpostoffice@niaid.nih.gov

National Institute of Diabetes and Digestive and Kidney Diseases (NIDDK)
Office of Communications and Public Liaison (OCPL)
Bldg. 31 Rm. 9A06
31 Center Dr. MSC 2560
Bethesda, MD 20892
Toll-Free: 800-891-5390
Phone: 301-496-3583
Website: www2.niddk.nih.gov
E-mail: healthinfo@niddk.nih.gov

National Institute of Neurological Disorders and Stroke (NINDS)
NIH Neurological Institute
P.O. Box 5801
Bethesda, MD 20824
Toll-Free: 800-352-9424
Phone: 301-496-5751
TTY: 301-496-5981
Website: www.ninds.nih.gov
E-mail: braininfo@ninds.nih.gov

National Institute on Aging (NIA)
Bldg. 31 Rm. 5C27
31 Center Dr., MSC 2292
Bethesda, MD 20892
Toll-Free: 800-222-2225
Phone: 301-496-1752
Toll-Free TTY: 800-222-4225
Fax: 301-496-1072
Website: www.nia.nih.gov
E-mail: niaic@nia.nih.gov

National Institutes of Health (NIH)
9000 Rockville Pike
Bethesda, MD 20892
Phone: 301-496-4000
TTY: 301-402-9612
Website: www.nih.gov
E-mail: NIHinfo@od.nih.gov

National Vaccine Injury Compensation Program
Parklawn Bldg. Rm. 8A-35
5600 Fishers Ln.
Rockville, MD 20857
Toll-Free: 800-338-2382
Website: www.hrsa.gov/vaccinecompensation
E-mail: healthit@hrsa.gov.

National Women's Health Information Center (NWHIC)
200 Independence Ave. S.W.
Washington, DC 20201
Toll-Free: 800-994-9662
Toll-Free TDD: 888-220-5446
Website: www.womenshealth.gov, or www.4woman.gov
E-mail: womenshealth@hhs.gov

Office of Dietary Supplements (ODS)
Rm. 3B01 MSC 7517
6100 Executive Blvd.
Bethesda, MD 20892
Phone: 301-435-2920
Fax: 301-480-1845
Website: dietary-supplements.info.nih.gov
E-mail: ods@nih.gov

U.S. Food and Drug Administration (FDA)
10903 New Hampshire Ave.
Silver Spring, MD 20993
Toll-Free: 888-463-6332
Phone: 301-796-8240
Fax: 301-443-9767
Website: www.fda.gov
E-mail: druginfo@fda.hhs.gov

U.S. Department of Health and Human Services (HHS)
200 Independence Ave. S.W.
Washington, DC 20201
Toll-Free: 877-696-6775
Website: www.hhs.gov

U.S. Environmental Protection Agency (EPA)
1200 Pennsylvania Ave. N.W.
Washington, DC 20460
Phone: 202-272-0167
TTY: 202-272-0165
Website: www.epa.gov
E-mail: r8eisc@epa.gov

U.S. National Library of Medicine (NLM)
8600 Rockville Pike
Bethesda, MD 20894
Toll-Free: 888-346-3656
Phone: 301-594-5983
Toll-Free TDD: 800-735-2258
Fax: 301-402-1384
Website: www.nlm.nih.gov
E-mail: r8eisc@epa.gov

Vaccine Adverse Event Reporting System (VAERS)
P.O. Box 1100
Rockville, MD 20849
Toll-Free: 800-822-7967
Website: www.vaers.hhs.gov
E-mail: info@vaers.org

Private Agencies That Provide Information about Contagious Diseases

American Academy of Allergy, Asthma, and Immunology (AAAAI)
555 E. Wells St. Ste. 1100
Milwaukee, WI 53202
Phone: 414-272-6071
Website: www.aaaai.org
E-mail: Info@aaaai.org

American Academy of Family Physicians (AAFP)
P.O. Box 11210
Shawnee Mission, KS 66207
Toll-Free: 800-274-2237
Phone: 913-906-6000
Website: www.aafp.org
E-mail: aafp@aafp.org

American Association of Blood Banks (AABB)
8101 Glenbrook Rd.
Bethesda, MD 20814
Phone: 301-907-6977
Fax: 301-907-6895
Website: www.aabb.org
E-mail: aabb@aabb.org

American Cancer Society (ACS)
1599 Clifton Rd. N.E.
Atlanta, GA 30329
Toll-Free: 800-227-2345
Toll-Free TTY: 866-228-4327
Website: www.cancer.org

American Liver Foundation (AAFP)
75 Maiden Ln., Ste. 603
New York, NY 10038
Toll-Free: 800-GO-LIVER (800-465-4837) / 888-4HEP-USA (888-443-7872)
Phone: 212-668-1000
Fax: 212-483-8179
Website: www.liverfoundation.org
E-mail: support@liverfoundation.org.

American Lung Association (ALA)
1301 Pennsylvania Ave N.W.
Ste. 800
Washington, DC 20004
Toll-Free: 800-586-4872 (for location of nearest ALA group); 800-548-8252 (to speak with a lung health professional)
Phone: 212-315-8700
Website: www.lungusa.org
E-mail: info@lung.org

American Medical Association (AMA)
515 N. State St.
Chicago, IL 60610
Toll-Free: 800-621-8335
Phone: 312-464-5000
Fax: 312-464-5600
Website: www.ama-assn.org
E-mail: profilescs@ama-assn.org

American Social Health Association (ASHA)
P.O. Box 13827
Research Triangle Park
NC 27709
Toll-Free: 800-656-4673
Phone: 919-361-8400
Fax: 919-361-8425
Website: www.ashastd.org
E-mail: info@ashasexualhealth.org

Hepatitis Foundation International (HFI)
8121 Georgia Ave.
Silver Spring, MD 20910
Toll-Free: 800-891-0707
Phone: 301-565-9410
Website: www.hepatitisfoundation.org
E-mail: Info@hepatitisfoundation.org

Immunization Safety Review Committee (ISR)
Institute of Medicine
500 Fifth St. N.W.
Washington, DC 20001
Phone: 202-334-2352
Fax: 202-334-1412
Website: www.iom.edu/imsafety
E-mail: iowww@nas.edu

National Foundation for Infectious Diseases (NFID)
Institute of Medicine
Bethesda, MD 20814
Phone: 301-656-0003
Fax: 301-907-0878
Website: www.nfid.org
E-mail: idcourse@nfid.org

National Network for Immunization Information (NNii)
301 University Blvd.
Galveston, TX 77555
Phone: 409-772-0199
Fax: 409-772-5208
Website: www. immunizationinfo.org
E-mail: nnii@i4ph.org

National Patient Advocate Foundation (NPAF)
725 15th St. N.W. 10th Fl.
Washington, DC 20005
Phone: 202-347-8009
Fax: 202-347-5579
Website: www.npaf.org
E-mail: caitlin.donovan@npaf.org

The Nemours Foundation
Center for Children's Health Media
1600 Rockland Rd.
Wilmington, DE 19803
Phone: 302-651-4000
Website: www.kidshealth.org or www.teenshealth.org
E-mail: info@kidshealth.org

World Health Organization (WHO)
Ave. Appia 20
1211 Geneva 27
Switzerland
Phone: (00 41 22) 791-21-11
Website: www.who.int

Index

Index

Page numbers followed by 'n' indicate a footnote. Page numbers in *italics* indicate a table or illustration.

NINDS *see* National Institute of
  Neurological Disorders and Stroke
nitazoxanide, *Cryptosporidium* 134
nits, described 214
NLM *see* U.S. National Library of
  Medicine
non-A–E hepatitis, viral
  hepatitis 172
"Non-Polio Enterovirus" (CDC) 245n
"Norovirus" (CDC) 249n
noroviruses, overview 249–53
Norwegian scabies 281
notifiable infectious diseases,
  overview 75–8
nymphs
  lice 217
  scabies 285

O

Office of Dietary Supplements (ODS),
  contact 639
"Office of Public Health Preparedness
  and Response" (CDC) 70n
Omnigraphics
  publications
       antibiotics, antivirals,
         and other prescription
         medicines 480n
       fever 411n
       Staphylococcus aureus and
         pregnancy 306n
       vaccine misinformation 597n
oophoritis, mumps 242
opportunistic infections, primary
  immunodeficiency 178
oral herpes, genital herpes 157
oral poliovirus vaccine (OPV) 269
oral rehydration solution,
  cholera 110
oral sex
  chlamydia 101
  condoms 46
  gonorrhea 162
  herpes 155
  HIV 183
orchitis
  defined 633
  mumps 242

oseltamivir
  antiviral resistance 499
  H1N1 flu 501
  influenza 483
oseltamivir resistance 500
osteomyelitis
  fever 412
  staph bacteria 310
"OTC Cough and Cold Products: Not
  for Infants and Children under 2
  Years of Age" (FDA) 424n
otitis media
  bacterial meningitis 232
  defined 633
  medical exam during adoption 61
  scarlet fever 318
  Streptococcus pneumoniae 324
outbreak, defined 633
over-the-counter (OTC) medications
  chickenpox 98
  mononucleosis 150
  pinworm 257
  see also medications
"Over-The-Counter Medicines: What's
  Right for You?" (FDA) 418n
oxacillin, staph infections 307
oxymatrine, chronic hepatitis 456
oxyuriasis, pinworm infection 255

P

palivizumab, respiratory syncytial
  virus 276
pandemic, defined 633
parainfluenza virus
  common cold 117
  pneumonia 261
parasites
  amebiasis 87
  Cryptosporidium 131
  defined 633
  lice 214, 216, 221
  pinworms 255
  scabies 281
  trichomoniasis 347
"Parasites-Amebiasis-*Entamoeba
  histolytica* Infection" (CDC) 87n
"Parasites-Cryptosporidium (Also
  Known As "Crypto")" (CDC) 131n

T

Tamiflu (oseltamivir)
  anti-influenza 483
  antiviral resistance 499
tampons, vaginal yeast infections 365
T cells
  defined 634
  depicted24
  human immunodeficiency virus 177
  immune system 17
  PI3 kinase disease 30
  subunit vaccines 531
Tdap vaccine, young adults 553
telbivudine, hepatitis B 170
temperature *see* fever
tetanus, defined 634
tetanus vaccine, vaccine
  adjuvants 570
tetracyclines, antibiotics 481
thermophiles, bacteria 5
thimerosal, defined 634
"Things to Know When Selecting
  a Complementary Health
  Practitioner" (NCCIH) 436n
threadworm *see* pinworm
throat culture (strep screen),
  described 466
thymus, immune system 22
thymus extract, hepatitis C 456
tinea infections, overview 343–6
"Tinea (Ringworm, Jock Itch, Athlete's
  Foot)" (The Nemours Foundation/
  KidsHealth®) 343n
tinidazole, trichomoniasis 349
tissue, defined 634
titer, defined 634
TNFRSF13B gene, common variable
  immunodeficiency 36
toll-like receptors (TLRs), innate
  immunity 23
tonsils, herpangina 128
toxic shock syndrome, staph
  infections 302
toxins
  defined 634
  pertussis 371
  staph infections 302
  toxoid vaccines 531

toxoid vaccines
  defined 634
  described 531
Toxoplasma gondii, protozoa 7
travel vaccine, adult immunization
  schedule 556
Treponema pallidum, syphilis 64
Trichomonas hominis, tabulated 7
Trichomonas vaginalis, sexually
  transmitted disease 347
trichomoniasis, overview 347–9
"Trichomoniasis—CDC Fact Sheet"
  (CDC) 347n
trimethoprim-sulfamethoxazole,
  antibiotic resistance 289
tuberculosis (TB)
  fever 412
  microbes 41
  overview 351–4
  quarantine 623
  tabulated *10*
"Tuberculosis (TB)" (CDC) 351n, 355n
"2015–Sexually Transmitted Diseases
  Treatment Guidelines" (CDC) 101n
Tylenol (acetaminophen), fever 413
typhoid fever
  overview 355–8
  salmonella serotype typhi 515
  vaccines 13

U

ultrasound, described 465
"Understand Quarantine and
  Isolation: Questions and Answers"
  (CDC) 623n
"Understanding How Vaccines Work"
  (CDC) 525n
"Understanding Microbes" (NIAID)
  12n, 15n, 529n
"Understanding Microbes in Sickness
  and in Health" (NIAID) 4n
upper gastrointestinal imaging
  (upper GI), described 465
urinary tract infections (UTI),
  antimicrobials 494
urine test
  described 466
  infectious diseases 16
  Zika 381

665